Perioperative Critical Care Cardiology

2nd edition

J. L. Atlee
A. Gullo
G. Sinagra
J.- L. Vincent

J. L. Atlee • A. Gullo • G. Sinagra • J.-L. Vincent (Eds)

Perioperative Critical Care Cardiology

2nd edition

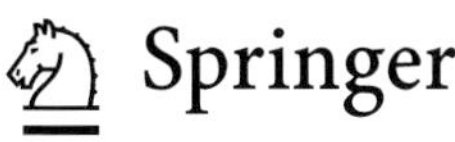

John L. Atlee
Department of Anesthesiology
University of Wisconsin (Madison)
Medical College of Wisconsin (Milwaukee)
Hartland, USA

Antonino Gullo
Department of Anaesthesia and
Intensive Care
Policlinic University Hospital
Catania, Italy

Gianfranco Sinagra
Cardiovascular Department
Ospedali Riuniti and University
of Trieste, Italy

Jean-Louis Vincent
Department of Intensive Care
Erasme University Hospital
Brussels, Belgium

Library of Congress Control Number: 2006937626

ISBN-10 88-470-0557-4 Springer Milan Berlin Heidelberg New York
ISBN-13 978-88-470-0557-0 Springer Milan Berlin Heidelberg New York

Springer is a part of Springer Science+Business Media
springer.com

Cover design: Simona Colombo, Milan, Italy
Typesetting: Graphostudio, Milan, Italy
Printer: Arti Grafiche Nidasio, Assago, Italy
Printed in Italy

Preface to the 2nd edition

Perioperative critical care cardiology (PCCC) includes the cardiovascular management of patients with any underlying diseases or imposed conditions (whether natural or iatrogenic) that involve or affect the heart–including, acute or chronic mechanical heart failure (HF). This can result from ischemic heart disease, diabetes mellitus, uncontrolled hypertension, arrhythmias that compromise heart function, circulatory shock, or dilated or obstructive cardiomyopathy. Patients needing therapy for HF are especially challenging to clinicians involved their perioperative care.

While PCCC has traditionally been within the context of anesthesia and surgery, we now must consider the implications of other therapeutic interventions outside of surgery in critically ill patients. Thus, we may become involved in any stage of their care, including specialized diagnostics, nonsurgical interventions, both during and after such intervention, all of which occur outside of traditional OR settings. Interventions can include percutaneous coronary angioplasty; aortic, endovascular or intracranial aneurysm repair; specialized imaging (magnetic resonance imaging and the like); radiation oncology; etc. Any of these "non-OR" interventions performed in a critically ill patient require the same level of care provided to surgical patients, including: 1) preprocedural patient evaluation and risk stratification; 2) periprocedural care; 3) post-procedural care (post-anesthetic care unit) and 4) any needed critical care (intensive care unit) for whatever reason. Also, as perioperative physicians, we must be able to anticipate and plan for any needed therapy that may improve our patient's well-being or physical status.

Professor Gullo generously provided me with the opportunity to organize the topics for this 2nd edition of Perioperative Critical Care cardiology. I gave this serious thought at the time of A.P.I.C.E. 20, and we agreed there to the Table of Contents. I hope this volume adequately addresses the "idealls" set forth above.

The first chapter addresses sudden death (SD) in HF, including strategies for stratifying risk and therapy. An important conclusion is that despite advances in therapy for improving the prognosis for these patients, SD remains a leading cause for death. As the authors suggest, new, non-pharmacologic strategies (discussed in more detail later in this book) may offer some hope. However, most, today, are ill-affordable to most of the world. Our best hope for now may be high-risk behavior modification, including more healthy diets and exercise. Next, two chapters address 1) the etiology and pathophysiology of HF, and 2) cardiac protection for non-cardiac surgery. The first of these is required reading for anyone who treats patients with or at risk for HF. The second addresses drug-protection against myocardial ischemia, arrhythmias and HF in noncardiac surgical patients. Prof. Gombotz and colleagues deal with anesthetic preconditioning as protection in a later chapter (CH 14) on prevention and management of cardiac dysfunction during and after cardiac surgery. Chapters 4-6 address hypertensive crises, atrial fibrillation and diabetes mellitus in patients with HF, and bedside monitoring for circulatory failure. CH 6 is especially interesting in that it discusses the merits and disadvantages of available, relatively noninvasive strategies for bedside hemodynamic monitoring, a field of technology that is rapidly evolving. CH 7 by Prof. Auler et al. on perioperative cardiac risk stratification was a "must" for this work, and is up to date and current with the available literature. CH 8 by Prof. Vincent and Holsten addresses invasive and noninvasive monitoring in patients with acute HF; including, an analysis of the advantages and disadvantages of pulmonary artery catheter (PAC) monitoring. A relatively noninvasive alternative is needed. Two chapters follow, one on electrocardiography in heart failure and another on pacemaker and internal cardioverter-defibrillator therapies in HF, interposed between which is an extremely relevant chapter on the management of patients with acute HF. In addition to monitoring and drugs for management of acute HF, this latter chapter also addresses devices as therapy for acute HF. Next, Prof. Weil and colleagues provide us with a up-to-date review of recent advances in cardiopulmonary resuscitation, a topic not addressed in the first edition of this work. The management of circulatory shock is discussed by Prof. Vincent and Rapotec in the following chapter. It describes four types of circulatory shock (hypovolemic, distributive, cardiogenic and obstructive), which dictates the diagnosis and management of each. Prevention and management of cardiac dysfunction after cardiac surgery follows (Prof. Gombotz and colleagues), and this in turn by a chapter on differential monitoring and therapy for systemic or pulmonary arterial hypertension. The last chapter, based on a registry of data in Trieste, Italy, reviews the natural history of dilated cardiomyopathy.

Again, I express my appreciation to Prof. Gullo for recruiting me to organize the topics for this edition of PCCC, and to my co-editors Profs. A. Gullo, G. Sinagra, and J-L Vincent for their valauable contributions and support in this collegial, international effort.

Milwaukee, November 2006

John L. Atlee, MS (Pharmacology)
MD, FACA, FACC, FAMA

Preface to the 1st edition

The peri-operative period represents a crucial phase not only for the patient, but also for the surgical and anaesthesiological team which must coordinate harmoniously to ensure the patient's rapid functional recovery. Therefore, an interdisciplinary approach to peri-operative care is essential, both in terms of clinical competency and of instrumental monitoring. Obviously, patient monitoring and all diagnostic and treatment procedures must be modulated in relation to the actual situation. Above all, the pre-operative evaluation of the patient's health conditions and surgical needs has to follow standardized protocols. It is important to determine the functional state of the patient and, in particular, the functional reserves of the cardiovascular system.

Determining the surgical indications and carrying out the intervention both depend on the rigorous control of the patient's homeostasis throughout the peri-operative phase. Anesthesiological protocols are by now codified and familiar to all experienced operators. On this basis, I wished to offer votaries of this field, in particular anesthesiologists, surgeons, cardiologists, internists and intensive care physicians, an update on the more relevant problems that arise during peri-operative care. The focus of this volume is on surgery patients (including those undergoing non-cardiac interventions) whose clinical conditions require special strategies for the prevention and eventual treatment of critical conditions.

Considering the innumerable pathophysiological and clinical situations that may develop in the peri-operative period, continuous education is essential. It is particularly opportune to stress the importance of first-hand experience and the ability to interpret the multiplicity of the hemodynamic complications that can occur in the delicate phase of the peri-operative period.

Sure progress has come from the availability of sophisticated means of hemodynamic monitoring, particularly the noninvasive techniques such as transesophageal echocardiography (TEE) and intra-esophageal echo Doppler ultrasound. In addition to methods for monitoring blood pressure, it is now routine to perform bedside monitoring of cardiac volumes, myocardial contractility, and organ perfusion based on entidal CO_2 levels. These methods are now commonplace in modern clinical practice.

In this context, the management of arrhythmias assumes an important role. The correct and timely diagnosis of arrhythmias and the appropriate use of the different anti-arrhythmic drugs depend on an accurate knowledge of current medical practices. Therefore, the chapter on temporary pacing for the treatment of dangerous arrhythmias is extremely important basically for the training process.

The contributions on monitoring for myocardial ischaemia in the peri-operative period and on the principal trials of novel clinical approaches to acute myocardial infarction are germane to this volume. Another interesting contribution focuses on dilated cardiomyopathy and on the different therapeutic options for this disorder. In addition, two chapters are dedicated to the care of patients undergoing surgical intervention for myocardial revascularization. These patients require different strategies of intervention to improve ventricular failure and to treat secondary complications due to cardiac dysfunction. Finally, this volume could not fail to include a chapter on cardiogenic pulmonary edema that often characterizes the clinical *iter* of patients with cardiac insufficiency.

In light of this brief preface, I have valid motives to retain that this volume will arouse interest in both researchers and experts of this subject. It will also be informative for young physicians who are completing their training.

I wish to thank all the authors for their valuable contributions and for helping to bring this initiative to a fulfillment. I particularly thank my friends and colleagues J.L. Atlee and J.-L. Vincent, with whose efforts this volume became possible.

Trieste, November 2000

Antonino Gullo
University Medical School
Trieste, Italy

Table of Contents

List of Contributors

A. Aleksova, 77
J. L. Atlee, 61, 145, 175
J.O.C. Auler jr., 109
B. Biagioli, 243
A. Di Lenarda, 267
P. Foëx, 21, 41
F.R.B.G. Galas,
G. Gemes, 159
P. Giomarelli, 243
H. Gombotz, 225
A. Gullo, 195
L. A. Hajjar, 109
A. Hofer, 225
R. Holsten, 135
G. Howard-Alpe, 21, 41
H. Metzler, 159
W. Moosbauer, 225
M. Moretti, 267
A. Perkan, 77
A. Rapotec, 211
G. Ristagno, 195
S. Romagnoli, 89
S.M. Romano, 89
A. Rossi, 89
S. Scolletta, 243
G. Sinagra, 1, 77, 267
C. Sorbara, 89
W. Tang, 195
W. G. Toller, 159
J.- L. Vincent, 135, 211
G. Vitrella, 1
M. H. Weil, 195
M. Zecchin, 1

1 Sudden Death in Heart Failure: Risk Stratification and Treatment Strategies

M. Zecchin, G. Vitrella and G. Sinagra

Definitions and Epidemiology

Attempting a careful evaluation of the incidence of sudden death (SD) in congestive heart failure is inevitably a complex and imprecise task. In particular, this is due to the difficulties in defining and understanding the baseline mechanisms underlying SD. "Sudden" death is commonly regarded as a synonym of "cardiac arrest due to ventricular fibrillation," which is in turn considered to be a merely arrhythmic phenomenon occurring during apparent wellbeing, and without any precipitating cause other than an extrasystole or a sustained ventricular tachycardia. Cardiac arrest may also be the terminal event during refractory pulmonary edema and/or cardiogenic shock in a patient with end-stage heart failure, a pulmonary embolism in a patient with severe biventricular dysfunction, bradyarrhythmia due to advanced atrioventricular (AV) block, electrical asystole, ventricular fibrillation secondary to myocardial ischemia or infarction, or secondary to a noncardiac event such as a cerebrovascular accident or a ruptured aortic aneurysm. Pratt et al. [1] analyzed a population of 834 patients with an automatic implantable cardioverter defibrillator (ICD) implanted for ventricular tachycardia or sustained ventricular tachycardia. During follow-up 109 patients died (17 died "suddenly"). Autopsy findings revealed a nonarrhythmic cause (pulmonary embolism, ruptured aortic aneurysm, stroke, acute myocardial infarction) in 7/17 patients. Postmortem analysis of the ICD memory revealed ventricular tachyarrhythmias preceding death in only 7/17 patients. Both cardiac and noncardiac events may cause SD, which may be indistinguishable from arrhythmic death.

Cardiovascular Department, "Ospedali Riuniti" and University of Trieste, Trieste, Italy

Before large pharmacologic trials in heart failure were published, the terminal mechanisms of death were never thoroughly evaluated. Hinkle and Thaler [2] provided a first classification: death was to be considered arrhythmic when pulselessness preceded cardiocirculatory collapse, and due to pump failure when cardiocirculatory collapse preceded pulselessness. This classification tends to overestimate the incidence of SD due to the aforementioned causes. Furthermore, it was not able to distinguish between the various mechanisms of SD.

When evaluating studies that have assessed the incidence of SD, it is of the first importance to take account of the definition of SD used, and, in particular, the time from symptom onset to SD. Classification was not always the same in all studies. In the SOLVD [3] study 23% of deaths were considered "arrhythmic, without worsening heart failure"; in VHeFT I [4] 43.8% of deaths were "sudden, witnessed as instantaneous, or considered instantaneous on a clinical basis when unwitnessed." In VHeFT II [5], an incidence of 36.5% of SD was found, with a similar definition of SD. In STAT-CHF [6] death was considered "sudden" in 49% and 52% of cases, respectively in the amiodarone and placebo groups, but individual cases were evaluated by a clinical events committee, not by the investigators. In conclusion, accurate evaluation of the epidemiology of SD must take into account the different definitions among studies, even if very similar populations were being analyzed [7].

Whether novel therapeutic interventions, improved diagnostic techniques, and increasing attention given to the problem in recent years have modified (and if so to what extent) the incidence of SD in addition to the improvement in the prognosis in patients with heart failure remains to be established. A study by Stevenson et al. [8] showed a reduction in the incidence of SD in patients with heart failure from diverse causes, from 20% (1986–1988) to 8% (1991–1993). Although a reduction in global mortality has been observed in patients with dilated cardiomyopathy, a reduction in SD remains to be established [9], even though it was found to be lower than expected in more recent trials. In the CAT [10] trial, expected mortality in the control group according to the literature [11] was 12%. However, none of 109 study patients suffered SD. A 2% annual incidence of SD was observed [12] in patients with dilated cardiomyopathy receiving optimized medical treatment. In more recent studies evaluating the use of β-blockers in patients with heart failure from different causes [13–15], the incidence of SD varied from 1.7% to 6.4% during follow-up (from 10 months to 1.3 years).

Lastly, the reduction in mortality in patients with heart failure may increase the number of patients at risk of SD. This may in part explain a persistently elevated risk of SD in paucisymptomatic patients with a long history of disease and persistent severe left ventricular dilatation and dysfunction, in whom SD is the first cause of mortality [12].

Mechanisms

Understanding the mechanisms underlying SD is the first step toward its prevention. Different etiologies and degrees of severity of heart failure may result in a wide variety of arrhythmias. In ischemic heart failure, cardiac arrest is frequently caused by tachyarrhythmias (ventricular tachycardia/fibrillation), while hypokinetic deaths (AV block, pulmonary embolism, pulseless electrical activity) cause only 5% of total deaths [16]. Conversely, in patients with advanced stages of dilated cardiomyopathy, nontachyarrhythmic SD is more common [17].

Ventricular arrhythmias may have various origins. In ischemic patients sustained VT are generally caused by reentry mechanisms, with an anatomic substrate of scarred myocardium (post myocardial infarction) and slow electrical conduction, which is necessary to initiate and maintain the arrhythmia [18]. Ventricular fibrillation may be primary (in around 10% of cases) or secondary to degeneration of sustained ventricular tachycardia [19]. In patients with heart failure from coronary artery disease, SD is in more than 50% of cases caused by an ischemic episode (myocardial infarction or transient myocardial ischemia), which very often goes unrecognized [20].

In patients with nonischemic dilated cardiomyopathy, monomorphic ventricular tachycardias are quite rare. Since the distribution of fibrosis is homogeneous, a slow conduction pathway may be recognizable in only 14% of cases [21].

In failing hearts, a suppression of potassium channels and consequent induction of early afterdepolarizations are observed. Early afterdepolarizations are thought to be the basis of triggered activity [22, 23], which is known to be the most frequent mechanism causing ventricular tachyarrhythmias in nonischemic dilated cardiomyopathy [24].

An additional subgroup of arrhythmias in patients with heart failure, especially in severe left ventricular dilation and dysfunction, are branch-to-branch tachyarrhythmias. These arrhythmias represent up to 20% of induced arrhythmias in nonischemic dilated cardiomyopathy. They may be found in patients with infra-His conduction abnormalities. They are characterized by a macro-reentry, which generally involves the right bundle branch as the orthodromic pathway and the left bundle branch as the antidromic pathway. This causes VT which are morphologically similar to left bundle branch block. It is important to recognize them, as their treatment is relatively simple: ablation of the right bundle branch prevents the arrhythmia from occurring and perpetuating [25].

Identifying Patients at Risk

Identifying patients at high risk is an important step in prevention of SD, and allows a cost-effective strategy in patient selection for ICD implantation. Unfortunately, no indicator sufficiently reliable in predicting SD has yet been found. The positive predictive value (ability to predict the event in the presence of the indicator) is generally low, whereas the negative predictive value (low risk of the event in the absence of the indicator) is quite high in some cases [26].

The indicators of severity of the functional status are also associated with a higher risk of SD. Patients in NYHA functional classes I–II have an incidence of SD of 0.5–2%, versus an incidence of 4–19% in patients in NYHA classes III–IV [27]. In addition, patients at higher risk of SD because they are in an advanced functional class are also at high risk of death due to pump failure. Conversely, in patients with few symptoms, who are the majority, SD represents the first cause of mortality, even though the relative risk is lower.

Syncopal episodes, independent of cause, are a marker of high risk of SD in patients with heart failure and left ventricular dysfunction [28]. According to the 2002 ACC/AHA/NASPE Pacemaker-ICD Guidelines [28a].Patients treated with ICD have a high incidence of ICD interventions for ventricular tachyarrhythmias, which are seldom induced during electrophysiological studies [29–31].

Survivors of cardiac arrest due to ventricular tachyarrhythmias, independent of etiology, are a subset of patients at high risk for SD [32]. The risk is particularly elevated (>10%) in the first months following the event, and tends to decrease in the following years [33]. However, in this population risk is also influenced by other factors, such as left ventricular ejection fraction (LVEF), which is significantly associated with a higher risk, especially in patients with ischemic heart disease [26, 34, 35]. Recent studies on primary and secondary prevention of SD showed how ICD is almost exclusively effective in patients with severe left ventricular dysfunction [36, 37]. According to ACC/AHA/NASPE guidelines, a LVEF of 30% of less alone identifies subjects who may benefit from this treatment (class IIa recommendation).

In order to accurately stratify the risk of arrhythmias, especially in patients with less than severe dysfunction, it is necessary to consider additional parameters that may facilitate or predict potentially lethal tachyarrhythmias and SD in patients with anatomic or functional substrates for reentry including: 1) evidence for the presence of late potentials, 2) spontaneous ventricular arrhythmias on Holter monitoring, 3) evidence for neurohumoral activation (e.g. heart rate variability) and 4) electrocardiographic (ECG) evidence for repolarization abnormalities (QT dispersion, T wave alternans). Pedretti et al. suggested a multistep approach, with invasive testing only in patients considered to be at high risk after stratification using noninvasive methods (LVEF, afterdepolarizations, arrhythmias) [35]. The positive predictive value of this approach increases from 30% to 60%, while maintaining a negative predictive value of 99%. Bailcy et al. [26] conducted a detailed analysis of data available in the literature, regarding the usefulness of tests for stratifying patients after myocardial infarction (post-MI patients). The authors found that the specificity of single tests [signal-averaged electrocardiography (SAECG), ventricular arrhythmias, heart rate variability, LVEF, and electrophysiologic studies (EPS)] varies from 77% to 85%, whereas the sensitivity varies from 42% to 62%. A multistep combined approach may be useful to distinguish a subgroup (12% of post-MI patients) of patients at higher risk (41% risk of major ventricular arrhythmias at 2-year follow-up) from patients (80%) of post-Mi patients) with lower risk of SD (2.9% risk of major ventricular arrhythmias). This type of approach may reduce the number of ICDs needed to save a single life (18 ICDs at 2 years in the MADIT II study) [38] and increase the number of patients who are correctly stratified. Patients enrolled in MADIT I, for example, had a high risk of arrhythmic events (66.5% at 2 years), but represented only 1.9% of the general post-MI population [26].

Risk stratification is, furthermore, complex in patients with heart failure and severe left ventricular dysfunction of nonischemic origin. This is due to the wide variety of mechanisms underlying SD and ventricular arrhythmias in this subset. The role of ejection fraction [10, 39] and ventricular arrhythmias [39–41] is controversial, and the role of EPS is inconclusive [42]. The association of various indicators, such as left ventricular function and geometry [12, 39], afterdepolarizations [43], or T wave alternans [44], may increase sensitivity and specificity in identifying patients who may benefit from ICD implantation.

Prevention

Cardiomyopathies that are associated with a high risk of SD are caused by a concurrence of genetic and environmental factors. Dyslipidemia, hypertension, cigarette smoking, obesity, and diabetes mellitus are important risk factors for ischemic heart disease, left ventricular dysfunction, and SD.

The increase in SD among the youth in the US [45] is (at least) in part due to the increase in obesity and type II diabetes mellitus. Treatment is thus based on achieving an appropriate body mass index (<25 kg/m^2) and lowering blood pressure, cholesterol, triglycerides, postprandial blood glucose, and glycosylated hemoglobin levels. Hypolipidemic agents are also thought to have a direct antiarrhythmic effect. In a subanalysis of the AVID study, patients who were receiving statins had a 40% reduction of their risk of recurrent ventricular tachycardia/fibrillation [46].

An important contributor in preventing SD in post-MI patients may be intake of polyunsaturated fatty acids, especially those containing omega-3 fatty acids, such as eicosapentaenoic acid (EPA) and docosahexaenoic acid (DHA). The primary sources of omega-3 fatty acids are phytoplankton and all the fish that eat it. The minimum recommended daily intake for man is 1.5 g EPA and DHA. The benefit of EPA and DHA in reducing mortality in post-MI patients, especially through a 45% reduction in SD, has been convincingly demonstrated [47]. Furthermore, the concentration in omega-3 fatty acids is inversely related to the risk of SD in apparently healthy subjects [48]. The protective mechanism of omega-3 fatty acids is unclear. A direct antiarrhythmic effect, through membrane stabilization and modulation of conduction through sodium and calcium channels [49, 50], and an antithrombotic and anti-inflammatory effect [51] are thought to play a role.

A high alcohol intake is associated with left ventricular dilation and dysfunction [52], especially in predisposed subjects, and is the cause of an increased mortality [53] due to SD in alcoholic patients. However, moderate alcohol consumption seems to be protective against global cardiovascular mortality and against SD in particular [54].

Pharmacologic Prevention

Evidence-based treatment of heart failure includes angiotensin-converting enzyme inhibitors (ACE-I), angiotensin II receptor blockers (ARB-II's), β-blockers, diuretics, aldosterone antagonists, and digitalis. They have shown their efficacy in improving the symptoms [55] and natural history of heart failure independently of its cause [5, 56–58]. ACE-I reduced mortality in all trials in which they were tested [59, 60]. Their benefit is greater in patients with severe heart failure (NYHA class IV, LVEF <25%), but is also seen in all other subgroups. However, the reduction in mortality is secondary to a reduction in myocardial infarction, mortality, and rehospitalization for heart failure, not to a significant reduction in arrhythmic death [59].

ARB-II's have an effect similar to that of ACE-I: a reduction in total mortality is not accompanied by a reduction in arrhythmic death [61].

Diuretic therapy is certainly effective in improving symptoms in heart failure patients. However, its use has been demonstrated to be associated with an increase in mortality [62] secondary to electrolyte imbalance and increased neurohumoral activation.

The DIG trial has contributed to clarifying the role of digitalis in the treatment of heart failure. This drug reduces rehospitalization for heart failure, but not total mortality. In addition, a slight but significant increase in cardiac death due to causes other than heart failure (almost certainly arrhythmic death) was seen in the treatment group versus the placebo group (15% vs 13%; $P = 0.04$) [55].

Another category of drugs that have beneficial effects on mortality are the aldosterone receptor antagonists. The RALES study [63] enrolled 1635 patients who were in NYHA class IV with a LVEF below 35%. The study showed a significant reduction in cardiac mortality, by 31%, caused by both a reduction in death due to heart failure and a reduction in SD (RR 0.71; $P = 0.02$). More recently, the EPHESUS [64] study enrolled 6642 post-MI patients with heart failure and a LVEF below 40%. Eplerenone was shown to be effective in reducing all cause of mortality and mortality due to SD (RR 0.79; $P = 0.03$).

β-blockers

In recent years, β-blockers, which were contraindicated in the past, have become a cornerstone of treatment of heart failure [13–15, 65]. The reduction in mortality in patients with ischemic and nonischemic left ventricular dysfunction is similar to that of ACE-I and cumulative with that of ACE-I. The neutralization of circulating catecholamines leads to an improvement in left ventricular function and prognosis. Unlike ACE-I, β-blockers may also counteract proarrhythmic effects of increased neurohumoral activation, and have a direct antiarrhythmic effect which is protective against SD. The US carvedilol trial [13] enrolled 1094 patients with heart failure and left ventricular dysfunction (LVEF <35%) on ACE-I, digitalis, and diuretic treatment. A 65% reduction in total mortality in the carvedilol group was observed compared to the placebo group. The incidence of SD at 10-month follow-up was 1.7% in the carvedilol group, and 3.8% in the placebo group. The MERIT-HF [15] study randomized 3991 patients with heart failure and LVEF below 40% to metoprolol or placebo (in addition to digitalis and ACE-I). A 41% reduction in SD was observed in the metoprolol group compared to the placebo group.

The reduction in the incidence of SD seems even more impressive in patients in a higher functional class and at higher risk. In CIBIS II [14], which randomized patients in NYHA classes III–IV (and LVEF <35%) to receive bisoprolol or placebo, showed a 42% reduction in the incidence of SD and a reduction in total mortality. The COPERNICUS trial [65] evaluated patients with a LVEF below 25% and dyspnea on minimal exertion or at rest despite optimization of medical treatment with diuretics and ACE-I. The incidence of SD in the metoprolol group was 3.9%, versus 6.1% in the control group ($P = 0.016$).

Antiarrhythmic Drugs

Although sustained ventricular tachycardia/fibrillation is the primary cause of SD, "pure" antiarrhythmic drugs (i.e., sodium and potassium channel blockers), which are effective in reducing ventricular extrasystole and non-sustained ventricular arrhythmias, are not effective in reducing SD or total mortality.

Conversely, sodium channel-blocking drugs may even reduce survival in post-MI patients with left ventricular dysfunction and frequent ventricular extrasystole, as observed in the CAST and CAST II trials [66, 67]. The CASH study tested the effect of propafenone, metoprolol, and amiodarone versus ICD in patients who suffered from a prior cardiac arrest. The propafenone group showed an excess mortality and this arm of the trial was thus prematurely interrupted [68].

The negative experiences with class I antiarrhythmic drugs prompted an increasing focus on class III drugs: potassium channel blockers. Agents in this class, unlike class I agents, do not carry negative inotropic effects, and thus seem ideal for patients with heart failure. The ESVEM study [69] suggested that sotalol was more effective than class I agents. However, the absence of a placebo group make it impossible to rule out the possibility that sotalol was simply less harmful than class I drugs. In addition, sotalol is a racemic mixture of D-sotalol (with class III effects), and L-sotalol (with β-blocker effects), and the benefit might be attributable to only one of the isomers. In the SWORD study [70], which enrolled patients with prior myocardial infarction, heart failure (NYHA classes II–III), and LVEF below 40%, D-sotalol was associated with higher total and arrhythmic mortality.

The effectiveness of dofetilide–an inhibitor of a single potassium channel which is commercially available in the US but not in Europe–was evaluated in the DIAMOND-CHF study [71]. Patients with heart failure (NYHA classes III–IV) and LVEF below 35% were enrolled. Dofetilide did not worsen heart failure, reduced the incidence of atrial fibrillation, and increased the rate of successful cardioversion to normal sinus rhythm. However, no effect, favorable or unfavorable, was seen on total or arrhythmic mortality.

The lack of success of antiarrhythmic drugs in preventing SD is difficult to explain. Class I agents have a negative inotropic effect which may favor an increase in mortality in patients with heart failure. Furthermore, a subanalysis of CAST and CAST II studies showed a higher risk of arrhythmic death, especially in subgroups of patients with non-Q-wave myocardial infarction, suggesting that class Ic drugs may favor the occurrence of lethal arrhythmias especially in patients with ischemic instability [72].

As stated above, a "fetospecific" reinduction of genetic programs, with a suppression of potassium channels, has been shown in patients with heart failure [22]. This leads to an increase in QT interval, with consequent increased risk of polymorphous ventricular tachycardia. This effect may vary according to the area of the heart, and thus lead to an increased QT interval dispersion and areas of block and/or reentry. This may in part explain why potassium channel blockers have failed to show a beneficial effect. In the DIAMOND-CHF study, 3% of patients developed torsades de pointes. This was especially true for patients with severe heart failure, and during the initial days of treatment. Although class III agents may reduce ICD shocks [73], and amiodarone is the most effective drug in treating refractory ventricular fibrillation [74], the use of agents of this class remains controversial due to their lack of effect on total and arrhythmic mortality.

Of all drugs that affect the action potential, amiodarone appears to be the only one to have an effect, although limited, in reducing arrhythmic mortality, (possibly also because it has no effect on QT dispersion although increasing PT interval [75]) but not in reducing total mortality. A meta-analysis [76] of 13 studies and 6553 patients showed that amiodarone reduced arrhythmic mortality by 29%, and had a neutral effect on nonarrhythmic mortality, with a 13% decrease of total mortality. After the publication of studies showing not univocal results [77-79] data from SCD-HeFT (which enrolled 2521 patients with heart failure and LVEF <35%) definitely ruled out an effect on mortality by amiodarone in patients with heart failure. This is independent of the organic heart disease (ischemic or nonischemic) that caused the heart failure [80]. In addition, there was a significant worsening of survival in the subgroup of patients with NYHA class III heart failure.

Internal Cardioverter-Defibrillator (ICD)

The goal of ICD implantation, unlike that of treatment with antiarrhythmic drugs, is not the prevention of arrhythmias, but their quick interruption. Modern ICDs are able to recognize ventricular tachyarrhythmias with nearly 100% sensitivity and more than 90% specificity, and to effectively treat them in almost 100% of cases. The operative risk of implanting an ICD is low (similar to the risk of a pacemaker implant). ICD is thus the ideal tool in preventing SD from purely arrhythmic events, such as ventricular tachycardia or ventricular fibrillation. This has led to extensive use of ICDs. Even though the relative risk of SD is very high in a selected subset of patients with defined characteristics [81], most subjects who die suddenly belong to lower risk categories. Theoretically, if the cost and risk of ICD implantation were nil, the whole population would benefit from it. Unfortunately, ICD is still a very expensive and invasive treatment, with potential complications and limits, especially in the long term. The current matter of concern is not whether ICD reduces SD, but whether this effect is clinically relevant and economically sustainable.

ICD for Primary Prevention

Patients with heart failure have a high incidence of life-threatening ventricular tachyarrhythmias and a low probability of surviving such arrhythmic events [82]. It is thus necessary to correctly identify patients at high risk of SD, who may benefit from ICD implantation as a primary prevention procedure.

The MADIT and MUSTT [83, 84] studies, respectively published in 1996 and 1999, showed a superiority of ICD in patients with ischemic heart disease, severe left ventricular dysfunction (LVEF ≤35% in MADIT, and ≤40% in MUSTT), nonsustained ventricular tachycardia on Holter monitoring, and inducible sustained ventricular tachycardia at EPS. The effect of ICD was similar in the two studies, with a hazard ratio of 0.46 ($P = 0.009$) in MADIT and 0.49 ($P = 0.001$) in MUSTT. These studies suggested the appropriateness of a selectively invasive approach (initially with noninvasive testing, then with EPS). However, subanalysis of the MUSTT study suggested that EPS testing added little prognostic value in patients with LVEF <30% compared to patients with LVEF between 30% and 40% [85].

These impressions were later confirmed when the MADIT II study was published in 2002. The authors showed that ICD implantation as primary prevention led to a 31% reduction in total mortality in post-MI patients with LVEF ≤30% [86].

An important question raised by a subanalysis of MADIT II [86] and by the DINAMIT study [87] was timing the ICD implantation. In particular, excessively early implantation (within 40 days of the MI), was found to reduce lethal arrhythmias but not total mortality. Similarly, the main benefit in terms of survival was seen in patients with a more remote diagnosis of MI (more than 18 months prior to ICD implantation) [88]. These data underscored the importance of implanting ICDs in patients with a stabilized left ventricular dysfunction, after completion of the myocardial remodeling process.

The data on ICD implantation for primary prevention in nonischemic cardiomyopathies are controversial. The CAT and AMIOVIRT [10, 41] studies failed to demonstrate a beneficial effect in patients with LVEF ≤30% [10], and in patients with LVEF ≤35% and nonsustained ventricular tachycardia [41]. However, the CAT study enrolled only 104 instead of the 1348 projected patients. In addition, study patients had a recent (<9 months) diagnosis of heart failure, and it was demonstrated how variable the long-term outcome may be, and how over 50% of patients may radically improve over the following months or years, when on optimized medical treatment [89]. Furthermore, the incidence of SD in the first years after diagnosis is lower than the incidence of death caused by pump failure. The risk of SD increases in patients with a long history of disease, and persistent severe left ventricular dilation and dysfunction, regardless of their functional status [90].

While the CAT study was interrupted due to the paucity of arrhythmic mortality (which made it impossible to interpret the results), AMIOVIRT was interrupted because of the lack of evidence that continuing the analysis would be able to demonstrate differences between the ICD and amiodarone groups. The cutoff value for LVEF (35%) that was chosen as a criterion for enrolling patients may not have been low enough to select high-risk patients. Grimm et al. [30] observed a similar incidence of appropriate ICD interventions in patients treated with the device for secondary prevention because of prior ventricular tachycardia/fibrillation or syncope and in those treated for primary prevention because of LVEF ≤30% and nonsustained ventricular tachycardia.

The DEFINITE [91] study randomized 458 patients with dilated cardiomyopathy, LVEF ≤35%, and nonsustained ventricular tachycardia (ventricular tachycardia or frequent premature ventricular beats), to ICD implantation or conventional treatment. The incidence of arrhythmic death was 74% lower in the ICD group ($P<0.05$). However, SD only accounted for one-third of total mortality, and the reduction in total mortality in the ICD group was not statistically significant ($P = 0.06$).

Data from SCD-HeFT confirmed that in a large population of subjects (2521 patients) with heart failure and LVEF of 35% or less, ICD reduces 5-year mortality by 23% ($P = 0.007$) compared to conventional treatment. The reduction in mortality in patients affected by dilated cardiomyopathy (HR = 0.73) was similar to that in patients with ischemic heart disease (HR = 0.79) [80].

ICD for Secondary Prevention

Patients who survive a cardiac arrest are at high risk of recurrence. In this subgroup of patients, revascularization and pharmacologic interventions, including amiodarone and β-blockers, have failed to significantly reduce the risk of SD. Conversely, the role of ICD is supported by three randomized, controlled studies published in the late 1990s. The AVID study was published in 1997 [92]. One thousand and thirteen patients who survived a cardiac arrest from ventricular fibrillation, had ventricular tachycardia with syncope or hemodynamically relevant ventricular tachycardia associated with LVEF ≤40%, were randomized to receive ICD or antiarrhythmic drugs (amiodarone or sotalol). Most patients had signs and symptoms of heart failure at enrollment. At 1-year follow-up the group that received an ICD had 39% lower mortality than the control group. Long-term results confirmed these data (37% at

2 years and 31% at 3 years). Similar results were found in two later studies, CASH and CIDS [68, 93]. The former enrolled patients with similar characteristics to those in the AVID study (except for the cutoff of LVEF, which was 35%, and the inclusion of patients with prior syncope and inducible sustained ventricular tachycardia on electrophysiologic testing). A nonsignificant reduction in total mortality by 23%, and significant reduction of SD by 38%), was found in the ICD group compared to the amiodarone group. The CASH study compared ICD to metoprolol and amiodarone (the propafenone arm was stopped prematurely due to excess mortality) in survivors from cardiac arrest. A significant reduction in total mortality by 37%, and in arrhythmic mortality by 63%, were found in patients in the ICD group.

These studies also suggest that the benefit of ICD increases with increasing left ventricular dysfunction and functional limitation. A post-hoc analysis of the AVID [94] study showed lack of benefit in patients with LVEF greater than 35%. These data were later confirmed in a meta-analysis which included the CASH and CIDS studies among others [37]. The reduction in mortality in the CIDS study was more evident in patients with a greater functional class according to a score based on a LVEF of 35% or more, NYHA class III–IV, and age 70 years or over [95]. These data underscore the importance of LVEF in the risk stratification in patients surviving cardiac arrest. Furthermore, they mandate careful evaluation of comorbidities, the possibility of heart transplantation, and the risk of death due to pump failure.

Role of Myocardial Revascularization for the Prevention of Sudden Death

The role of myocardial revascularization in reducing total mortality in patients with coronary artery disease and severe left ventricular dysfunction has been well established since the 1980s [96, 97]. Surgical revascularization was shown to be superior to medical treatment in preventing SD, especially in patients with heart failure [98].

Sudden death may often be caused by acute coronary syndrome [20]. Susceptibility to major ventricular arrhythmias during ischemia has been experimentally demonstrated [99]. Large primary and secondary prevention trials have generally excluded patients with evidence of ischemia, and a direct randomized comparison between myocardial revascularization and ICD has never been performed. The CABG-PATCH trial [100] enrolled 1055 patients with left ventricular dysfunction (LVEF ≤35%) and late afterdepolarizations on SAECG, indication for revascularization, and who were treated with coronary artery bypass graft surgery. Patients were randomized to receive ICD versus no antiarrhythmic treatment. ICD was found not to have any additional benefit over revascularization alone. This may have been due to the ability of myocardial revascularization to reduce SD in a theoretically high-risk population. Actually, ICD reduced arrhythmic mortality by 45%, but since 77% of deaths were not arrhythmic, total mortality was not significantly affected [101]. On the other hand, the low incidence of arrhythmic mortality may be secondary to an improvement in left ventricular function after revascularization.

Myocardial revascularization alone does not seem to favorably improve the prognosis in patients with coronary artery disease who survive a cardiac arrest. A study by Trappe et al. [102] enrolled 139 patients with coronary artery disease who survived a cardiac arrest from ventricular fibrillation or sustained ventricular tachycardia. Patients were treated with ICD and bypass surgery in the presence of inducible ischemia, and with ICD alone in the absence of inducible ischemia. The incidence of appropriate ICD shocks was similar in the two groups (respectively 81% and 82% at 26 ± 20 months). These results suggest that myocardial revascularization did not have any benefit in preventing recurrent tachyarrhythmias in this population. Other uncontrolled studies have had similar results [103, 104].

Conclusions

The widespread use of pharmacologic treatment, which has proven effective in improving the prognosis in patients with heart failure, has increased the population at risk of sudden death (SD). SD remains the leading cause of death, especially in paucisymptomatic patients. Although the recent introduction of effective treatments such as β-blockers and omega-3 fatty acids has reduced arrhythmic mortality, preventing SD in patients with heart failure remains a challenge due to the difficulty in identifying patients at greater risk, and the poor effect of the majority of treatments. The only real exception to this is represented by ICD, which is, however, an invasive and expensive solution. In the future, technological advances, the reduction of device costs, and systematic selection of patients who will benefit from ICD will be necessary to achieve effective prevention of SD in the wide and heterogeneous population of patients with heart failure.

References

1. Pratt CM, Greenway PS, Schoenfeld MH et al (1996) Exploration of the precision of classifying sudden cardiac death. Implications for the interpretation of clinical trials. Circulation 93:519–524

2. Hinkle LE, Thaler HT (1982) Clinical classification of cardiac deaths. Circulation 65:457–464
3. The SOLVD Investigators (1992) Effect of enalapril mortality and the developement of heart failure in asymptomatic patients with reduced left ventricular ejection fractions. N Engl J Med 327:685–691
4. Cohn J N, Archibald DG, Ziesche S et al (1986) Effect of vasodilator therapy on mortality in chronic congestive heart failure. Results of a Veterans Administration Cooperative Study. N Engl J Med 314:1547–1552
5. The Vasodilatator-Heart failure Veterans Affairs Cooperative Study Group (1991) A comparison of enalapril with hydralazine-isosorbide dinitrate in the treatment of chronic congestive heart failure. N Engl J Med 325:303–310
6. Singh SN, Fletcher RD, Fisher SG et al for the Survival Trial of Antiarrhythmic Therapy in Congestive Heart Failure (1995) Amiodarone in patients with congestive heart failure and asymptomatic ventricular arrhythmia. N Engl J Med 333:77–82
7. Ziesche S, Rector T, Cohn J (1995) Interobserver discordance in the classification of mechanism of death in studies of heart failure. J Card Fail 1:127–132
8. Stevenson WG, Stevenson LW, Middlekauff HR et al (1995) Improving survival for patients with advanced heart failure: a study of 737 consecutive patients. J Am Coll Cardiol 26:1417–1423
9. Di Lenarda A, Hlede S, Sabbadini G et al (1999) Improvement of prognosis in idiopathic dilated cardiomyopathy: role of early diagnosis and optimized medical treatment. Study Group on Heart Muscles Diseases. G Ital Cardiol 29:1452–1462
10. Bänsch D, Antz M, Boczor S et al for the CAT Investigators (2002) Primary prevention of sudden cardiac death in idiopathic dilated cardiomyopathy: the Cardiomyopathy Trial (CAT). Circulation 105:1453–1458
11. Tamburro P, Wilber DJ (1992) Sudden death in idiopathic dilated cardiomyopathy. Am Heart J 124:992–997
12. Zecchin M, Di Lenarda A, Gregori D et al (2005) Prognostic role of non-sustained ventricular tachycardia in a large cohort of patients with idiopathic dilated cardiomyopathy. Ital Heart J 6:721-727
13. Packer M, Bristow MR, Cohn JN et al (1996) The effect of carvedilol on morbidity and mortality in patients with chronic heart failure. US Carvedilol Heart Failure Study Group. N Engl J Med 334:1349–1355
14. No authors listed (1999) The Cardiac Insufficiency Bisoprolol Study II (CIBIS II) a randomized trial. Lancet 353:9–13
15. No authors listed (1999) Effect of metoprolol CR/XL in chronic heart failure: Metoprolol CR/XL Randomized Intervention Trial in Congestive Heart Failure (MERIT-HF). Lancet 353:2001–2007
16. Uretsky BF, Sheahan RG (1997) Primary prevention of sudden cardiac death in heart failure: will the solution be shocking? J Am Coll Cardiol 30:1589–1597
17. Luu M, Stevenson LW, Brunken RC et al (1989) Diverse mechanisms of unexpected cardiac arrest in advanced heart failure. Circulation 80:1675–1680
18. Gardner PI, Ursell, PC, Fenoglio JJ Jr et al (1985) Electrophysiologic and anatomic basis for fractioned electrograms recorded from healed myocardium infarcts. Circulation 72:596–611
19. Raitt MH, Dolack GL, Kudenchuk PJ et al (1995) Ventricular arrhythmias detected after transvenous defibrillator implantation in patients with a clinical history of only ventricular fibrillation: implications for use of implantable defibrillator. Circulation 91:1996–2001
20. Uretsky BF, Thygesen K, Armstrong PW et al (2000) Acute coronary findings at

autopsy in heart failure patients with sudden death. Results from the assessment of treatment with lisinopril and survival (ATLAS) study. Circulation 102:611–616

21. Roberts WC, Siegel RJ, McManus BM (1989) Idiopathic dilated cardiomyopathy: analysis of 152 necropsy patients. Am J Cardiol 64:1063–1066
22. Armoundas AA, Wu R, Juang G et al (2001) Electrical and structural remodeling in the failing ventricle. Pharmacol Ther 92:213–239
23. Pacifico A, Henry PD (2003) Structural pathways and prevention of heart failure and sudden death. J Cardiovasc Electrophysiol 14:764–775
24. Pogwizd SM, McKenzie JP, Cain ME (1998) Mechanisms underlyng spontaneous and induced ventricular arrhythmias in patients with idiopathic dilated cardiomyopathy. Circulation 98:2404–2414
25. Delacretaz E, Stevenson WG, Eleison KE et al (2000) Mapping and radiofrequency catheter ablation of the three types of sustained ventricular tachycardia in nonischemic heart disease. J Cardiovasc Electrophysiol 11:11–17
26. Bailey JJ, Berson AS, Handelsman H et al (2001) Utility of current risk stratification tests for predicting major arrhythmic events after myocardial infarction. J Am Coll Cardiol. 38:1902–1911
27. Zoni Berisso M, Delfino L, Viani S (2002) Nei pazienti con insufficienza cardiaca il cardioverter-defibrillatore impiantabile ritarda la morte o salva la vita? Ital Heart J Suppl 3:36–44
28. Middlekauff HR, Stevenson WG, Stevenson LW et al (1993) Syncope in advanced heart failure: high risk of sudden death regardless of origin of syncope. J Am Coll Cardiol 21:110–116

28a. Gregoratos G, Abrams J, Epstein AE et al (2002) American College of Cardiology, American Heart Association Task Force on Practice Guidelines, North American Society for Pacing and Electrophysiology Committee to Update the 1998 Pacemaker Guidelines. Circulation 106(16)2145-2161

29. Knight BP, Goyal R, Pelosi F et al (1999) Outcome of patients with nonischemic dilated cardiomyopathy and unexplained syncope treated with an implantable defibrillator. J Am Coll Cardiol 33:1964–1970
30. Grimm W, Hoffmann J, Muller HH et al (2002) Implantable defibrillator event rates in patients with idiopathic dilated cardiomyopathy, nonsustained ventricular tachycardia on Holter and a left ventricular ejection fraction below 30%. J Am Coll Cardiol 39:780–787
31. Zecchin M, Di Lenarda A, Proclemer A (2004) ICD for primary and secondary prevention of sudden death in patients with dilated cardiomyopathy. Europace 6:400-406
32. Ehlert FA, Cannom DS, Renfroe EG (2001) Comparison of dilated cardiomyopathy and coronary artery disease in patients with life-threatening ventricular arrhythmias: differences in presentation and outcome in the AVID registry. Am Heart J 142:816–822
33. Myerburg RJ, Castellanos A (2001) Cardiac arrest and sudden cardiac death. In: Braunwald E, Zipes DP Libby P (eds) Heart disease. Saunders, Philadephia, pp 908
34. McClements BM, Adgey AAJ (1993) Value of signal-averaged electrocardiography, radionuclide ventriculography, Holter monitoring and clinical variables for prediction of arrhythmic events in survivors of acute myocardial infarction in the thrombolitic era. J Am Coll Cardiol 21:1419–1427
35. Pedretti R, Etro M, La porta A et al (1993) Prediction of late arrhythmic events after acute myocardial infaction from combined use of noninvasive prognostic variables and inducibility of sustained monomorphic venticular tachycardia. Am J

Cardiol 71:1131–1141

36. Moss AJ (2000) Implantable cardioverter defibrillator therapy. The sickest patients benefit the most. Circulation 101:1638–1640
37. Connolly SJ, Hallstrom AP, Cappato R et al (2000) Meta-analysis of the implantable cardioverter defibrillator secondary prevention trials. AVID, CASH and CIDS studies. Antiarrhythmics Vs Implantable Defibrillator study. Cardiac Arrest Study Hamburg. Canadian Implantable Defibrillator Study. Eur Heart J 21:2071–2078
38. Ezekowitz JA, Armstrong PW, McAlister FA (2003) Implantable cardioverter defibrillators in primary and secondary prevention: a systematic review of randomized, controlled trials. Ann Intern Med 138:445–452
39. Grimm W, Glaveris C, Hoffmann J et al (2000) Arrhythmia risk stratification in idiopathic dilated cardiomyopathy based on echocardiography, 12-lead electrocardiogram, signal-averaged electrocardiogram and 24-hour Holter electrocardiogram. Am Heart J 140:43–51
40. Meinertz T, Hoffmann T, Kasper W et al (1984) Significance of ventricular arrhythmias in idiopathic dilated cardiomyopathy. Am J Cardiol 53:902–907
41. Strickberger SA, Hummel JD, Bartlett TG et al for the AMIOVIRT Investigators (2003) Amiodarone Versus Implantable Cardioverter-Defibrillator: Randomized Trial in Patients With Nonischemic Dilated Cardiomyopathy and Asymptomatic Nonsustained Ventricular Tachycardia–AMIOVIRT. J Am Coll Cardiol 41:1707–1712
42. Brembilla-Perrot B, Donetti J, Terrier de la Chaise A et al (2001) Diagnostic value of ventricular stimulation in patients with idiopathic dilated cardiomyopathy. Am Heart J 121:1124–1131
43. Fauchier L, Babuty D, Cosnay P et al (2000) Long-term prognostic value of time domain analysis of signal-averaged electrocardiography in idiopathic dilated cardiomyopathy. Am J Cardiol 85:618–623
44. Hohnloser SH, Klingenheben T, Bloomfield D et al (2003) Usefulness of microvolt T-wave alternans for prediction of ventricular tachyarrhythmic events in patients with dilated cardiomyopathy: results from a prospective observational study. J Am Coll Cardiol 41:2220–2224
45. Zheng ZJ, Croft JB, Giles WH (2001) Sudden cardiac death in the United States, 1989–1998. Circulation 104:2158–2163
46. Mitchell LB, Powell JL, Gillis AM, and the AVID Investigators (2003) Are lipid-lowering drugs also antiarrhythmic drugs? An analysis of the Antiarrhythmics Versus Implantable Defibrillators (AVID) trial. J Am Coll Cardiol 42:81–87
47. Marchiali R, Barzi F, Bomba E et al on behalf of the GISSI-Prevenzione Investigators (2002) Early protection against sudden death by n-3 polyunsaturated fatty acids after myocardial infarction. Circulation 105:1897–1903
48. Albert CM, Campos H, Stampefer MJ et al (2002) Blood levels of long chain n-3 fatty acids and the risk of sudden death. N Engl J Med 346:1113–1118
49. Xiao YF, Wright SN, Wang GK et al (1998) n-3 fatty acids suppress voltage-gated Na currents in HEK293t cells transfected with the alpha-subunit of the human cardiac Na channel. Proc Natl Acad Sci USA 95:2680–2685
50. Xiao YF, Gomez AM, Morgan JP et al (1997) Suppression of voltage-gated L-type Ca currents by polyunsatured fatty acid in neonatal and adult cardiac myocytes. Proc Natl Acad Sci USA 94:4182–4187
51. Chinetti G, Fruchart JC, Staels B (2000) Peroxisome proliferator-activated receptors: nuclear receptors at the crossroads between lipid metabolism and inflammation. Inflamm Res 49:497–505

52. Fuster V, Gersh BJ, Giuliani ER et al (1981) The natural history of idiopathic dilated cardiomyopathy. Am J Cardiol 47:525–531
53. Rosengren A, Wilhelmsen L, Pennert K et al (1987) Alcoholic intemperance, coronary heart disease and mortality in middle-aged Swedish men. Acta Med Scand 222:201–213
54. Albert CM, Manson JE, Cook NR et al (1999) Moderate alcohol consumption and the risk of sudden cardiac death among US male physicians. Circulation 100:944–950
55. The Digitalis Investigation Group (1997) The effect of digoxin on mortality and morbidity in patients with heart failure. N Engl J Med 336:525–533
56. The SOLVD Investigators (1991) Effect of enalapril on survival in patients with reduced left ventricular ejection fractions and congestive heart failure. N Engl J Med 325:293–302
57. The CONSENSUS Trial Study Group (1987) Effects of enalapril on mortality in severe congestive heart failure: results of the Cooperative North Scandinavian Enalapril Survival Study (CONSENSUS). N Engl J Med 316:1429–1435
58. Packer M, Poole-Wilson PA, Armstrong PW et al on behalf of the ATLAS Study Group (1999) Comparative effects of low and high doses of the angiotensin-converting enzyme inhibitor, lisinopril, on morbidity and mortality in chronic heart failure. Circulation 100:2312–2318
59. Garg R, Yusuf S (1995) Overview of randomized trial of angiotensin-converting enzyme inhibitors on mortality and morbidity in patients with heart failure. JAMA 273:1450–456
60. Flather M, Yusuf S, Kober L et al for the ACE-Inhibitors Myocardial Collaborative Group (2000) Long term ACE-inhibitor therapy in patients with heart failure or left ventricular dysfunction: a systematic overview of data from individual patients. Lancet 355:1575–1581
61. Cohn JN, Tognoni G; Valsartan Heart Failure Trial Investigators (2001) A randomized trial of the angiotensin-receptor blocker valsartan in chronic heart failure. N Engl J Med. 345:1667–1675
62. Cooper HA, Dries DL, Davis CE et al (1999) Diuretics and risk of arrhythmic death in patients with left ventricular dysfunction. Circulation 100:1311–1315
63. Pitt B, Zannad F, Remme WJ et al for the Randomized Aldosterone Evauation Study Investigators (1999) The effect of spironolactone on morbidity and mortality in patients with severe heart failure. N Engl J Med 341:709–717
64. Pitt B, Remme W, Zannad F et al for the Eplerenone Post-Acute Myocardial Infarction Heart Failure Efficacy and Survival Study Investigators (2003) Eplerenone, a selective aldosterone blocker, in patients with left ventricular dysfunction after myocardial infarction. N Engl J Med 348:1309–1321
65. Packer M, Coats AJS, Fowler MB et al, the Carvedilol Prospective Randomized Cumulative Survival Study Group (2001) Effect of carvedilol on survival in severe chronic heart failure. N Engl J Med 344:1651–1658
66. The Cardiac Arrhythmia Suppression Trial (CAST) Investigators (1989) Preliminary report: effect of encainide and flecainide on mortality in a randomized trial of arrhythmia suppression after myocardial infarction. N Engl J Med 321:406–412
67. The Cardiac Arrhythmia Suppression Trial II Investigators (1992) Effect of the antiarrhythmic agent moricizine on survival after myocardial infarction. N Engl J Med 327:227–233
68. Kuck KH, Cappato R, Siebels J, Ruppel R for the CASH investigators (2000)

Randomized comparison of antiarrhythmic drug therapy with implantable cardioverter defibrillators in patients resuscitated from cardiac arrest. The Cardiac Arrest Study Hamburg (CASH). Circulation Am Heart J 102:748-754
69. Mason JW for The Electrophysiologic Study versus Electrocardiographic Monitoring Investigators (1993) A comparison of seven antiarrhythmic drugs in patients with ventricular tachyarrhythmias. N Engl J Med 329:452–458
70. Hohnloser SH, Meinertz T, Stubbs P et al for the d-Sotalol PVC Study Group (1995) Efficacy and safety of d-sotalol, a pure class III antiarrhythmic compound, in patients with symptomatic complex ventricular ectopy. Circulation 92:1517–1525
71. Kober L, Bloch Thomsen PE, Moller M et al; Danish Investigations of Arrhythmia and Mortality on Dofetilide (DIAMOND) Study Group (2000) Effect of dofetilide in patients with recent myocardial infarction and left-ventricular dysfunction: a randomised trial. Lancet 356:2052–2058
72. Anderson JL, Platia EV, Hallstroim A et al for the Cardiac Arrhythmia Suppression Trial (CAST) Investigators (1994) Interaction of baseline characteristics with the hazard of encainide, flecainide, and moricizine therapy in patients with myocardial infarction. A possibile explanation for increased mortality in the Cardiac Arrhythmia Suppression Trial (CAST). Circulation 90:2843–2852
73. Pacifico A, Hohnloser SH, Williams JH et al for the d,l-Sotalol Implantable Cardioverter Defibrillator Study Group (1999) Prevention of implantable defibrillator shocks by treatment with sotalol. N Engl J Med 340:1855–1862
74. Dorian P, Mangat I (2003) Role of amiodarone in the era of the implantable cardioverter defibrillator. J Cardiovasc Electrophysiol 14(Suppl 9):S78-S81
75. Cui G, Sen L, Sager P et al (1994) Effects of amiodarone, sematilide and sotalol on QT dispersion. Am J Cardiol 74:896–900
76. No author listed (1997) Effect of prophylactic amiodarone on mortality after acute myocardial infarction and in congestive heart failure: meta-analysis of individual data from 6500 patients in randomised trials. Amiodarone Trials Meta-Analysis Investigators. Lancet 350:1417–1424
77. Julian DG, Camm AJ, Frangin G et al (1997) Randomised trial of effect of amiodarone on mortality in patients with left-ventricular dysfunction after recent myocardial infarction: EMIAT. Lancet 349:667–674
78. Doval HC, Nul DR, Grancelli HO et al (1994) Randomised trial of low-dose amiodarone in severe congestive heart failure. Grupo de Estudio de la Sobrevida en la Insuficiencia Cardiaca en Argentina (GESICA). Lancet 344:493–498
79. Cairns JA, Connolly SJ, Roberts R et al (1997) Randomised trial of outcome after myocardial infarction in patients with frequent or repetitive ventricular premature depolarisations: CAMIAT. Lancet 349:675–682
80. Bardy GH, Lee KL, Mark DB et al (2005) Amiodarone or an implantable cardioverter-defibrillator for congestive heart failure. N Engl J Med 352:225–237
81. Myerburg RJ, Mitrani R, Interian A Jr et al (1998) Interpretation of outcomes of antiarrhythmic clinical trials: design features and population impact. Circulation 97:1514–1521
82. Myerburg RJ, Kessler KM, Castellanos A (1992) Sudden cardiac death. Structure, function, and time-dependence of risk. Circulation 85:I2–10
83. Moss AJ, Hall WJ, Cannom DS et al (1996) Improved survival with an implanted defibrillator in patients with coronary disease at high risk for ventricular arrhythmia. N Engl J Med 335:1933–1940
84. Buxton AE, Lee KL, Fisher JD et al (1999) A randomized study of the prevention of sudden death in patients with coronary artery disease. Multicenter Unsustained

Tachycardia Trial Investigators. N Engl J Med 341:1882–1890
85 Buxton AE, Lee KL, HafleyGE et al; for the MUSTT Investigators (2002) Relation of ejection fraction and inducible ventricular tachycardia to mode of death in patients with coronary artery disease. An analysis of patients enrolled in the Multicenter Unsustained Tachycardia Trial. Circulation 106:2466–2472
86. Moss AJ, Zareba W, Hall WJ et al (2002) Prophylactic implantation of a defibrillator in patients with myocardial infarction and reduced ejection fraction. N Engl J Med 346:877–883
87. Hohnloser SH, Kuck KH, Dorian P et al on behalf of the DINAMIT Investigators (2004) Prophylactic use of an implantable cardioverter–defibrillator after acute myocardial infarction. N Engl J Med 351:2481–2488
88. Wilber DJ, Zareba W, Hall J et al (2004) Time dependence of mortality risk and defibrillator benefit after myocardial infarction. Circulation 109:1082–1084
89. Di Lenarda A, Hlede S, Sabbadini G et al (1999) Improvement of prognosis in idiopathic dilated cardiomyopathy: role of early diagnosis and optimized medical treatment. Study Group on Heart Muscles Diseases. G Ital Cardiol 29:1452–1462
90. Zecchin M, Di Lenarda A, Bonin M et al (2001) Incidence and predictors of sudden cardiac death during long-term follow-up in patients with dilated cardiomyopathy on optimal medical therapy. Ital Heart J 2:213–222
91. No authors listed (2003) Expanding use of ICDs in nonischemic cardiomyopathy patients: no DEFINITE answers yet. HeartWire, News Nov 11
92. The Antiarrhythmics versus Implantable Defibrillators (AVID) Investigators (1997) A comparison of antiarrhythmic-drug therapy with implantable defibrillators in patients resuscitated from near-fatal ventricular arrhythmias. N Engl J Med 337:1576–1583
93. Connolly SJ, Gent M, Roberts RS et al (2000) Canadian Implantable Defibrillator Study (CIDS): a randomized trial of the implantable cardioverter defibrillator against amiodarone. Circulation 101:1297–1302
94. Domanski MJ, Saksena S, Epstein AE et al for the AVID Investigators (1999) Relative effectiveness of the implantable cardioverter-defibrillator and antiarrhythmic drugs in patients with varying degrees of left ventricular dysfunction who have survived malignant venticular arrhythmias. J Am Coll Cardiol 34:1090–1095
95. Sheldon RS, Connolly S, Krahn A, on behalf of the CIDS Investigators (2000) Identification of patients most likely to benefit from implantable cardioverter-defibrillator therapy. The Canadian Defibrillator Study. Circulation 191:1660–1664
96. Holmes DR Jr, David KB, Mock MB et al (1986) The effect of medical and surgical treatment on subsequent cardiac death in patients with coronary artery disease: a report from the Coronary Artery Surgery Study. Circulation 73:1254–1263
97. The Veterans Administration Coronary Artery Bypass Surgery Cooperative Study Group (1984) Eleven-year survival in the Veterans Administration randomized trial of coronary bypass surgery for stable angina. N Engl J Med 311:1333–1339
98. Holmes DR, Jr, Davis KB, Mock MB et al (1986) The effect of medical and surgical treatment and subsequent sudden cardiac death in patients with coronary artery disease: a report from the Coronary Artery Surgery Study. Circulation 73:1254–1263
99. Janse MJ, Wils-Schopman FJG, Opthof T (1990) Mechanism of antifibrillatory action of Org 7797 in regionally ischemic pig heart. J Cardiovasc Pharmacol 15:633–643
100. Bigger JT Jr (1997) Prophylactic use of implanted cardiac defibrillators in patients at high risk for ventricular arrhythmias after coronary-artery bypass graft surgery.

Coronary Artery Bypass Graft (CABG) Patch Trial Investigators. N Engl J Med 337:1569–1575
101. Bigger JT, Whang W, Rottman JN et al (1999) Mechanisms of death in the CABG Patch Trial: a randomized trial of implantable cardiac defibrillator prophylaxis in patients at high risk of death after coronary artery bypass graft surgery. Circulation 99:1416–1421
102. Trappe HJ, Klein H, Wahlers T et al (1994) Risk and benefit of additional aortocoronary bypass grafting in patients undergoing cardioverter-defibrillator implantation. Am Heart J 127:75–82
103. Natale A, Sra J, Axtell K et al (1994) Ventricular fibrillation and polymorphic ventricular tachycardia with critical coronary artery stenosis: does bypass surgery suffice? J Cardiovasc Electrophysiol 5:988–994
104. Geelen P, Primo J, Wellens F et al (1999) Coronary artery bypass grafting and defibrillator implantation in patients with ventricular tachyarrhythmias and ischemic heart disease. Pacing Clin Electrophysiol 22:1132–1139

2 Etiology and Pathophysiology of Heart Failure

P. Foëx and G. Howard-Alpe

Introduction

In the United States there are 4.9 million people with heart failure, 50% of whom will be dead within 5 years. There are also over 400 000 new cases reported annually [1], with approximately 43 000 deaths. The number of hospital admissions resulting from heart failure approaches 900 000 per annum and represents 20% of all admissions of patients over 65 years of age. Over the past four decades, the number of deaths caused by heart failure has increased from 10 in 1000 to 50 in 1000 [2].

A similar prevalence of heart failure exists in Northern Europe, while the prevalence of heart disease, particularly coronary heart disease, is lower in Southern Europe. As coronary heart disease is a major cause of cardiac failure, it can be assumed that heart failure and ventricular dysfunction are also somewhat less common in Southern Europe than in Northern Europe or in North America. However, because of the prevalence of heart failure, a large number of patients present for surgery with impaired cardiac function. These patients are at risk for major complications of anesthesia and surgery. Indeed, heart failure is one of the major predictors of cardiac complications of anesthesia and surgery [3–5].

Etiology of Heart Failure

Heart failure may result from four main categories of cause:

- Failure related to work overload or mechanical abnormalities (valvular

Nuffield Department of Anaesthetics, University of Oxford, Oxford, UK

heart disease, other anatomical abnormalities)
- Failure related to myocardial abnormalities
- Failure related to abnormal cardiac rhythm or conduction disturbances
- Failure resulting from myocardial ischemia and infarction

Cardiomyopathies

Primary cardiomyopathies include idiopathic dilated cardiomyopathy, familial dilated cardiomyopathy, and hypertrophic cardiomyopathy.
- *Idiopathic dilated cardiomyopathy* is generally biventricular without inflammation, family history, or coronary artery disease. It is characterized by myocyte loss and patchy fibrosis.
- *Familial dilated cardiomyopathy* is more common than is generally believed [6]. It may progress more rapidly than idiopathic cardiomyopathy to the need for heart transplant [7]. As many as 30% of patients with dilated cardiomyopathy may have an inherited disorder [8].
- *Hypertrophic obstructive cardiomyopathy* (HOCM) and nonobstructive hypertrophic cardiomyopathies are often familial, but many mutations have been described for at least seven abnormal sarcomeric proteins.

Secondary cardiomyopathies include:
- *Alcoholic and viral cardiomyopathies* (secondary to inflammatory myocarditis), which may be overdiagnosed. There are no specific markers of alcoholic cardiomyopathy except the history of excessive alcohol intake. Viral myocarditis can only be diagnosed with certainty by cardiac biopsy. Only 5–10% of biopsies of patients deemed to have viral myocarditis test positive for inflammatory reaction. Inflammatory myocarditis can improve spontaneously [9]. However, there is risk of severe rejection in patients with viral cardiomyopathies if cardiac transplantation is necessary.
- *Toxic heart failure.* A considerable variety of drugs can induce toxic heart failure [10]. Doxorubicin may cause toxic heart failure long after its administration [10]. Herceptin (used in the treatment of breast cancer) associated with doxorubicin or paclitaxel is more likely to cause toxic heart failure than doxorubicin or paclitaxel alone. Other agents can cause cardiomyopathies, including cocaine, cytotoxic drugs, interferons, interleukin-2, and anabolic steroids [10].
- *Chronic obstructive airway disease (COPD).* Although generally associated with right ventricular dysfunction secondary to pulmonary hypertension, COPD may cause systolic left ventricular dysfunction, probably secondary to hypercapnia and hypoxia. Moreover, it can cause diastolic left ventricular dysfunction as right ventricular dilatation and hypertrophy force the interventricular septum to bulge toward the cavity of the left ventricle.

Myocardial Overload

Pressure overload causes the myocytes to hypertrophy and to contract and relax more slowly. Myocytes are subjected to metabolic limitations and have a shorter life span. Generally diastolic dysfunction precedes systolic dysfunction. Pressure overload and hypertrophy increase wall stress; eventually contractility decreases.

Volume overload (high output syndromes) causes left ventricular dysfunction because of a noncardiac circulatory overload. Left ventricular end-diastolic pressure and volume are increased and the ejection fraction remains normal or is even increased. Volume overload can occur because of hypervolemia, excessive venous return (arteriovenous fistulae), or decreased peripheral vascular resistance. It is also observed in conditions such as beriberi (vitamin B_1 deficiency), liver cirrhosis, severe anemia or large, highly vascularized tumors. As volume overload results in left ventricular dilatation, functional mitral regurgitation can develop.

Myocardial Ischemia and Infarction

Coronary artery disease is a major cause of cardiac failure. Acutely, ischemia causes a very rapid reduction of contraction in the compromised myocardium. Dysfunction is both systolic and diastolic with paradoxical wall motion. When the mass of ischemic muscle is large, pump failure occurs. Paradoxical wall motion (early systolic dilatation) results in loss of efficiency as part of the energy is expended in shifting blood within the ventricle into a "functional" ventricular aneurysm. With prolonged ischemia myocardial necrosis occurs and the myocytes are replaced by scar tissue. This may result in the development of a true anatomical ventricular aneurysm.

Pathophysiology of Heart Failure

Heart failure is a process in which the venous return to the heart is normal but the heart is unable to pump sufficient blood to meet the body's metabolic needs at normal filling pressures. Heart failure may be caused by myocyte death, myocyte dysfunction, ventricular remodeling or a combination of these factors [11, 12]. Abnormal energy utilization, ischemia and neurohormonal disturbances occur. Heart failure may result from systolic dysfunction, diastolic dysfunction or both.

In the presence of disturbed myocardial contractility or excessive hemodynamic burden, the heart depends on adaptive mechanisms to maintain its pump function (Fig. 1). The following mechanisms play an important role:

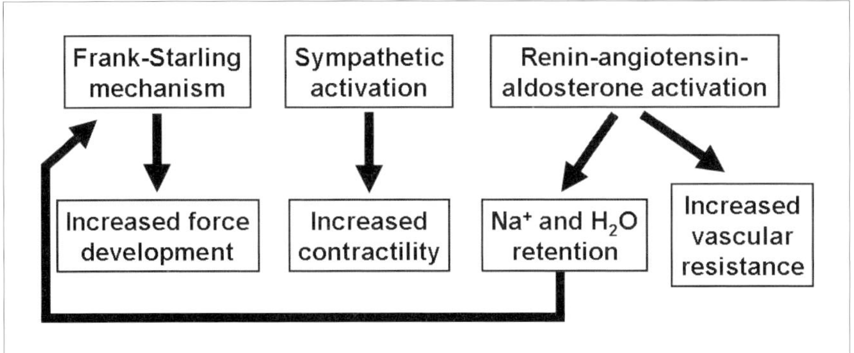

Fig. 1. Adaptive mechanisms in heart failure showing the relationships between Frank-Starling mechanism, sympathetic activation, and activation of the renin-angiotensin-aldosterone system

1. The Frank-Starling mechanism: an increase in fiber length increases the force of contraction developed.
2. Activation of the sympathetic nervous system: augments contractility.
3. Activation of the renin–angiotensin–aldosterone system: increases sodium and water retention and increases vascular resistance, thereby increasing the perfusion pressure of the tissues.
4. Myocardial remodelling with or without chamber dilatation (remodeling and hypertrophy occur slowly).

With heart failure, cardiac output is often reduced and oxygenation of the tissues relies on an increased oxygen extraction: the arteriovenous oxygen content difference widens even in the resting state. With mild heart failure, resting cardiac output is normal but fails to rise appropriately with exercise. In a normal subject, exercise is associated with an increase in sympathetic activity that causes an increase in contractility so that the ventricle functions on a left-shifted starling curve. In addition, muscle vasodilatation facilitates output to skeletal muscle. By contrast, in moderately severe heart failure output is maintained because of an increased end-diastolic volume and the dysfunctional myocytes do not respond adequately to adrenergic stimulation. In addition, as there is permanent sympathetic stimulation, β-adrenoceptor downregulation occurs. This limits the efficacy of further increases in sympathetic activity in response to exercise or stress to augment cardiac output.

Vascular redistribution is a "defensive" feature of heart failure. Vasoconstriction limits blood supply to skin, muscle, gut and kidney. In addition to sympathetically induced vasoconstriction, there are contributions from the renin–angiotensin–aldosterone system and from endothelin. An increased sodium content of the vascular wall contributes to thickening and stiffening of the vessel wall. There is also attenuation of ischemia-induced and exercise-induced vasodilatation, partly because of endothelial dysfunction. Impaired endothelial receptor function and deficiency in L-arginine substrate and in endothelial cell NO synthase (eNOS) contribute to a limited vasodilatory response.

Ventricular remodeling involves changes in the mass, volume, shape and composition of the ventricular muscle. Pressure overload causes more hypertrophy (parallel replication of myofibrils) than volume overload (replication in series with elongation of myocytes). Ventricular remodeling is characterized by activation of genes for several peptide growth factors [13], synthesis of additional mitochondria to meet the increased metabolic ATP requirements, and alterations of the extracellular matrix. These alterations have a profound effect on the mechanical behavior of heart muscle, as was demonstrated as early as in 1967 in isolated cardiac muscle: the maximum velocity of fiber shortening is decreased [14]. The possibility of cell necrosis and apoptosis cannot be discounted. With hypertrophy there is risk of subendocardial ischemia with necrosis. In addition, a number of neurohumoral factors present in heart failure are known to cause apoptosis. Similarly, cytokines may cause apoptosis [15]. It is likely that some of the beneficial effects of angiotensin-converting enzyme (ACE) inhibitors and β-blockers result from blockade of the adverse effects of angiotensin and catecholamines.

The excitation–contraction coupling is altered in heart failure. Calcium handling is profoundly altered in end-stage heart failure where action potential and force development are prolonged while relaxation is impaired [16]. The blunted rise of the intracellular calcium transport (calcium transient) reflects the slower delivery of Ca^{2+} to the contractile apparatus, thus reducing contractility. The function of the sarcoplasmic reticulum is altered as shown by an altered force–frequency relationship. Instead of an increase in rate causing an increase in inotropy, in the failing heart tachycardia does not increase contractility. This indicates that the cycling of Ca^{2+} is altered. In addition, other functions of the sarcoplasmic reticulum are altered: the activity and expression of SERCA-2 (the mediator of Ca^{2+} reuptake by the sarcoplasmic reticulum) are reduced. The Ca^{2+} release channel (CRC) located on the sarcoplasmic reticulum is hyperphosphorylated by protein kinase A, resulting in Ca^{2+} leakage. This decreases the sarcoplasmic reticulum Ca^{2+} content, as well as Ca^{2+} release and uptake [17]. In addition, the mRNA and protein levels of the voltage-dependent Ca^{2+} channel are decreased [18].

Alterations of contractile proteins occur in heart failure. This is expressed as reduced myofibrillar ATPase, actomyosin ATPase, and myosin ATPase activity. This reduces contractility by decreasing the rate of interaction of actin and myosin filaments. Hemodynamic overload enhances protein synthesis, resulting in different isoforms of cardiac proteins. Changes in α- and β-myosin heavy chains (MHC) have been documented in humans with dilated cardiomyopathies [19]. Another cause of decreased contractile force is a change in the myosin light chain and the troponin–tropomyosin complex [20]; in particular, there is an increased level of the T_2 isoform of troponin [21] in heart failure, whereas in the normal heart the T_1 isoform represents almost the totality of the troponin content.

In addition to the changes observed in the myocytes, there are changes in the connective tissue. Excess collagen may interfere with ventricular relaxation and filling; this contributes to diastolic dysfunction. Excess collagen is observed in response to pressure overload. ACE inhibitors are beneficial as they prevent the increase in muscle stiffness, minimize interstitial fibrosis and prevent the induction of collagen [22].

Energy is required for both contraction and relaxation, as reuptake of Ca^{2+} by the sarcoplasmic reticulum and extrusion of Ca^{2+} from the cell are against a concentration gradient. They need energy. This is particularly relevant to severe ischemia.

In chronic heart failure, oxygen consumption is normal or increased. However, cytochromes of the mitochondrial membrane that are coupling oxidation to the synthesis of chemical energy may be decreased, causing an imbalance between energy delivery and energy requirements. In addition, creatine kinase (CK) activity can be reduced, probably because of alterations in the isoforms of CK. The reduction of high-energy phosphates in heart failure has an effect on the contractile apparatus, thereby decreasing contractility, and on the sarcoplasmic reticulum, reducing Ca^{2+} uptake so that diastolic function is also impaired with a detrimental effect on overall cardiac function.

Systolic Dysfunction

Ventricular systolic dysfunction is characterized by a loss of contractile strength of the myocardium accompanied by compensatory ventricular remodeling and activation of the sympathetic system and the renin–angiotensin–aldosterone (RAS) systems. In the face of increased preload and afterload, there is necessarily a decrease in ventricular emptying. An ejection fraction less than 45% is usually associated with an increase in diastolic volume, constituting a dilated cardiomyopathy.

In the early stages, overall pump function may be maintained at rest but the exercise capacity is impaired. At more advanced stages, cardiac output is reduced even at rest and there is an inability for systemic vascular resistance to decrease when metabolic demands increase.

Systolic dysfunction is not necessarily irreversible. It may be present where some myocardium is hibernating [23, 24]. This condition was considered to result from downregulated function in response to decreased myocardial blood flow. However, more recently myocardial hibernation has been attributed to a decrease of the coronary flow reserve such that episodes of ischemia occur in the face of increased demand. These episodes of ischemia cause repetitive myocardial stunning[24]. The hibernating myocardium can recover after myocardial revascularization. The presence of hibernating myocardium can be detected by dobutamine echocardiography and other techniques of myocardial imaging [25]. In this situation, coronary revascularization may cause a significant improvement of cardiac function [26].

The factors that precipitate systolic dysfunction include uncontrolled hypertension, atrial fibrillation, noncompliance with medical treatment, myocardial ischemia, anemia, renal failure, nonsteroidal anti-inflammatory drugs and excess sodium.

A recent UK study of patients with stable heart failure has shown that the 5-year mortality was 41.5% in those with systolic dysfunction (ejection fraction <50%) and 25.2% of those with diastolic dysfunction alone (ejection fraction >50%) [27]. This clearly demonstrates the impact of systolic dysfunction on the patient's prognosis.

Diastolic Dysfunction

Approximately one-third or more of patients with heart failure suffer predominantly from diastolic dysfunction with pulmonary venous congestion, while their systolic function is normal or almost normal as evidenced by the ejection fraction [28]; symptoms of failure may be absent [29].

Ventricular diastolic dysfunction is characterized by altered relaxation of the cardiac fibers, resulting in slower pressure decline, reduced rapid filling and increased myocardial stiffness. In many patients, diastolic dysfunction may exist while systolic function remains essentially normal. Gandhi and colleagues found that during acute episodes of hypertensive pulmonary edema left ventricular ejection fraction and the extent of regional motion were similar to those measured after resolution of the acute episode, which further supports the role of diastolic dysfunction [30].

Diastolic dysfunction may result from a thickened ventricular wall, as in restrictive or infiltrative cardiomyopathies, and/or from tachycardia, as the latter decreases the filling time resulting in elevated diastolic ventricular pressure. Indeed, pacing-induced tachycardia is used to create experimental models of heart failure.

Advancing age, hypertension, diabetes, left ventricular hypertrophy and coronary artery disease are the main risk factors for diastolic dysfunction.

Diastolic heart failure affects women particularly frequently [28]. This may be due to an increased remodeling in response to pressure overload [31].

The annual mortality from diastolic heart failure is estimated to be between 5–8% [29]. It is four times the mortality of persons without heart failure but half that of patients with systolic heart failure [32].

The presence of significant diastolic dysfunction has several major implications for patients with acute illnesses or presenting for major surgery during which fluid shifts are an issue: as diastolic distensibility is reduced, inadequate fluid replacement causes an exaggerated reduction in cardiac output. Conversely, fluid overload causes exaggerated increases in end-diastolic left ventricular pressure and pulmonary artery occluded pressure: this may result in acute pulmonary edema with volume loads that would be well tolerated in the absence of diastolic dysfunction. The onset of atrial fibrillation–a frequent complication of heart failure–is poorly tolerated as it decreases the atrial contribution to filling.

Diastolic characteristics of the heart represent two distinct phenomena: relaxation and wall stiffness. The former is a dynamic process that is controlled by the rate of uptake of Ca^{2+} by the sarcoplasmic reticulum and the efflux of Ca^{2+} from the cell. SERCA-2 and sarcolemmal calcium pumps control these energy-requiring processes. Reduction in ATP concentration impairs relaxation and results in reduced filling. In the failing heart there are regional variations in onset, rate and magnitude of fiber lengthening (diastolic asynergy); these abnormalities may also impair early filling. Later during diastole, ventricular stiffness is the major determinant of filling, as the compliance curve may be shifted upwards so that much higher pressures are observed for the same ventricular volume (Fig. 2).

Diagnosis of Diastolic Dysfunction and Diastolic Heart Failure

A diagnosis of diastolic heart failure requires symptoms and signs of heart failure associated with a normal left ventricular ejection fraction and no valvular abnormalities on echocardiography.

Echocardiography can provide information on left ventricular filling including two-dimensional evaluation of the cardiac chamber dimensions and Doppler recordings of left ventricular inflow and pulmonary venous flow. All of these parameters are necessary to assess fully diastolic function.

Left Ventricular Inflow

Left ventricular inflow (Fig. 3) can be divided into four periods:

Isovolumetric relaxation time (IVRT): Interval between closure of the aortic valve and the onset of mitral inflow.

E wave: Early rapid diastolic filling. Peak E velocity is influenced by atrial

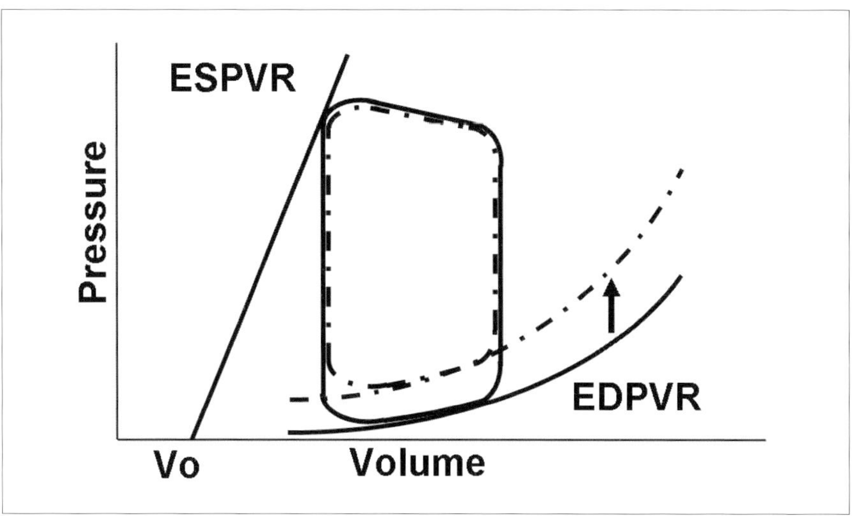

Fig. 2. Pure diastolic dysfunction is characterized by an increase in the stiffness of the ventricle such that the compliance curve (end-diastolic pressure–volume relationship, EDPVR) is shifted upwards, while the end-systolic pressure–volume relationship (ESPVR) and the volume at zero pressure (Vo) are unchanged. Only the diastolic part of the dynamic pressure–volume loop is altered

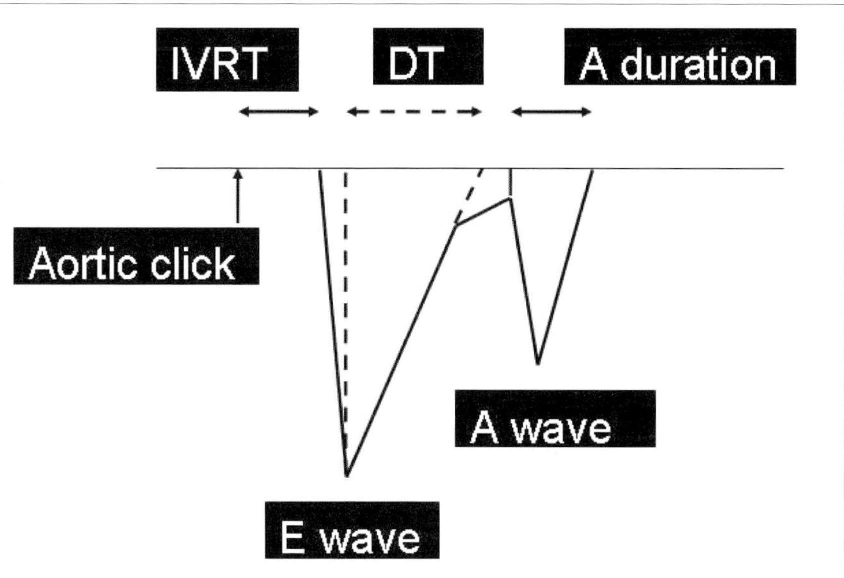

Fig. 3. Left ventricular inflow. Isovolumetric relaxation time (IVRT), early diastolic filling (E wave), deceleration time (DT), the slow filling phase (interval between E and A wave), and the late filling and its atrial contribution (A wave) are represented as well as the duration of the A wave

pressure. The deceleration time (DT) is influenced by left ventricular diastolic pressures and stiffness.

Interval between the E wave and A wave: Reflects slow filling phase.

A wave: Reflects the late diastolic filling and the atrial contribution. Peak A velocity is influenced by atrial contractility, residual atrial pressure and left ventricular end-diastolic pressure (LVEDP).

The E:A ratio is normally greater than 1. Three primary diastolic dysfunction patterns are seen: impaired relaxation, pseudonormal and restrictive. In early diastolic dysfunction the E:A ratio decreases to less than 1 (E to A re-versal) due to impaired relaxation, and the DT and IVRT are prolonged. The trace then normalizes as rising left atrial pressure compensates for impaired left ventricular relaxation. Finally, the restrictive pattern develops, characterized by a supranormal E:A ratio and a decreased DT and IVRT.

Pulmonary Venous Flow

The normal pattern of pulmonary venous flow (Fig. 4) has four peaks:

PVS_1: Active atrial relaxation during early systole.

PVS_2: Left atrial filling and descent of the mitral annulus during left ventricular contraction.

D: Early diastole, immediately after mitral valve opening.

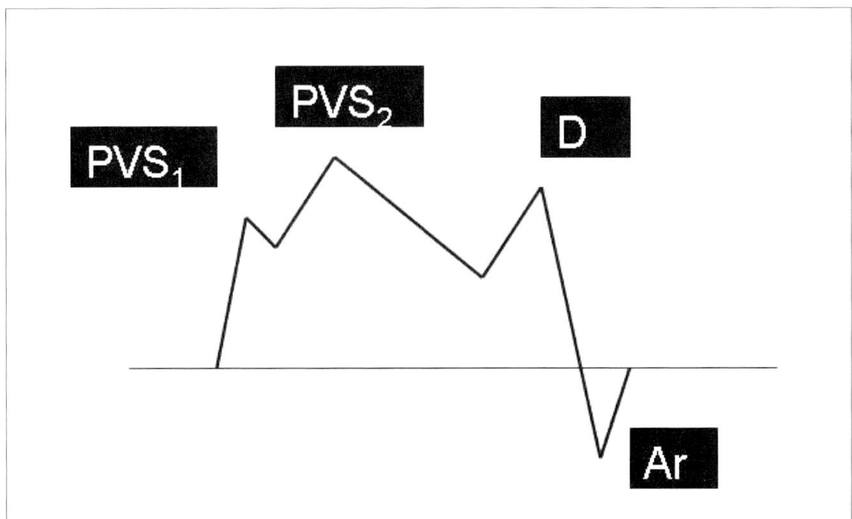

Fig. 4. Pulmonary venous flow. Active atrial relaxation during early systole (PVS_1), left atrial filling and descent of the mitral annulus during LV contraction (PVS_2), early diastole immediately after mitral valve opening (D), and late diastole when reverse flow is seen as a consequence of atrial contraction (Ar)

Ar: Late diastole, on atrial contraction.

In diastolic dysfunction the PVS_1 and PVS_2 velocity ratio reverses and becomes less than the D component.

Assessment of these characteristic flow patterns along with the cardiac chamber dimensions can provide diagnostic evidence of diastolic dysfunction.

Management of Diastolic Heart Failure

The initial aim in the management of diastolic heart failure is to reduce pulmonary venous congestion. Diuretics and nitroglycerin supplemented by morphine and additional oxygen are needed. However, aggressive diuresis may cause severe hypotension because of excessive reduction of atrial pressure. Nitroglycerin is particularly indicated if there is myocardial ischemia, as acute ischemia has a profound effect on early relaxation and on myocardial stiffness [33].

While there have been many large studies of the pharmacological treatment of systolic heart failure, there is little data on that of diastolic heart failure [34]. The controlled studies Candesartan in Heart Failure [35] and Perindopril for Elderly People with Chronic Heart Failure [36] are still addressing this issue. However, before gene therapy is introduced some time in the future [37], the treatment of left ventricular diastolic dysfunction remains empirical with avoidance of excessive sodium intake, cautious use of diuretics (lest reduced preload reduces cardiac output), restoration and maintenance of sinus rhythm at a heart rate that optimizes ventricular filling, and the correction of precipitating factors such as myocardial ischemia and arterial hypertension. Calcium channel blockers, ACE inhibitors, or angiotensin receptor antagonists are used for their effect mostly on surrogate outcomes.

Because treatment of diastolic dysfunction is difficult, it is very important to prevent its development. As arterial hypertension is a major cause of diastolic dysfunction, early detection and treatment of hypertension is critical. However, stage 3 hypertension (>180 mmHg/>110 mmHg) remains common and is very frequently poorly controlled.

Right Ventricular Dysfunction

While in most instances circulatory failure results from acute or acute-on-chronic left ventricular failure, it can also be caused by acute or acute-on-chronic right ventricular failure. The latter may seem to be a rather uncommon event, and as a result it may not be recognized, resulting in potentially preventable deaths.

The reason why right ventricular failure is often overlooked as a cause of circulatory failure is that for many years experimental studies showed that extensive damage of the right side of the heart caused only minimal changes in venous pressure and cardiac output [38, 39]. Thus, the right ventricle was regarded as unimportant for the maintenance of adequate circulatory function. However, this is only true so long as the pulmonary circulation is normal and contraction of the septum and of neighboring areas of the left ventricle is intact. However, in critically ill patients, acute right ventricular failure may be the main determinant of acute circulatory failure.

Etiology of Acute Right Ventricular Failure

Inferior myocardial infarction often includes part of the right ventricle [40]. When associated with permanent dysfunction, the presence of right ventricular myocardial infarction worsens the long-term prognosis ten-fold [41]. However, dysfunction is not always present. When the free wall of the right ventricle is damaged and is replaced by a poorly compliant scar, contraction of the left ventricle pulls on this noncontractile wall. As the septum still bulges into the cavity of the right ventricle, pressure increases and ejection occurs even though the right ventricle is essentially passive. However, when the right ventricular wall adjacent to the left ventricle and the septum is damaged, such compensation cannot occur and right ventricular output is reduced (Fig. 5).

Cardiopulmonary bypass is a known cause of acute right ventricular failure. Inflammatory mediators, free radicals, episodes of hypoxia, hypercapnia and acidosis, as well as mechanical shear stresses may result in endothelial injury in the pulmonary circulation [42]. These in turn cause an imbalance between vasorelaxing mediators [NO, endothelium-derived hyperpolarizing factor (EDHF), and prostacyclin] and vasoconstrictors (thromboxane A_2, angiotensin, endothelins).

Acute pulmonary embolism may be associated with a significant reduction in the ejection characteristics of the right ventricle which can be substantially reversed by thrombolysis [43].

Acute respiratory distress syndrome can cause pulmonary vascular obstruction and pulmonary hypertension, probably mediated by thromboxanes and leukotrienes, activation of the complement, extravascular compression, and thickening of the media of the arterial wall. In addition, the need to use positive end-expiratory pressure to maintain oxygenation may further increase pulmonary vascular resistance, thus causing pulmonary hypertension [44].

Hypoxia in the presence of a compromised pulmonary circulation and right ventricular dysfunction may precipitate acute right ventricular failure by causing right ventricular ischemic wall dysfunction at a time when high afterload requires a dynamic wall to maintain right ventricular (and, therefore, left ventricular) output.

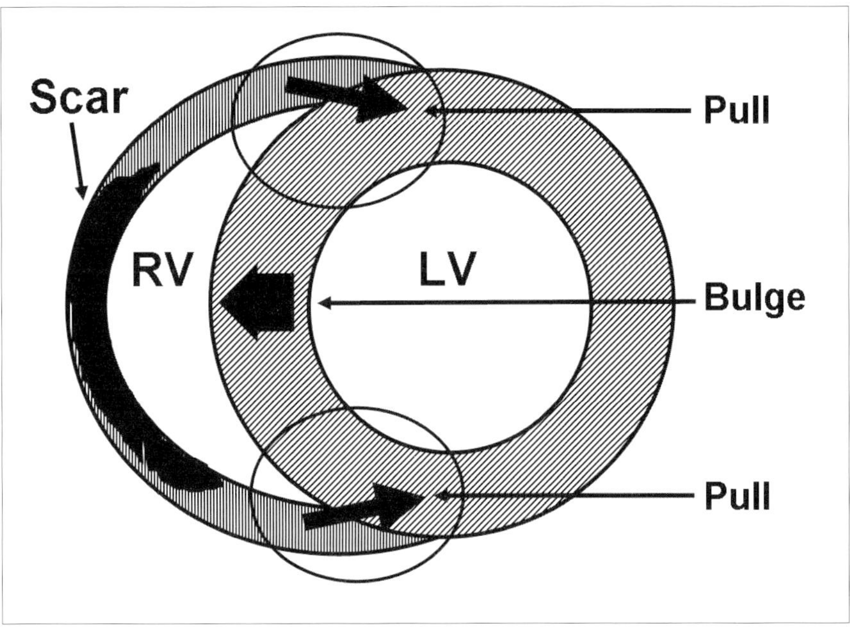

Fig. 5. Possible interactions between right and left ventricle in the presence of right ventricular infarction. Two major factors influence the reduction of right ventricular volume in the presence of myocardial scar tissue: the pull of the adjacent left ventricular wall and the bulge of the left ventricle as its muscle thickens during systole. *RV* and *LV* denote right and left ventricular cavities respectively. Clearly, scars that extend from the right ventricle to the left ventricle (*circled areas*) prevent the effect of the pull from the left ventricle and cause ejection failure even in the presence of a normal pulmonary circulation

Pathophysiology of Right Ventricular Failure

Dysfunction is generally caused by pressure overload: and may result from ischemia with normal coronary arteries. The ability of the right ventricle to eject is a function of its preload, contractility and afterload [45]. Because of its thin wall, the right ventricle is very sensitive to an increase in afterload (e.g., acute pulmonary hypertension, acute-on-chronic pulmonary hypertension). Sudden increases in afterload because of hypoxia or hypercapnia may reduce right ventricular stroke volume. However, increases in afterload may also exert a detrimental effect through their influence on the coronary circulation.

Blood supply to the right ventricle is by the right and left anterior descending coronary arteries. Coronary flow to the wall of the right ventricle occurs during both systole and diastole because a pressure gradient exists between aortic pressure and right ventricular intramural pressure during systole and diastole.

In response to acute pulmonary hypertension, pressure increases in the right ventricle, the ventricle dilates and wall tension increases. This reduces the effective coronary pressure gradient: systolic coronary blood flow is reduced or suppressed. This creates a mismatch between impaired oxygen supply and augmented oxygen demand [46]. Note that this imbalance does not imply the presence of coronary artery lesions. Ischemia of the wall of the right ventricle can occur in acute or acute-on-chronic pulmonary hypertension in the presence of completely normal coronary arteries, as demonstrated in experimental models. As the afterload mismatch causes myocardial ischemia, ischemic wall dysfunction develops. While this ischemic dysfunction can be tolerated if the pulmonary pressure is normal, it results in acute failure when pulmonary hypertension is present.

Treatment of Acute Right Ventricular Failure

As acute right ventricular failure can be overlooked, it is useful to consider how its treatment may differ from that of left ventricular failure especially in the presence of afterload mismatch.

In the case of acute myocardial infarction, the treatment is that of infarction, with particular attention paid to preventing the development of pulmonary hypertension. When right ventricular extension of left ventricular infarction is the primary cause of circulatory failure, optimization of volume loading, inotropic support and mechanical right ventricular assistance may be needed [47].

When failure is caused primarily by an increase in pulmonary vascular resistance associated with pulmonary hypertension, raised afterload and reduced right ventricular coronary perfusion play an important role [48]. The intravenous administration of pulmonary vasodilators such as prostacyclin or nitroglycerin usually also causes peripheral vasodilatation and, therefore, the benefit of right ventricular afterload reduction may be offset by a further reduction in the coronary perfusion pressure gradient. Dopexamine has been advocated and may be more effective than prostacyclin [49]. When pulmonary vasodilators, including phosphodiesterase inhibitors, are used, the addition of a systemic vasopressor may be necessary. Indeed, there is good experimental evidence that a vasopressor can restore right ventricular coronary perfusion, increase contractility and restore cardiac output simply by increasing the coronary pressure gradient[50]. The use of a vasopressor in the presence of acute cardiogenic circulatory failure may seem paradoxical. However, there is little doubt that it is effective when acute right ventricular wall ischemia is present. Another new approach is to use vasopressin. Vasopressin causes pulmonary vasodilation, thus reducing right ventricular afterload, and increases peripheral vascular resistance so that coronary perfusion of the right ventricle improves [51, 52].

A significant advance has been the introduction of inhaled NO [53] and inhaled prostacyclin [48]. Inhaled NO and prostacyclin allow pulmonary vascular resistance to be lowered with minimal effect on the systemic circulation. As a result, the coronary perfusion of the right ventricle is not decreased and the reduction of pulmonary vascular resistance facilitates right ventricular ejection. However, the addition of a systemic vasopressor may further enhance recovery by improving coronary perfusion. With NO there is the possibility of rebound pulmonary hypertension on its discontinuation. At least experimentally, the addition of dipyridamole allows lower concentrations of NO to be used and prevents rebound hypertension [54].

By contrast with acute syndromes, the long-term management of pulmonary hypertension and its consequences in terms of right ventricular failure rests mainly on various forms of prostanoids (continuous infusion, subcutaneous, inhaled and oral administration) and on endothelin-1 blockers (bosentan).

Cardiac Failure and Perioperative Risk

All the studies of risk factors for perioperative cardiac complications of anesthesia and surgery include heart failure, even in its incipient forms, as the most important factor [3, 4].

A clear association exists between low ejection fraction and increased risk of postoperative acute left ventricular failure [55–57]. In addition, patients with reduced cardiac function may tolerate anesthesia poorly. This is not surprising as inhalation anesthetics exhibit strong negative inotropic properties because they reduce both transmembrane calcium flux and activated calcium release from the myocyte sarcoplasmic reticulum [58–60]. Even nitrous oxide exhibits negative inotropic properties [61]. Intravenous induction agents such as thiopentone and propofol [62] have strong negative inotropic properties. Of the drugs in the current anesthetic armamentarium, only etomidate is devoid of negative inotropy. Similarly, benzodiazepines and opioids do not depress contractility. This is advantageous as, in the presence of an already depressed myocardium, further negative inotropy is poorly tolerated. Unlike other agents, xenon does not cause myocardial depression [63], but its high cost precludes its widespread use.

Postoperatively, many other factors contribute to worsening of cardiac function: silent ischemia, especially in hypertensive patients [64] and nocturnal hypoxemia [65] are frequently observed. They have an adverse effect on cardiac function. In addition fluid overload may precipitate acute left ventricular failure.

Conclusion

Heart failure has multiple etiologies, the two most common being coronary artery disease and hypertensive heart disease. Heart failure may result from systolic or diastolic dysfunction. The latter is not always recognized, and yet in the long-term it has serious implications, especially in hypertensive patients. Both systolic and diastolic dysfunction can be exaggerated by anesthesia and perioperative events. While left ventricular failure is very frequent, right ventricular failure should not be overlooked as a cause of overall circulatory failure, especially acute or acute-on-chronic right ventricular failure caused by afterload mismatch and right ventricular ischemia in the presence of normal coronary arteries. The management of this condition may be very different from that of left ventricular failure.

References

1. Rich MW, Nease RF. Cost-effectiveness analysis in clinical practice: the case of heart failure. Arch Intern Med 1999;159:1690–700
2. Minino AM, Arias E, Kochanek KD, et al. Deaths: Final data for 2000. Hyattsville, Maryland: National Center for Health Statistics; 2002. National Vital Statistics Reports, vol 50, no 15
3. Goldman L, Caldera DL, Nussbaum SR, et al. Multifactorial index of cardiac risk in noncardiac surgical procedures. N Engl J Med 1977;297:845–50
4. Lee TH, Marcantonio ER, Mangione CM, et al. Derivation and prospective validation of a simple index for prediction of cardiac risk of major noncardiac surgery. Circulation 1999;100:1043–9
5. Detsky AS, Abrams HB, Forbath N, et al. Cardiac assessment for patients undergoing noncardiac surgery. A multifactorial clinical risk index. Arch Intern Med 1986;146:2131–4
6. Mestroni L, Rocco C, Gregori D, et al. Familial dilated cardiomyopathy: evidence for genetic and phenotypic heterogeneity. Heart Muscle Disease Study Group. J Am Coll Cardiol 1999;34:181–90
7. Valantine HA, Hunt SA, Fowler MB, et al. Frequency of familial nature of dilated cardiomyopathy and usefulness of cardiac transplantation in this subset. Am J Cardiol 1989;63:959–63
8. Grunig E, Tasman JA, Kucherer H, et al. Frequency and phenotypes of familial dilated cardiomyopathy. J Am Coll Cardiol 1998;31:186–94
9. Mason JW, O'Connell JB, Herskowitz A, et al. A clinical trial of immunosuppressive therapy for myocarditis. The Myocarditis Treatment Trial Investigators. N Engl J Med 1995;333:269–75
10. Feenstra J, Grobbee DE, Remme WJ, Stricker BH. Drug-induced heart failure. J Am Coll Cardiol 1999;33:1152–62
11. Houser SR, Margulies KB. Is depressed myocyte contractility centrally involved in heart failure? Circ Res 2003;92:350–8
12. Alpert NR, Mulieri LA, Warshaw D. The failing human heart. Cardiovasc Res 2002;54:1–10

13. Calderone A, Takahashi N, Izzo NJ, et al. Pressure- and volume-induced left ventricular hypertrophies are associated with distinct myocyte phenotypes and differential induction of peptide growth factor mRNAs. Circulation 1995;92:2385–90
14. Spann JF, Jr., Buccino RA, Sonnenblick EH, Braunwald E. Contractile state of cardiac muscle obtained from cats with experimentally produced ventricular hypertrophy and heart failure. Circ Res 1967;21:341–54
15. Ing DJ, Zang J, Dzau VJ, et al. Modulation of cytokine-induced cardiac myocyte apoptosis by nitric oxide, Bak, and Bcl-x. Circ Res 1999;84:21–33
16. Piacentino V, 3rd, Weber CR, Chen X, et al. Cellular basis of abnormal calcium transients of failing human ventricular myocytes. Circ Res 2003;92:651–8
17. Marks AR, Reiken S, Marx SO. Progression of heart failure: is protein kinase A hyperphosphorylation of the ryanodine receptor a contributing factor? Circulation 2002;105:272–5
18. Chen X, Piacentino V, Furukawa S, et al. L-type Ca2+ channel density and regulation are altered in failing human ventricular myocytes and recover after support with mechanical assist devices. Circ Res 2002;91:517–24
19. Abraham WT, Gilbert EM, Lowes BD, et al. Coordinate changes in myosin heavy chain isoform gene expression are selectively associated with alterations in dilated cardiomyopathy phenotype. Mol Med 2002;8:750–60
20. Solaro RJ, Rarick HM. Troponin and tropomyosin: proteins that switch on and tune in the activity of cardiac myofilaments. Circ Res 1998;83:471–80
21. Anderson PA, Malouf NN, Oakeley AE, et al. Troponin T isoform expression in the normal and failing human left ventricle: a correlation with myofibrillar ATPase activity. Basic Res Cardiol 1992;87 Suppl 1:117–27
22. Brooks WW, Bing OH, Robinson KG, et al. Effect of angiotensin-converting enzyme inhibition on myocardial fibrosis and function in hypertrophied and failing myocardium from the spontaneously hypertensive rat. Circulation 1997;96:4002–10
23. Wijns W, Vatner SF, Camici PG. Hibernating myocardium. N Engl J Med 1998;339:173–81
24. Camici PG, Wijns W, Borgers M, et al. Pathophysiological mechanisms of chronic reversible left ventricular dysfunction due to coronary artery disease (hibernating myocardium). Circulation 1997;96:3205–14
25. Afridi I, Kleiman NS, Raizner AE, Zoghbi WA. Dobutamine echocardiography in myocardial hibernation. Optimal dose and accuracy in predicting recovery of ventricular function after coronary angioplasty. Circulation 1995;91:663–70
26. Louie HW, Laks H, Milgalter E, et al. Ischemic cardiomyopathy. Criteria for coronary revascularization and cardiac transplantation. Circulation 1991;84(5 Suppl):III290–5
27. MacCarthy PA, Kearney MT, Nolan J, et al. Prognosis in heart failure with preserved left ventricular systolic function: prospective cohort study. BMJ 2003;327:78–9
28. Vasan RS, Benjamin EJ, Levy D. Prevalence, clinical features and prognosis of diastolic heart failure: an epidemiologic perspective. J Am Coll Cardiol 1995;26:1565–74
29. Aurigemma GP, Gaasch WH. Clinical practice. Diastolic heart failure. N Engl J Med 2004;351:1097–105
30. Gandhi SK, Powers JC, Nomeir AM, et al. The pathogenesis of acute pulmonary edema associated with hypertension. N Engl J Med 2001;344:17–22
31. Weinberg EO, Thienelt CD, Katz SE, et al. Gender differences in molecular remodeling in pressure overload hypertrophy. J Am Coll Cardiol 1999;34:264–73
32. Vasan RS, Larson MG, Benjamin EJ, et al. Congestive heart failure in subjects with

normal versus reduced left ventricular ejection fraction: prevalence and mortality in a population-based cohort. J Am Coll Cardiol 1999;33:1948–55

33. Marsch SC, Wanigasekera VA, Ryder WA, et al. Graded myocardial ischemia is associated with a decrease in diastolic distensibility of the remote nonischemic myocardium in the anesthetized dog. J Am Coll Cardiol 1993;22:899–906
34. Vasan RS, Benjamin EJ. Diastolic heart failure–no time to relax. N Engl J Med 2001;344:56–9
35. Yusuf S, Pfeffer MA, Swedberg K, et al. Effects of candesartan in patients with chronic heart failure and preserved left-ventricular ejection fraction: the CHARM-Preserved Trial. Lancet 2003;362:777–81
36. Cleland JG, Tendera M, Adamus J, et al. Perindopril for elderly people with chronic heart failure: the PEP-CHF study. The PEP investigators. Eur J Heart Fail 1999;1:211–7
37. Webster KA, Bishopric NH. Molecular aspects and gene therapy prospects for diastolic failure. Cardiol Clin 2000;18:621–35
38. Starr I, Jeffers WA, Meade JR. The absence of conspicuous increments of venous pressure after severe damage to the right ventricle of the dog, with a discussion of the relation between clinical congestive failure and heart disease. Am Heart J 1943;26:291–301
39. Brooks H, Kirk ES, Vokonas PS, et al. Performance of the right ventricle under stress: relation to right coronary flow. J Clin Invest 1971;50:2176–83
40. Kinch JW, Ryan TJ. Right ventricular infarction. N Engl J Med 1994;330:1211–7
41. Sakata K, Yoshino H, Kurihara H, et al. Prognostic significance of persistent right ventricular dysfunction as assessed by radionuclide angiocardiography in patients with inferior wall acute myocardial infarction. Am J Cardiol 2000;85:939–44
42. Kaul TK, Fields BL. Postoperative acute refractory right ventricular failure: incidence, pathogenesis, management and prognosis. Cardiovasc Surg 2000;8:1–9
43. Nass N, McConnell MV, Goldhaber SZ, et al. Recovery of regional right ventricular function after thrombolysis for pulmonary embolism. Am J Cardiol 1999;83:804–6, A10
44. Foex P. Right ventricular function during ARDS. Acta Anesthesiol Scand Suppl 1991;95:72–9; discussion 80
45. Weber KT, Janicki JS, Shroff SG, et al. The right ventricle: physiologic and pathophysiologic considerations. Crit Care Med 1983;11:323–8
46. Fixler DE, Archie JP, Jr., Ullyot DJ, Hoffman JI. Regional coronary flow with increased right ventricular output in anesthetized dogs. Am Heart J 1973;86:788–97
47. Chen JM, Levin HR, Rose EA, et al. Experience with right ventricular assist devices for perioperative right-sided circulatory failure. Ann Thorac Surg 1996;61:305–10
48. Riedel B. The pathophysiology and management of perioperative pulmonary hypertension with specific emphasis on the period following cardiac surgery. Int Anesthesiol Clin 1999;37:55–79
49. Honkonen EL, Kaukinen L, Kaukinen S, et al. Dopexamine unloads the impaired right ventricle better than iloprost, a prostacyclin analog, after coronary artery surgery. J Cardiothorac Vasc Anesth 1998;12:647–53
50. Vlahakes GJ, Turley K, Hoffman JI. The pathophysiology of failure in acute right ventricular hypertension: hemodynamic and biochemical correlations. Circulation 1981;63:87–95
51. Holmes CL, Patel BM, Russell JA, Walley KR. Physiology of vasopressin relevant to management of septic shock. Chest 2001;120:989–1002
52. Leather HA, Segers P, Berends N, et al. Effects of vasopressin on right ventricular

function in an experimental model of acute pulmonary hypertension. Crit Care Med. 2002;30:2548–52
53. Hillman ND, Cheifetz IM, Craig DM, et al. Inhaled nitric oxide, right ventricular efficiency, and pulmonary vascular mechanics: selective vasodilation of small pulmonary vessels during hypoxic pulmonary vasoconstriction. J Thorac Cardiovasc Surg 1997;113:1006–13
54. Foubert L, De Wolf D, Mareels K, et al. Intravenous dipyridamole enhances the effects of inhaled nitric oxide and prevents rebound pulmonary hypertension in piglets. Pediatr Res 2002;52:730–6
55. Lazor L, Russell JC, DaSilva J, Radford M. Use of the multiple uptake gated acquisition scan for the preoperative assessment of cardiac risk. Surg Gynecol Obstet 1988;167:234–8
56. Baron JF, Mundler O, Bertrand M, et al. Dipyridamole-thallium scintigraphy and gated radionuclide angiography to assess cardiac risk before abdominal aortic surgery. N Engl J Med 1994;330:663–9
57. Godet G, Riou B, Bertrand M, et al. Does preoperative coronary angioplasty improve perioperative cardiac outcome? Anesthesiology 2005;102:739–46
58. Huneke R, Fassl J, Rossaint R, Luckhoff A. Effects of volatile anesthetics on cardiac ion channels. Acta Anesthesiol Scand 2004;48:547–61
59. Housmans PR, Bartunek AE. Effects of volatile anesthetics on ryanodine-treated ferret cardiac muscle. J Cardiovasc Pharmacol 2001;38:211–8
60. Lee DL, Zhang J, Blanck TJ. The effects of halothane on voltage-dependent calcium channels in isolated Langendorff-perfused rat heart. Anesthesiology 1994;81:1212–9
61. Messina AG, Yao FS, Canning H, et al. The effect of nitrous oxide on left ventricular pump performance and contractility in patients with coronary artery disease: effect of preoperative ejection fraction. Anesth Analg 1993;77:954–62
62. Hamilton DL, Boyett MR, Harrison SM, et al. The concentration-dependent effects of propofol on rat ventricular myocytes. Anesth Analg 2000;91:276–82
63. Goto T, Hanne P, Ishiguro Y, et al. Cardiovascular effects of xenon and nitrous oxide in patients during fentanyl-midazolam anesthesia. Anesthesia 2004;59:1178–83
64. Allman KG, Muir A, Howell SJ, et al. Resistant hypertension and preoperative silent myocardial ischaemia in surgical patients. Br J Anesth 1994;73:574–8
65. Reeder MK, Goldman MD, Loh L, et al. Postoperative hypoxaemia after major abdominal vascular surgery. Br J Anesth 1992;68:23–6

3 Cardiac Protection for Noncardiac Surgery

P. Foëx and G. Howard-Alpe

Introduction

Cardiovascular complications of anesthesia and surgery remain, unfortunately, very frequent. In the USA, Mangano and Goldman concluded that approximately 27 million anesthetics were given every year, including 8 million to patients with coronary artery disease. They estimated the number of cardiovascular complications to be approximately 1 million per annum, including 500 000 postoperative myocardial infarctions [1]. This represents one cardiovascular complication for every 27 anesthetics. The complications considered in this context include myocardial infarction, unstable angina, life-threatening arrhythmias, and acute left ventricular failure.

In the UK the number of anesthetics is estimated at 3 million per annum. The number of perioperative cardiac deaths has been found to be approximately 20 000 per annum for many years [2]. Sixty percent of the patients who die within 30 days of surgery have evidence of coronary heart disease [3], and the number of cardiac deaths is approximately 9000 per annum [2]. A systematic review and meta-analysis of randomised controlled trials (2005) shows that for each cardiac death there are ten major cardiovascular complications [4], therefore, the total number of cardiac deaths and cardiovascular complications is likely to be in the region of 100 000 per annum, or one cardiovascular complication for every 30 anesthetics. It is known that perioperative cardiac complications are associated with a significant reduction of the patient's life expectancy [5], and these complications represent a major health problem.

Postoperative myocardial infarction is one of the major complications of

Nuffield Department of Anaesthetics, University of Oxford, Oxford, UK

anesthesia and surgery. It occurs in 2.5% of unselected patients aged over 40 years and 8.6% of patients in whom suspicion of coronary artery disease is sufficiently strong to justify myocardial perfusion scintigraphy [6]. In patients with confirmed significant coronary artery disease on dobutamine-sensitized echocardiography or myocardial perfusion scintigraphy, vascular surgery may be associated with a 30% risk of myocardial infarction or cardiac death [7, 8]. In the face of such a major health risk, active steps must be taken to protect patients as there are very large health costs associated with the treatment of perioperative adverse cardiac events.

Mechanisms of Myocardial Ischemia and Its Complications

Ischemic complications result from the presence of underlying cardiac disease and the stress of surgery with its associated increase in sympathetic activity and other stress hormones such as corticosteroids.

In the presence of fixed coronary artery stenoses with limited coronary flow reserve, myocardial ischemia can occur because increases in myocardial oxygen requirements cannot be met by commensurate increases in coronary blood flow. In the presence of dynamic coronary stenoses, myocardial ischemia is caused by sudden increases in coronary vascular tone. α-adrenergic stimulation, release of endothelins, and thromboxane, as well as inhibition of vasodilators such as nitrous oxide, cause vasoconstriction and curtail oxygen supply. In addition, the probability of vasoconstriction is increased because of endothelial damage. This tends to alter the local balance of vasodilators and vasoconstrictors in favor of vasoconstrictors. Thus, many factors contribute to myocardial ischemia (Fig. 1).

Myocardial ischemia causes an immediate reduction in regional cardiac function. Depending upon its duration, myocardial ischemia may be followed by complete recovery, albeit after a period of stunning, or by myocardial infarction. Repeated episodes of ischemia followed by stunning may result in myocardial hibernation, a prolonged, but potentially reversible, depression of function. Paradoxically, myocardial ischemia may also be protective; short episodes of ischemia can reduce the extent of damage after coronary occlusion, as shown in ischemic preconditioning.

Over the past decade, however, it has become increasingly obvious that acute coronary syndromes may be caused by the release of inflammatory mediators. Indeed, in patients with elevated C-reactive protein (CRP), the prognosis of coronary artery disease is worse than in those with normal CRP, especially in acute coronary syndromes [9, 10]. Other inflammatory markers are also elevated. Major surgery causes the release of inflammatory mediators. This can be followed by adverse cardiac events resulting from unstable

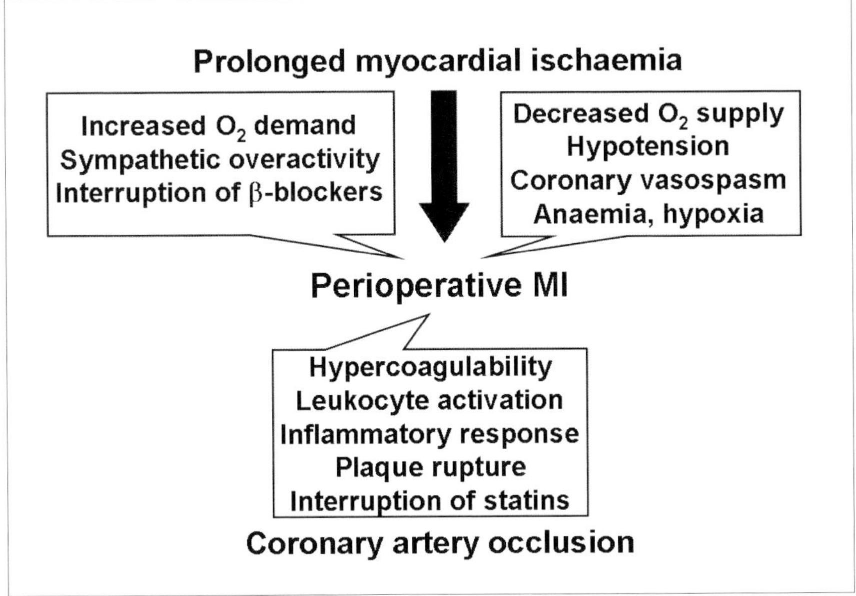

Fig. 1. Causes of perioperative myocardial infarction. Perioperative myocardial infarction may be caused by acute coronary occlusion or result from prolonged myocardial ischemia. In both situations many factors contribute to myocardial damage

coronary syndromes. Indirectly, the protective effect of statins confirms the involvement of inflammatory mediators in perioperative cardiovascular complications. Further confirmation of the role of inflammatory mediators is the observation of plaque disruption (hemorrhage, rupture) as a cause of acute myocardial infarction in daily life and during the perioperative period.

Currently, perioperative ischemia and its complications can be considered under three headings (Figs. 1, 2):

- Increased oxygen demand, including sympathetic overactivity and, possibly, the untimely interruption of β-blockers.
- Decreased oxygen supply including hypotension, vasospasm, anemia, and hypoxia.
- Hypercoagulability, leukocyte activation, the inflammatory response, and plaque rupture, including the interruption of statins.

Identification of High-Risk Patients

In order to prevent cardiovascular complications, patients at risk must be identified preoperatively. This can be difficult as the medical history may be unrevealing and obvious clinical manifestations of coronary artery disease

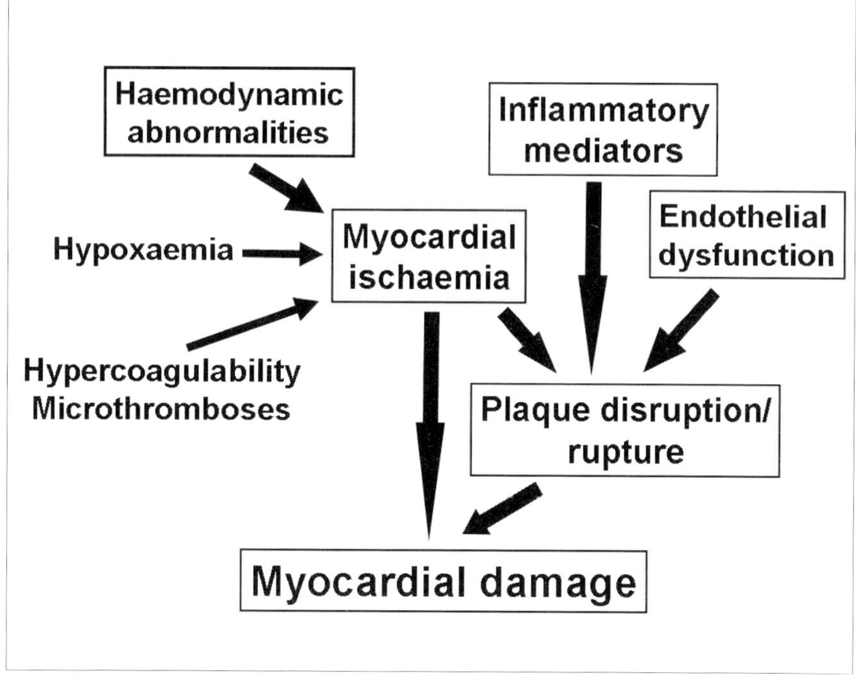

Fig. 2. Causes of perioperative myocardial damage. The *left side* of the diagram emphasizes the role of hemodynamic disorders as causes of myocardial ischemia. The *right side* shows factors that have been recognized more recently, namely the role of inflammatory mediators and endothelial dysfunction

may be absent. The electrocardiogram can also be normal at rest. Many patients with coronary artery lesions are asymptomatic as their ischemia is silent. Myocardial infarction can also be totally or almost totally silent, especially in diabetic patients.

While coronary angiography is the gold standard for the evaluation of coronary heart disease, it is impractical to carry it out in all patients presenting for major noncardiac surgery who are at risk for coronary artery disease because of costs and risks. Noninvasive screening tests are useful; they are based on the imposition of a physical (exercise test) or pharmacological challenge (dobutamine, dipyridamole, or adenosine) together with electrocardiography, echocardiography, radionuclide angiography (multiple-gated acquisition scan), or myocardial scintigraphy (thallium, technetium-99m sestamibi). Stress is used to elicit reversible ischemia (ST-segment depression, reduced ejection fraction, new wall motion abnormalities, or reversible defect of thallium or technetium-99m sestamibi uptake). Reversible ischemia indicates the presence of significant coronary artery lesions and justifies coronary angiography.

Coronary Revascularization or Pharmacological Prophylaxis?

In the presence of significant coronary lesions, should coronary revascularization be offered or medical treatment? If the extent of coronary lesions or symptoms constitutes in its own right a clear indication for coronary revascularization, independently of impending noncardiac surgery, revascularization should precede noncardiac operations [11]. By contrast, purely prophylactic coronary revascularization should be limited to patients with significant coronary disease undergoing high risk major surgery, as stated in the 2002 American College of Cardiology/American Heart Association (ACC/AHA) guideline [11].

This approach has been called into question recently because a prospective study has shown no benefit of coronary revascularization (coronary bypass surgery or angioplasty) before vascular surgery [12]. However, in this study patients with severe coronary disease (left main stem coronary artery) or severe cardiac failure were excluded. Clearly a full cardiological evaluation had been carried out in all these patients. Moreover, all patients were on maximum medication including β-blockers (85%), statins (55%), and antiplatelet drugs (70%). This study does not prove that revascularization is ineffective in all patients, because those likely to benefit had been excluded after careful evaluation. In addition, the majority of patients underwent coronary angioplasty, an intervention of little value for the prevention of adverse cardiac outcome in surgical patients [13, 14].

In the face of these uncertainties regarding coronary revascularization, an alternative approach is to consider that all eligible patients with risk factors for coronary artery disease should be treated with cardioprotective drugs during the perioperative period and beyond [15]. The emphasis on the prevention of myocardial ischemia and its consequences is legitimate as the majority of complications result from underlying coronary artery disease.

Prophylaxis Based on Hemodynamic Stabilization

For many years the main pharmacological approach has been the modulation of hemodynamic responses.

The prophylactic administration of drugs that decrease oxygen demand, make the circulation more stable, or improve coronary blood flow and its distribution, should reduce the risk of ischemia and its consequences. Several classes of drugs must be considered: nitrates, calcium channel blockers, α_2-adrenoceptor agonists, adenosine modulators, ATP-dependent potassium channel openers, sodium-proton (Na^+/H^+) exchanger inhibitors, angiotensin-converting enzyme (ACE) inhibitors, and, more importantly, β-blockers. Many of these drugs have been reviewed systematically by Stevens and colleagues [16].

Nitrates

There is no evidence that nitrates protect against cardiovascular complications of anesthesia and surgery [16].

Calcium Channel Blockers

The acute administration of calcium antagonists is of limited efficacy [16], even though calcium antagonists cause coronary vasodilatation, relieve exercise-induced vasoconstriction, reduce left ventricular afterload, and improve the oxygen balance. Benefits can be expected from the perioperative administration of verapamil and diltiazem, but not of a dihydropyridine calcium channel blocker (e.g., nifedipine, nicardipine). In addition, there is no evidence that chronic treatment by dihydropyridines offers any protection [17].

α2-Adrenoceptor Agonists

α2-Adrenoceptor agonists decrease sympathetic activity by a central mechanism, improve hemodynamic stability and decrease the risk of ischemia. In addition, there is sedation and reduction in anesthetic and opioid requirements. α2-Adrenoceptor agonists have been used only to a limited extent and have proved effective in reducing ischemia and adverse cardiovascular events in relatively small groups of patients. Clonidine has been shown to reduce the risk of myocardial ischemia [18]. In a recent prospective study, clonidine was shown to protect against myocardial ischemia and adverse cardiac outcome [19]. Mivazerol, another α2-adrenoceptor agonist, was shown to protect vascular surgical patients against the risk of myocardial infarction and cardiac death but did not show this protective effect in a more general surgical population [20]. As a result, the development of mivazerol was stopped.

Adenosine Modulators

Adenosine modulators control the release of adenosine, a very strong coronary vasodilator, and by so doing increase flow in poorly perfused myocardium. A meta-analysis of five trials of acadesine showed a significant reduction of adverse cardiac outcomes [21]. Unfortunately, by the time the meta-analysis was published, the development of acadesine had stopped.

K_{ATP} Channel Openers

K_{ATP} channel openers mimic ischemic preconditioning and have been shown to protect against myocardial ischemia. Nicorandil is effective in the management of coronary artery disease and protects the heart against the effects of brief periods of ischemia during angioplasty. Nicorandil has been shown to decrease perioperative ischemia but not adverse outcomes [22], perhaps because of the small size of the study. Demonstration of an effect on cardiac outcomes would require a large study, which has not yet been undertaken.

Na^+/H^+ Exchanger Blockers

The Na^+/H^+ exchanger figures prominently in cardiac ischemia–reperfusion injury. Several experimental and clinical studies have demonstrated a cardioprotective effect of Na^+/H^+ exchanger inhibition. Cariporide, a Na^+/H^+ exchanger blocker, protects cardiomyocytes against oxidant-induced cell death by preserving intracellular ion homeostasis and mitochondrial integrity [23]. Cariporide has also been shown to improve left ventricular morphology and function after myocardial infarction. In addition, it suppresses inflammation and neurohormonal activation in congestive heart failure [24]. As pretreatment with the Na^+/H^+ exchanger inhibitor cariporide limits infarct size, its effects are similar to those of ischemic preconditioning [25]. This may make Na^+/H^+ exchanger inhibitors important for cardiac protection during the perioperative period because of the known role of inflammatory mediators and the potential benefits of pharmacological preconditioning.

ACE Inhibitors

ACE inhibitors improve outcomes among patients with left ventricular dysfunction, whether or not they have heart failure. Highly beneficial effects of the ACE inhibitor ramipril were shown in the HOPE (Heart Outcomes Prevention Evaluation) study [26]. This study focused on patients with a history of coronary artery disease, stroke, peripheral vascular disease, or diabetes plus at least one other cardiovascular risk factor. The study showed relative risks of adverse cardiac events ranging from 0.68 to 0.82 (risk reductions 32% to 18%). On the strength of such benefits, the effects of ACE inhibitors deserved to be considered in the perioperative period. However, two published studies showed no benefit of long-term treatment with ACE inhibitors [17, 27].

β-Adrenoreceptor Blockers

Unlike the agents discussed above, β-blockers have been used extensively for many years in surgical patients. β-Blockers reduce myocardial oxygen demand by reducing heart rate while bringing myocardial contractility to the level that exists in the unstimulated myocardium. Moreover, β-blockers prevent the cardiac effects of sympathetic overactivity and may reduce sympathetic overactivity itself. They can redistribute coronary flow towards the compromised myocardium and may also modulate dysregulated cytokines [28]. As there is increasing emphasis on the role of inflammatory mediators in the development of unstable coronary syndromes [29], this may contribute to their efficacy.

β-Blockade reduces mortality after acute myocardial infarction [30] and protects against the risk of reinfarction, with a mortality reduction as high as 36% [31]. β-Blockers reduce the incidence of silent ischemia in ambulatory patients; this is accompanied by a significant reduction in the relative risk of cardiac events [32]. Although β-blockers play an important role in the management of arterial hypertension, their efficacy is now in question [33–35].

The potential benefits of acute perioperative β-blockade were first demonstrated in 1973 in a detailed hemodynamic study of a small number of hypertensive patients who were given an intravenous β-blocker after induction of anesthesia or an oral β -blocker for two days before surgery, and compared to untreated hypertensive patients. The patients given the β-blocker exhibited more stable hemodynamics than the untreated patients and were unlikely to exhibit myocardial ischemia or ventricular arrhythmias [36]. Later, a prospective, randomized, placebo-controlled study showed that a β-blocker given with the premedication prevented perioperative myocardial ischemia in most patients. However, some patients became hypotensive after induction of anesthesia [37]. More recent studies have shown that β-blockers protect against myocardial ischemia [38], myocardial infarction, arrhythmias [39], and adverse cardiac outcomes [40]. Much enthusiasm for β-blockade followed the publication of a study by Mangano and colleagues [41]. In this study 200 patients with coronary artery disease or risk factors for the condition, and undergoing noncardiac surgery, were randomized to receive atenolol or a placebo starting just before surgery and continuing for seven days. The study showed that the group treated with atenolol had a higher event-free survival (91%) than those given the placebo (81%) for up to 2 years, while there was no difference in respect of immediate perioperative mortality or myocardial infarction.

In 1997, the American College of Physicians published a guideline for assessing and managing the perioperative risk of coronary artery disease associated with major noncardiac surgery and recommended that all eligible patients should receive a β-blocker (atenolol) during the perioperative period [42]. This recommendation was based on the large body of evidence of the efficacy of β-blockade in medical patients and the more limited evidence in surgical patients.

Later this recommendation was reinforced by the results of a study by Poldermans and colleagues [7]. These authors studied high-risk vascular surgical patients selected because of the presence of reversible ischemia on dobutamine-sensitized echocardiography (a finding indicative of significant coronary artery disease). Patients were randomized to receive active treatment or conventional management. The active treatment was with bisoprolol, started a week or more before surgery and continued for 30 days postoperatively. At 30 days the results were highly positive: β-blockade caused a large reduction in cardiac death (3.4% versus 17% in the control group) and nonfatal myocardial infarction (0% versus 17% in the control group). Significant benefits continued to be observed during a 2-year follow-up. As all patients were at a particularly high risk for coronary events (34% combined incidence of cardiac death and nonfatal myocardial infarction in the conventional treatment group), the efficacy of β-blockade in this study cannot be extrapolated to patients at risk for coronary disease, rather than with demonstrably severe coronary artery disease.

β-Blockade seems to be the logical answer to the perioperative drug management of patients with coronary artery disease or risk factors for coronary artery disease. Indeed, as early as 1988, an editorial in *Anesthesiology* was entitled "Should we all have a sympathectomy at birth, or at least preoperatively?" [43]. More importantly, several systematic reviews have concluded its efficacy [16, 44, 45]. Why, then, are β-blockers not used much more frequently?

There are perceived risks to β-blockade, such as worsening of conduction disorders or airway obstruction in patients with reactive airway disease. There is also the risk of worsening of left ventricular dysfunction. Although β-blockers are used successfully in the treatment of patients with heart failure, their introduction shortly before surgery may not be well tolerated (indeed, treatment of cardiac failure with β-blockers must start with extremely low doses, increased progressively over several weeks). Several studies have shown that these guidelines are not followed [46, 47].

The POISE study (PeriOperative Ischemic Evaluation study) [48] has been designed to answer the question of the safety and efficacy of perioperative β-blockade in patients with coronary artery disease or risk factors for coronary artery disease. With over 7500 patients already enrolled (of a planned total of 10 000), the study should provide a definitive answer to the efficacy of β-blockade.

The reason behind the POISE study is that while the studies by Poldermans and colleagues [7] and Mangano and colleagues [41] showed clear benefits, a meta-analysis of all randomized controlled trials of perioperative β-blockade did not show statistically significant cardiac protection [4, 49, 50] but a significant risk of bradycardia requiring treatment. This is at variance with previous systematic reviews based on fewer studies and a far smaller number of patients [16, 44, 45], but these were heavily weighted by the results of the study by Poldermans et al. [7].

Administration of β-blockers is still widely recommended, but it is not without possible hazards. In order to avoid the risk of hypotension at induction of anesthesia, it may be appropriate to start treatment a few days ahead of surgery rather than the day before surgery, and to have rigorous protocols for omitting a dose of the drug if bradycardia and hypotension (heart rate less than 50 bpm and blood pressure less than 100 mmHg) occur during the perioperative period.

Surprisingly, evidence for perioperative protection by chronic β-blockade is lacking except in coronary bypass surgery [51]. In noncardiac surgery, the incidence of perioperative silent myocardial ischemia is not reduced in patients on long-term β-blockers and the perioperative mortality is not reduced [17]. A systematic review of observational studies of outcome in patients on long-term β-blocker therapy did not show any benefit [52]. This may reflect the presence of more severe coronary disease in patients on chronic β-blockers, β-receptor up-regulation [53], increased number and sensitivity of β_2-adrenoceptors when selective β_1-blockers are used, or simply inadequate β-blockade. To date there is no clear approach to the management of patients on chronic β-blockers. Their medication must be continued and the dose of the β-blocker may need to be increased in order to improve the control of heart rate. As the heart rate at which ischemia develops is lower in chronically β-blocked patients [54], relatively small, apparently innocuous, increases in heart rate during the perioperative period could cause ischemia in chronically β-blocked patients, thereby negating the beneficial effects of these agents. Vigilance is essential.

As the prevention of cardiac complications of anesthesia and surgery is of such importance, a more recent guideline revisited this issue. The latest 2002 ACC/AHA guideline [11] states that "appropriately administered β-blockers may reduce the risk of myocardial infarction and death in high risk patients. Where possible β-blockers should be started days or weeks before elective surgery, with doses titrated to achieve a resting heart rate between 50–60 beats per minute." The latter statement echoes the major importance of heart rate control in the prevention of myocardial ischemia [55]. Why is this new recommendation much more guarded than the 1997 recommendation [42]? This is probably because a number of questions have been raised about the studies of Mangano et al. [41] and Poldermans et al. [7]. Several aspects of the study by Mangano and colleagues make its interpretation difficult:

1. Complications that occurred during the administration of the drug or placebo were not included in the final analysis.
2. There were more diabetics in the placebo than in the control group, yet it is known that the long-term prognosis of coronary artery disease is worse in diabetic than in nondiabetic subjects [56].
3. β-Blockers were withdrawn so that patients could be randomized for the study, yet this is regarded by many authors as hazardous [57].

For these reasons, the conclusions reached by Mangano and his colleagues may be weaker than originally thought. As to the study by Poldermans and colleagues, there are also some comments to make. The study addresses the management of a very small population of patients. Out of more than 1350 patients who could have been considered, only just over 100 fulfilled the criteria for inclusion in the randomization process. The results in the treated patients were so good that the monitoring group stopped the study at an interim analysis, but the reductions of mortality by 80% and myocardial infarction by 100% cent in the perioperative period are far higher than any figure ever observed in nonsurgical patients [31].

Recently, the results of the MaVS study (Metoprolol after Vascular Surgery) [58] and of the POBBLE study [59] did not show any benefit from perioperative β-blockade. It could be argued that absence of proof is not proof of absence of benefits. Careful selection of patients may show that some groups of patients could benefit from perioperative β-blockade (Fig. 3), while others could suffer some harm.

Clearly, β-blockade should not be initiated in patients with obstructive lung disease or conduction disorders. Although β-blockers are now part of the treatment of cardiac failure, their introduction immediately before surgery in patients with poor left ventricular function is contraindicated. If they are used, caution is essential, as in patients with cardiac failure β-blockade always starts with very low doses and titration takes several weeks [60]. It should also be noted that several recent studies were carried out in patients admitted to high dependency or intensive care units. In such environments adverse effects, if any, could be easily detected and corrected. This may not be the case if patients are admitted to an ordinary ward. Therefore, the safety of introducing perioperative β-blockade when patients are on the ward needs to be demonstrated.

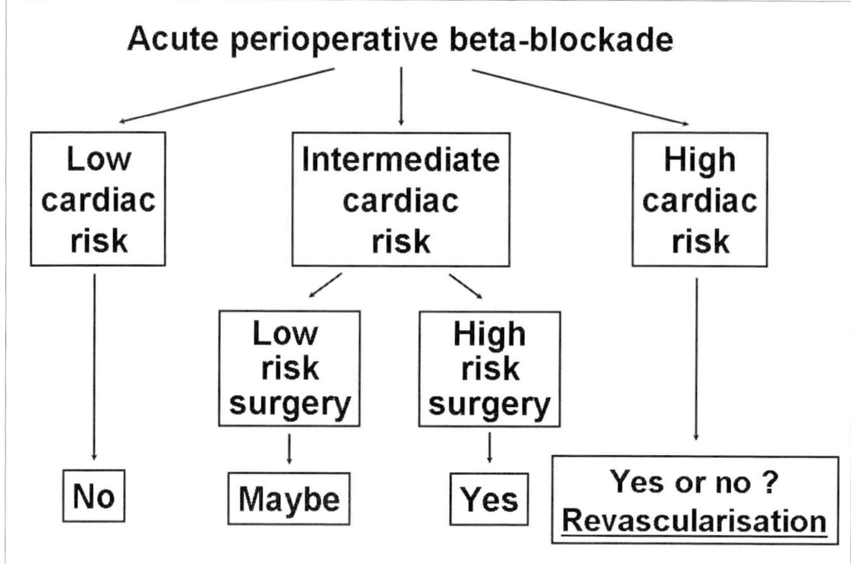

Fig. 3. Possible uses of β-blockers depending on the extent of coronary disease (severity of cardiac risk) and the type of surgery. This is the personal view of the authors

Statins

Statins block the biosynthesis of cholesterol, improve endothelial function by up-regulating nitric oxide synthase, reduce the levels of inflammatory mediators, scavenge superoxides, shift the fibrinolytic balance toward fibrinolysis, stabilize atherosclerotic plaques, and inhibit vascular smooth muscle proliferation. Statins reduce the risk of cardiac events and stroke in patients with coronary heart disease or cerebrovascular disease.

Over the past two decades it has become increasingly clear that myocardial damage often results from atheromatous plaque disruption (fissure, rupture, hemorrhage) with temporary or permanent occlusion. This may occur at the level of plaques that are hemodynamically insignificant but have a large lipid core and a thin fibrous cap–the so-called vulnerable plaques [61], which include plaques that are prone to rupture or erosion and plaques likely to develop intraplaque hemorrhage (Fig. 4). The extent of reduction of the lumen is in sharp contrast with critical stenosis. The risk of complications is already present with stenoses of the order of 30 % [61]. The concept of vulnerability extends to plaques, myocardium, and patient. Plaque disruption may result from inflammation. This can develop slowly with hypertension, smoking, and diabetes, or more acutely with injury, lipid peroxidation, and infection. Rupture and thrombosis may follow [62]. The presence of an underlying inflammatory response in coronary heart disease is exemplified

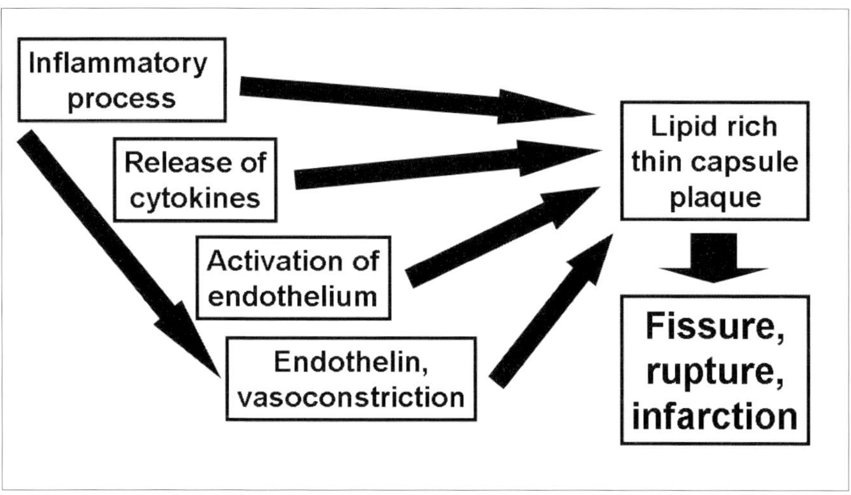

Fig. 4. Inflammatory and endothelial processes and their impact on lipid-rich, thin-capsule plaques, causing them to fissure and/or rupture

by the observation of an association between elevated CRP (>0.38 mg/dl) and inducible ischemia [9]. It is in this context that statins play an important role.

Statins are known to have pleiotropic effects, over and above the reduction of plasma lipids. They increase the stability of plaques of atheroma, inhibit neovascularization, modulate and moderate inflammatory responses, decrease subendothelial basement membrane degradation, decrease smooth muscle apoptosis, improve endothelial function, inhibit platelet activation, and promote fibrinolysis.

The evidence for protection in noncardiac surgery was first proposed by Poldermans and colleagues at a meeting of the American Heart Association in 2002: in a retrospective analysis of data on 123 802 surgical patients, they found that 26 264 had a least one risk factor for coronary heart disease. There were 1032 perioperative deaths. Eight hundred and seventy-three patients were receiving statins: mortality in the statins group was 2.3% versus 4.0% among patients not treated with statins. In another study Poldermans and colleagues [63] focused on patients undergoing vascular surgery: there were 160 deaths in the cohort. From the survivors, the authors identified 320 matched controls. Mortality was substantially reduced in patients on statins [odds ratio 0.22 (95% CI 0.10-0.47)]. Other studies have confirmed reduced adverse cardiac events in patients treated chronically with statins [27, 64–66]. It is only in cardiac surgery that statins do not seem to confer protection once data is adjusted for propensity scores [67].

By contrast with studies in patients chronically treated with statins, there are few studies of the deliberate administration of statins as prophylactic perioperative medication. Durazzo and colleagues [68] gave atorvastatin or a placebo to 100 patients undergoing vascular surgery, with surgery at day 30 of treatment. Cardiac events within 6 months were far fewer in statins-treated patients (8%) as opposed to untreated patients (26%). In the study of Schouten et al. [69] protection was evident, but only 22% of patients included in the study had been started on statins before surgery; the others were on chronic statin medication. These observations suggest that statin administration during the perioperative period and chronic treatment with statins offer cardiac protection.

There is of course, as with any medication, the possibility of side effects. The most common in nonsurgical patients are headaches, gastrointestinal disturbances, and myalgia. Side effects are responsible for a withdrawal rate of 3%. Rhabdomyolysis occurs in one in 100 000 patients [70, 71] and is responsible for less than one death in 1 million patients treated. The risk of statins withdrawal has been clearly demonstrated in acute coronary syndromes (PRISM study), with and odds ratio for cardiac events of 2.93 (95% CI 1.64–6.27) [72].

The UK guideline for the administration of statins, if applied, should see a considerable increase in the administration of statins and should result in a significant reduction of perioperative adverse cardiac events. The perioperative period with its stress can be compared with percutaneous coronary interventions where statins are beneficial [73].

Aspirin

Aspirin is the prototype nonsteroidal anti-inflammatory agent. Aspirin blocks the synthesis of thromboxane A_2 (TxA_2) for the lifetime of the platelet (about 10 days), while the synthesis of PGI_2 is quickly restored where low-dose aspirin is used. Long-term aspirin prophylaxis is protective in patients with coronary and cerebrovascular disease. Aspirin has been shown to reduce cardiac mortality after coronary artery bypass surgery [74, 75]. However, administration of aspirin may increase the risk of bleeding during surgery [76].

Conclusion

For several decades, protection against perioperative adverse cardiac outcome has been based almost exclusively on the concept of prevention of hemodynamic disturbances likely to cause an imbalance between oxygen demand and restricted oxygen supply in patients with coronary artery disease. More recent understanding of the role of the endothelium and of inflammatory mediators in the development of unstable coronary syndromes means that such factors are now regarded as important determinants of perioperative myocardial damage including acute myocardial infarction. Therefore, the future of drug-based cardiac protection is likely to be multimodal, including agents that minimize hemodynamic changes, protect the ischemic myocardium, and reduce the release or activity of inflammatory mediators. However, the availability of protective drugs does not mean that thorough assessment of the patient and further investigations are no longer necessary, as drug prophylaxis cannot replace coronary revascularization where the latter would be required irrespective of impending noncardiac surgery. To this day, there is little evidence that percutaneous coronary interventions are as effective in the prevention of perioperative cardiac events as coronary bypass surgery.

References

1. Mangano DT (1995) Preoperative risk assessment: many studies, few solutions. Is a cardiac risk assessment paradigm possible? Anesthesiology 83:897–901
2. National Confidential Enquiry into Perioperative Deaths (1999) Extremes of age. The 1999 Report of the National Confidential Enquiry into Perioperative Deaths. The National Confidential Enquiry into Perioperative Deaths
3. National Confidential Enquiry into Perioperative Deaths (2001) Then and now: the 2000 report of the National Confidential Enquiry into Postoperative Deaths. The National Confidential Enquiry into Postoperative Deaths
4. Devereaux PJ, Beattie WS, Choi PT et al (2005) How strong is the evidence for the use of perioperative beta blockers in non-cardiac surgery? Systematic review and meta-analysis of randomised controlled trials. BMJ 331:313–321
5. Mangano DT, Browner WS, Hollenberg M et al (1992) Long-term cardiac prognosis following noncardiac surgery. The Study of Perioperative Ischemia Research Group. JAMA 268:233–239
6. Mangano DT (1998) Adverse outcomes after surgery in the year 2001–a continuing odyssey. Anesthesiology 88:561–564
7. Poldermans D, Boersma E, Bax JJ et al (1999) The effect of bisoprolol on perioperative mortality and myocardial infarction in high-risk patients undergoing vascular surgery. N Engl J Med 341:1789–1794
8. Mamode N, Docherty G, Lowe GD et al (2001) The role of myocardial perfusion scanning, heart rate variability and d-dimers in predicting the risk of perioperative cardiac complications after peripheral vascular surgery. Eur J Vasc Endovasc Surg 22:499–508
9. Beattie MS, Shlipak MG, Liu H et al (2003) C-reactive protein and ischemia in users and nonusers of beta-blockers and statins: data from the Heart and Soul Study. Circulation 107:245–250

10. Blake GJ, Ridker PM (2003) C-reactive protein and other inflammatory risk markers in acute coronary syndromes. J Am Coll Cardiol 41(4 Suppl S):37S-42S
11. Eagle KA, Berger PB, Calkins H et al (2002) ACC/AHA guideline update for perioperative cardiovascular evaluation for noncardiac surgery. Circulation 105:1257–1267
12. McFalls EO, Ward HB, Moritz TE et al (2004) Coronary-artery revascularization before elective major vascular surgery. N Engl J Med 351:2795–2804
13. Posner KL, Van Norman GA, Chan V (1999) Adverse cardiac outcomes after noncardiac surgery in patients with prior percutaneous transluminal coronary angioplasty. Anesth Analg 89:553–560
14. Godet G, Riou B, Bertrand M et al (2005) Does preoperative coronary angioplasty improve perioperative cardiac outcome? Anesthesiology 102:739–746
15. Grayburn PA, Hillis LD (2003) Cardiac events in patients undergoing noncardiac surgery: shifting the paradigm from noninvasive risk stratification to therapy. Ann Intern Med 138:506–511
16. Stevens RD, Burri H, Tramer MR. Pharmacologic myocardial protection in patients undergoing noncardiac surgery: a quantitative systematic review. Anesth Analg 2003;97:623–633
17. Sear JW, Howell SJ, Sear YM et al (2001) Intercurrent drug therapy and perioperative cardiovascular mortality in elective and urgent/emergency surgical patients. Br J Anaesth 86:506–512
18. Nishina K, Mikawa K, Uesugi T et al (2002) Efficacy of clonidine for prevention of perioperative myocardial ischemia: a critical appraisal and meta-analysis of the literature. Anesthesiology 96:323–329
19. Wallace AW, Galindez D, Salahieh A et al (2004) Effect of clonidine on cardiovascular morbidity and mortality after noncardiac surgery. Anesthesiology 101:284–293
20. Oliver MF, Goldman L, Julian DG, Holme I (1999) Effect of mivazerol on perioperative cardiac complications during non-cardiac surgery in patients with coronary heart disease: the European Mivazerol Trial (EMIT). Anesthesiology 91:951–961
21. Mangano DT (1997) Effects of acadesine on myocardial infarction, stroke, and death following surgery. A meta-analysis of the 5 international randomized trials. JAMA 277:325–332
22. Kaneko T, Saito Y, Hikawa Y et al (2001) Dose-dependent prophylactic effect of nicorandil, an ATP-sensitive potassium channel opener, on intra-operative myocardial ischaemia in patients undergoing major abdominal surgery. Br J Anaesth 86:332–337
23. Teshima Y, Akao M, Jones SP et al (2003) Cariporide (HOE642), a selective Na+-H+ exchange inhibitor, inhibits the mitochondrial death pathway. Circulation 108:2275–2281
24. Rungwerth K, Schindler U, Gerl M et al (2004) Inhibition of Na+-H+ exchange by cariporide reduces inflammation and heart failure in rabbits with myocardial infarction. Br J Pharmacol 142:1147–1154
25. Xu Z, Jiao Z, Cohen MV, Downey JM (2002) Protection from AMP 579 can be added to that from either cariporide or ischemic preconditioning in ischemic rabbit heart. J Cardiovasc Pharmacol 40:510–518
26. Yusuf S, Sleight P, Pogue J et al (2000) Effects of an angiotensin-converting-enzyme inhibitor, ramipril, on cardiovascular events in high-risk patients. The Heart Outcomes Prevention Evaluation Study Investigators. N Engl J Med 342:145–153
27. Kertai MD, Boersma E, Westerhout CM et al (2004) Association between long-term statin use and mortality after successful abdominal aortic aneurysm surgery. Am J

Med 116:96–103
28. Ohtsuka T, Hamada M, Hiasa G et al (2001) Effect of beta-blockers on circulating levels of inflammatory and anti-inflammatory cytokines in patients with dilated cardiomyopathy. J Am Coll Cardiol 37:412–417
29. Vallance P, Collier J, Bhagat K (1997) Infection, inflammation, and infarction: does acute endothelial dysfunction provide a link? Lancet 349:1391–1393
30. ISIS-1 (1986) Randomised trial of intravenous atenolol among 16 027 cases of suspected acute myocardial infarction: ISIS-1. First International Study of Infarct Survival Collaborative Group. Lancet 2:57–66
31. Owen A (1998) Intravenous beta blockade in acute myocardial infarction. Should be used in combination with thrombolysis. BMJ 317:226–227
32. Pepine CJ, Cohn PF, Deedwania PC et al (1994) Effects of treatment on outcome in mildly symptomatic patients with ischemia during daily life. The Atenolol Silent Ischemia Study (ASIST). Circulation 90:762–768
33. Carlberg B, Samuelsson O, Lindholm LH (2004) Atenolol in hypertension: is it a wise choice? Lancet 364:1684–1689
34. Dahlof B, Sever PS, Poulter NR et al (2005) Prevention of cardiovascular events with an antihypertensive regimen of amlodipine adding perindopril as required versus atenolol adding bendroflumethiazide as required, in the Anglo-Scandinavian Cardiac Outcomes Trial–Blood Pressure Lowering Arm (ASCOT-BPLA): a multicentre randomised controlled trial. Lancet 366:895–906
35. Poulter NR, Wedel H, Dahlof B et al (2005) Role of blood pressure and other variables in the differential cardiovascular event rates noted in the Anglo-Scandinavian Cardiac Outcomes Trial–Blood Pressure Lowering Arm (ASCOT-BPLA). Lancet 366:907–913
36. Prys-Roberts C, Foex P, Biro GP, Roberts JG (1973) Studies of anaesthesia in relation to hypertension. V. Adrenergic beta-receptor blockade. Br J Anaesth 45:671–681
37. Stone JG, Foex P, Sear JW et al (1988) Myocardial ischemia in untreated hypertensive patients: effect of a single small oral dose of a beta-adrenergic blocking agent. Anesthesiology 68:495–500
38. Wallace A, Layug B, Tateo I et al (1988) Prophylactic atenolol reduces postoperative myocardial ischemia. McSPI Research Group. Anesthesiology 88:7–17
39. Pasternack PF, Imparato AM, Baumann FG et al (1987) The hemodynamics of beta-blockade in patients undergoing abdominal aortic aneurysm repair. Circulation 76(3 Pt 2):III1–7
40. Yeager RA, Moneta GL, Edwards JM et al (1995 Reducing perioperative myocardial infarction following vascular surgery. The potential role of beta-blockade. Arch Surg 130:869–872; discussion 72–73
41. Mangano DT, Layug EL, Wallace A, Tateo I (1996) Effect of atenolol on mortality and cardiovascular morbidity after noncardiac surgery. Multicenter Study of Perioperative Ischemia Research Group. N Engl J Med 335:1713–1720
42. Palda VA, Detsky AS (1997) Perioperative assessment and management of risk from coronary artery disease. Ann Intern Med 127:313–328
43. Roizen MF (1988) Should we all have a sympathectomy at birth? Or at least preoperatively? Anesthesiology 68:482–484
44. Auerbach AD, Goldman L (2002) beta-blockers and reduction of cardiac events in noncardiac surgery: scientific review. JAMA 287:1435–1444
45. Schouten O, Shaw LJ, Boersma E et al (2006) A meta-analysis of safety and effectiveness of perioperative beta-blocker use for the prevention of cardiac events in dif-

ferent types of noncardiac surgery. Coron Artery Dis 17:173–179
46. Taylor RC, Pagliarello G (2003) Prophylactic beta-blockade to prevent myocardial infarction perioperatively in high-risk patients who undergo general surgical procedures. Can J Surg 46:216–222
47. Rapchuk I, Rabuka S, Tonelli M (2004) Perioperative use of beta-blockers remains low: experience of a single Canadian tertiary institution. Can J Anaesth 51:761–767
48. POISE Trial Investigators, Devereaux PJ, Yang H, Guyatt GH et al (2006) Rationale, design, and organization of the PeriOperative ISchemic Evalutaion (POISE) trial: a randomized controlled trial of metoprolol versus placebo in patients undergoing noncardiac surgery. Am Heart J S2:223-230
49. Devereaux PJ, Leslie K (2004) Best evidence in anesthetic practice. Prevention: alpha2- and beta-adrenergic antagonists reduce perioperative cardiac events. Can J Anaesth 51:290–292
50. Devereaux PJ, Yusuf S, Yang H et al (2004) Are the recommendations to use perioperative beta-blocker therapy in patients undergoing noncardiac surgery based on reliable evidence? Can Med Assoc J 171:245–247
51. ten Broecke PW, De Hert SG, Mertens E, Adriaensen HF (2003) Effect of preoperative beta-blockade on perioperative mortality in coronary surgery. Br J Anaesth 90:27–31
52. Giles JW, Sear JW, Foex P (2004) Effect of chronic beta-blockade on peri-operative outcome in patients undergoing non-cardiac surgery: an analysis of observational and case control studies. Anaesthesia 59:574–583
53. Yndgaard S, Lippert FK, Berthelsen PG (1997) Are patients chronically treated with beta 1-adrenoceptor antagonists in fact beta-blocked? J Cardiothorac Vasc Anesth 11:32–36
54. Tzivoni D, Medina A, David D et al (1998) Effect of metoprolol in reducing myocardial ischemic threshold during exercise and during daily activity. Am J Cardiol 81:775–777
55. Raby KE, Brull SJ, Timimi F et al (1999) The effect of heart rate control on myocardial ischemia among high-risk patients after vascular surgery. Anesth Analg 88:477–482
56. Juul AB, Wetterslev J, Kofoed Enevoldsen A et al (2004) The Diabetic Postoperative Mortality and Morbidity (DIPOM) trial: rationale and design of a multicenter, randomized, placebo-controlled, clinical trial of metoprolol for patients with diabetes mellitus who are undergoing major noncardiac surgery. Am Heart J 147:677–683
57. Shammash JB, Trost JC, Gold JM et al (2001) Perioperative beta-blocker withdrawal and mortality in vascular surgical patients. Am Heart J 141:148–153
58. Yang H, Raymer K, Butler R et al (2004) Metoprolol after vascular surgery (MaVS). Can J Anaesth 51:A7
59. Brady AR, Gibbs JS, Greenhalgh RM et al (2005) Perioperative beta-blockade (POBBLE) for patients undergoing infrarenal vascular surgery: results of a randomized double-blind controlled trial. J Vasc Surg 41:602–609
60. Gottlieb SS, McCarter RJ, Vogel RA (1998) Effect of beta-blockade on mortality among high-risk and low-risk patients after myocardial infarction. N Engl J Med 339:489–497
61. Naghavi M, Libby P, Falk E et al From vulnerable plaque to vulnerable patient: a call for new definitions and risk assessment strategies: Part II. Circulation 2003;108:1772–8
62. Willerson JT, Ridker PM (2003) Inflammation as a cardiovascular risk factor. Circulation 109[21 Suppl 1]:II2–10

63. Poldermans D, Bax JJ, Kertai MD et al (2003) Statins are associated with a reduced incidence of perioperative mortality in patients undergoing major noncardiac vascular surgery. Circulation 107:1848–1851
64. Lindenauer PK, Pekow P, Wang K et al (2004) Lipid-lowering therapy and in-hospital mortality following major noncardiac surgery. JAMA 291:2092–2099
65. O'Neil-Callahan K, Katsimaglis G, Tepper MR et al (2005) Statins decrease perioperative cardiac complications in patients undergoing noncardiac vascular surgery: the Statins for Risk Reduction in Surgery (StaRRS) study. J Am Coll Cardiol 45:336–342
66. Ward RP, Leeper NJ, Kirkpatrick JN et al (2005) The effect of preoperative statin therapy on cardiovascular outcomes in patients undergoing infrainguinal vascular surgery. Int J Cardiol 104:264–268
67. Ali IS, Buth KJ (2005) Preoperative statin use and outcomes following cardiac surgery. Int J Cardiol 103:12–18
68. Durazzo AE, Machado FS, Ikeoka DT et al (2004) Reduction in cardiovascular events after vascular surgery with atorvastatin: a randomized trial. J Vasc Surg 39:967–975
69. Schouten O, Kertai MD, Bax JJ et al Safety of perioperative statin use in high-risk patients undergoing major vascular surgery. Am J Cardiol 95:658–660
70. Staffa JA, Chang J, Green L (2002) Cerivastatin and reports of fatal rhabdomyolysis. N Engl J Med 346:539–540
71. Shepherd J, Hunninghake DB, Stein EA et al (2004) Safety of rosuvastatin. Am J Cardiol 94:882–888
72. Heeschen C, Hamm CW, Laufs U et al Withdrawal of statins increases event rates in patients with acute coronary syndromes. Circulation 2002;105:1446–52
73. Chan AW, Bhatt DL, Chew DP et al (2002) Early and sustained survival benefit associated with statin therapy at the time of percutaneous coronary intervention. Circulation 105:691–696
74. Mangano DT (2002) Aspirin and mortality from coronary bypass surgery. N Engl J Med 347:1309–1317
75. Lim E, Ali Z, Ali A et al (2003) Indirect comparison meta-analysis of aspirin therapy after coronary surgery. BMJ 327:1309
76. Rodgers A et al (2000) The Pulmonary Embolism Prevention (PEP) Trial Collaborative Group. Prevention of pulmonary embolism and deep vein thrombosis with low dose aspirin: Pulmonary Embolism Prevention (PEP) trial. Lancet 355: 1295–1302

4 Hypertensive Urgencies and Emergencies

J. L. Atlee

Hypertension: Perspectives and Definitions

Perspectives

As persons age, their life styles change, and they become more affluent and obese. If this trend continues, the incidence of associated hypertension (HTN) will continue to increase worldwide [1]. At the same time, despite widely recognized dangers of uncontrolled HTN, it is still under-treated in most patients. Such inadequate HTN control is seen not only in closely followed populations, but also in closely monitored anti-HTN drug trials [1]. Moreover, cardiovascular risk remains high in the majority of people with HTN, whether they are treated or not.

HTN control is elusive for the first 15–20 years after its onset, mainly due to its asymptomatic nature, even as it progressively damages the cardiovascular system and vital end organs [1]. In addition, affected but still asymptomatic patients, especially with early HTN, may be unwilling to alter their life styles or to take medications to forestall some danger perceived as "remote" (stroke, heart or renal failure, etc.), especially given the adverse side effects of many drugs used to treat HTN.

Definition

Blood pressure (BP) is distributed as a bell-shaped curve within the population as a whole. As observed in the 22-year follow-up of around 350 000 men

Department of Anesthesiology, Medical College of Wisconsin, Milwaukee, WI 53226, USA

screened for the Multiple Risk Factor Intervention Trial (MRFIT), the long-term risks for cardiovascular mortality associated with various levels of BP rose progressively over the entire range of BP, with no threshold that clearly identified a potential danger [2]. Thus, the definition of HTN is somewhat arbitrary, and usually is taken as that level of BP that doubles long-term risk for related adverse cardiovascular events [1]. Still, as Kaplan remarks, "perhaps the best operational definition for HTN is the level at which the benefits (minus the risks and costs) of action exceed the risks and costs (minus the benefits) of inaction".

For individuals, HTN is diagnosed if most BP readings are at a level known to be associated with significantly higher cardiovascular risk without therapy. Recommendations of the Sixth Joint National Committee (JNC-6) are shown in Table 1 [3]. Thus, when a person's consecutive BP readings (≥ 2 separate visits/occasions after their first visit/occasion) are in a high-normal range, that person has a significant increased risk of cardiovascular events over time (approx. 9% at 12 years) [1]. For persons with optimal or normal BP readings, the 12-year risk for cardiovascular events is approx. 1% or 4%, respectively. In view of this heightened risk, the JNC-7 report defines BP levels above 120/80 mmHg to as high as 140/90 mmHg as "prehypertension" [4].

Table 1. JNC-6 classification of blood pressure for adults aged 18 years and older

Category	**Blood pressure (mmHg)** **Systolic**		**Diastolic**
Optimal[a]	< 120	and	< 80
Normal	< 130	and	< 85
High-normal	130–139	or	85–89
Hypertension[b]			
Stage 1	140–159	or	90–99
Stage 2	160–179	or	100–109
Stage 3	≥ 180	or	≥ 110

Adapted from [3]. These definitions apply to individuals not taking anti-HTN drugs or who are acutely ill. If repeated blood pressure (BP) readings fall into different categories, the higher category is used to classify an individual's BP status

[a] Optimal BP with respect to cardiovascular risk. However, unusually low BP readings should be evaluated for clinical significance

[b] Based on the average of at least two readings taken on each of at least two visits after initial screening

Primary vs. Secondary Hypertension

Once HTN is recognized, it is helpful to know if some identifiable or secondary process–possibly, curable by surgery (e.g., pheochromocytoma), or more easily controlled with specific drugs–may be present [1]. Studies for the causes of HTN (primary vs. secondary) in increasingly suspect populations, including those resistant to conventional therapy and referred to specialists for evaluation of causes, find that in around 90% of cases HTN is primary (i.e., essential or idiopathic, with no identifiable cause). Renal parenchymal disease is the most common secondary cause, followed by renovascular disease or various adrenal disorders. Other causes of HTN are often overlooked (but, nonetheless, suspect), and include medications that patients may be taking, and "alternative" medications or herbals [5].

Complications of Hypertension

The higher the risk of complications with HTN, the more likely it is that cardiovascular diseases will develop prematurely due to acceleration of atherosclerosis [1]. Atherosclerosis progression is the pathologic hallmark of uncontrolled HTN. Unless treated, about one-half of patients with HTN die from coronary heart disease or congestive heart failure (CHF), another one-third from stroke, and the rest from renal failure. Those with rapidly accelerating HTN die more often from renal failure (especially diabetics), once proteinuria or other evidence of nephropathy develops. Finally, the biological aggressiveness of any degree of HTN varies among persons. Its propensity to cause vascular damage is best assessed by examination of the eyes, heart and kidneys [1].

- *Fundoscopic examination.* Ocular fundoscopic changes reflect retinopathy with HTN and atherosclerosis. First, these cause arteriolar narrowing (*grade 1*); then, adventitial sclerosis and/or thickening of the arteriolar wall–arteriovenous "nicking" (*grade 2*). Progressive HTN leads to small vessel rupture with hemorrhages and exudates (*grade 3*); and, ultimately, to papilledema (*grade 4*). Grade 3 and 4 changes are indicative of accelerated ("malignant") HTN, while grade 1 or 2 changes have been correlated with increased risk of coronary heart disease [6].
- *Cardiac involvement.* HTN increases left ventricular (LV) wall tension, which leads to increased LV wall stiffness and hypertrophy (LVH). It also accelerates the development of coronary atherosclerosis. If coronary atherosclerosis develops in patients with increased LV wall tension, combined increased myocardial O_2 demand and lower supply increases the risk for myocardial ischemia.

- *Abnormalities of LV function.* Yet, before LVH occurs, there may be altered *systolic function,* manifest as subnormal LV midwall fractional shortening [7]. This suggests a reduced LV functional reserve in patients with asymptomatic HTN, and may also help to identify those with extracardiac target-organ damage. Altered LV *diastolic function* may be predictive as well [1]. For example, normotensive offspring of young men at moderate genetic risk of HTN (vs. matched offspring of normotensive parents) had Doppler echocardiographic evidence of LV diastolic dysfunction before that of systolic dysfunction (i.e., lower E/A ratios and longer isovolemic relaxation times) [8].
- *LV hypertrophy.* LVH with increased afterload with high systemic vascular resistance is necessary and protective to a point [1]. However, in hypertensives, any deviation in LV mass from compensatory values for increased cardiac workload reduces coronary vasodilator capacity and LV wall mechanics, and leads to abnormal LV diastolic filling patterns [9]. Also, while LVH is identified by electrocardiography (ECG) in 5–10% of hypertensives, it is identified by echocardiography in around 30% of *unselected* hypertensive adults, but in up to 90% of persons with severe HTN [10]. Also, patterns of LVH differ according to the type of hemodynamic load [1]. Volume overload causes *eccentric* hypertrophy, while pressure overload causes increased LV wall thickness (without increased LV volume)–or *concentric* hypertrophy. In addition, the pattern of LVH is modified by increased arterial stiffness, pulse wave velocity, and blood viscosity. Thus, the presence of LVH may connote many deleterious effects of HTN on cardiac function [1]. This has led to efforts to show that treatment for HTN causes LVH to regress, and in fact all anti-HTN drugs, except those that increase sympathetic activity (e.g., direct vasodilators such as hydralazine–alone), do cause LVH regression [1]. With LVH regression, LV function often improves and cardiovascular morbidity declines [11].
- *Congestive heart failure.* Various alterations of systolic and diastolic LV function with HTN may lead to CHF. Most CHF in HTN is due to systolic dysfunction, manifest by a reduced ejection fraction. Still, about 40% of CHF episodes are *associated* with diastolic dysfunction, irrespective of LV systolic function. Regardless, in the Framingham study, a 20-mmHg increment in systolic BP conferred a 56% increased risk of CHF [12]. Thus, HTN is still a major preventable factor in CHF, the leading cause of hospitalization in the US for people aged 65 years or over [1]. In addition, while anti-HTN treatment does not fully prevent CHF, it probably postpones the development of CHF for several decades.

- *Coronary heart disease.* HTN is a known major risk factor for myocardial ischemia and infarction (MI). Moreover, the prevalence of "silent" MI is significantly increased in patients with HTN [13], and such patients are at higher risk of death after their first infarction [14]. Thus, HTN may play an even greater role in the pathogenesis of coronary heart disease than is commonly recognized, since preexistent HTN may go unrecognized in patients first seen after an MI [1]. How so? While an acute rise in BP may occur with ischemic pain, it will decline shortly thereafter if cardiac pump function is significantly impaired. Also, once an MI has occurred, the patient's prognosis is affected by both the preexisting and subsequent changes in BP.
- *Renal dysfunction.* Undetected, subtle renal dysfunction may underlie many cases of primary ("essential") HTN [1]. Increased renal retention of salt and water may even be the mechanism initiating it, but is so small that it escapes detection. However, detailed study reveals structural damage and functional derangements reflecting intraglomerular HTN (i.e., microalbuminuria) in most hypertensive persons. Microalbuminuria in patients with HTN correlates with LVH and carotid artery thickness.[1] As HTN-nephrosclerosis proceeds, plasma creatinine begins to rise, and ultimately renal insufficiency develops. Yet, despite epidemiological evidence for an association between HTN and renal disease, some question it [1]. Instead, they postulate that any renal damage in HTN is more often due to underlying renal disease, which is merely aggravated by the presence of HTN.
- *Cerebral involvement.* HTN, especially if systolic, is a major risk factor for ischemic stroke and intracerebral hemorrhage (ICH). BP often rises during acute stroke or ICH (i.e., during the first 24 h). However, BP must not be lowered too rapidly [1]. Why? Cerebral white matter lesions are common, and identified by brain magnetic resonance imaging in 41% of untreated, middle-aged asymptomatic persons with essential HTN [15]. Also, brain atrophy is more common after age 67 years in patients with HTN vs. normotensives [16]. Lastly, evidence supports the idea that HTN (especially, high diastolic BP) in late midlife leads to decline in the spatial performance of cognitive functions [17].

---

[1] The reference cited by Kaplan [1]; namely, Leoncini G, Sacchi G, Ravera M, et al (2002) Microalbuminuria is an integrated marker of subclinical organ damage in primary hypertension. J Hum Hypertens 16:399-404

Hypertensive Crises: Urgencies and Emergencies

Definitions

HTN crises require a severe (≥ stage 2 increase in BP; Table 1) *acute* elevation of BP [3], and are further subdivided by JNC-7 into HTN *urgencies* and *emergencies* [4]. With the former, the BP increase is subacute or chronic, but without evidence of end-organ damage. With the latter, the BP increase is acute, with evidence of end-organ damage. Also, with emergencies, an immediate reduction in BP (≤ 1 h) is needed [1, 4]. With HTN urgencies, BP reduction may take hours to days. "True" HTN emergencies are listed in Table 2 [1, 18].

Table 2. Clinical circumstances that represent "true" hypertensive emergencies, and thus demand an immediate reduction in BP over a time period of within 1 h

Ophthalmologic findings with *uncontrolled* HTN:
- Accelerated malignant HTN with papilledema

Cardiovascular conditions or findings with *uncontrolled* HTN:
- Acute aortic dissection
- Acute left ventricular failure
- Acute or impending myocardial infarction (e.g., unstable angina)
- Following coronary artery bypass or other cardiac surgery
- Following percutaneous coronary angioplasty/intervention (e.g., stent placement)

Cerebrovascular findings with *uncontrolled* HTN:
- HTN encephalopathy
- Intracranial hemorrhage–e.g., aneurysm rupture with uncontrolled bleeding
- Subarachnoid hemorrhage–e.g., traumatic or spontaneous cerebrovascular rupture in patients with severe (stage 2[a]) HTN
- Stroke (brain infarction) with severe (stage 2[a]) HTN

Eclampsia of pregnancy with *uncontrolled* HTN:
- Pregnancy-associated, stage 2[a] HTN with target (end) organ dysfunction

Excessive circulating catecholamines in *uncontrolled* HTN:
- Pheochromocytoma with stage 2[a] HTN and target (end) organ dysfunction
- Food/drug interactions with monoamine oxidase inhibitors → stage 2[a] HTN
- Sympathomimetic drug abuse (e.g., amphetamines, cocaine, methylphenidate)[b]
- Relative overdose with some herbals (e.g., ephedra, capsicum, ginseng, goldenseal, licorice)[c]
- Rebound HTN after sudden withdrawal of an anti-HTN drug

Renovascular changes with *uncontrolled* HTN:
- Acute glomerulonephritis
- Renal crises from collagen-vascular diseases
- Severe (stage 2[a]) HTN after renal transplantation

continue →

Table 2 *continue*

Surgery-associated *uncontrolled* HTN:
- Severe (stage 2[a]) HTN in patients requiring emergency surgery
- Severe (stage 2[a]) postoperative HTN *despite* adequate pain relief and sedation
- Postoperative bleeding from vascular suture lines with severe (stage 2[a]) HTN

Miscellaneous conditions associated with *uncontrolled* stage 2[a] HTN:
- Severe epistaxis
- Severe thermal injury
- Thrombotic thrombocytopenic purpura

[a] As defined in Table 1
[b] More probable in patients with unrecognized or poorly controlled essential HTN
[c] See the following websites: for research publication summaries http://herbmed.org; for fact sheets, consensus reports, and databases http://nccam.nih.gov; for abstracts of the peer-reviewed literature www.ods.od.nih.gov. Adapted from [1], p. 983

Incidence and Causes

Fewer than 1% of patients with primary HTN progress to an accelerated, malignant phase [1]. The incidence is falling due to more widespread HTN treatment. Any HTN condition can initiate a crisis. Some, including pheochromocytoma and renovascular HTN, do so at a higher rate than seen with primary HTN. However, since HTN is of unknown cause in more than 90% of all patients, most HTN crises appear in the setting of preexisting primary HTN.

Pathophysiology

When BP rises and remains above a critical level, various processes set off a series of local and systemic effects to cause further rises in BP and vascular damage that lead to accelerated malignant HTN (i.e., that associated with target end-organ damage, often manifest as encephalopathy [1]. Investigations in animals and humans (by Strandgaard and Paulsen [19]) have elucidated the mechanism for HTN-induced encephalopathy. First, they measured the caliber of cortical pial arterioles in cats, with BP varied over a wide range by vasodilator and angiotensin II infusions. As the BP declined, the arterioles dilated. As it rose, they constricted. Thus, cerebral blood flow (CBF) remained constant (was autoregulated) over a wide range of mean arterial BP (MAP). Autoregulation depends on cerebral sympathetic tone. However, if MAP rose above 180 mmHg, the tightly constricted pial arterioles no longer withstood the pressure, and suddenly dilated irregularly–first in areas with less muscle tone, then diffusely, causing generalized vasodilation. This "breakthrough" in CBF hyperperfused the brain under high pressure, leading to leakage of fluid into perivascular tissue, cerebral edema, and hypertensive encephalopathy. In humans, CBF was measured with an isotope technique, while BP was reduced or increased with vasodilators or vasoconstrictors. Curves of CBF as a function of MAP showed autoregulation over MAP of 60–120 mmHg (normotensives), and from about 110–180 mmHg in patients with HTN. The latter rightward shift in patients with HTN was attributed to structural thickening of the arterioles as an adaptation to chronically elevated BP. If BP was raised beyond the upper limit of autoregulation, the same "breakthrough" in CBF occurred as in cats. However, in normotensive persons, whose vessels had not been altered by prior exposure to high BP, "breakthrough" occurred at a MAP of about 120 mmHg.

Thus, acute HTN encephalopathy may be due to failure of autoregulatory vasoconstriction, with focal or generalized dilatation of small cerebral arteries and arterioles [1]. This is associated with a high CBF, dysfunction of the blood–brain barrier, and the formation of brain edema, which is thought to cause the clinical symptoms with acute hypertensive encephalopathy.

The above studies also confirm clinical observations [1]. In previously normotensive persons, severe encephalopathy occurs with relatively little HTN. In woman with eclampsia of pregnancy and in children with acute glomerulonephritis, convulsions may occur with BP as low as 150/100 mmHg. Yet, patients with chronic HTN withstand such pressures without difficulty. If their BP increases significantly, however, signs of encephalopathy can develop even in these patients.

Manifestations and Course

The symptoms and signs of HTN crises are usually dramatic (Table 3) [1], probably reflecting acute damage to endothelium and platelet activation [20]. Yet, some patients may be relatively asymptomatic despite markedly high BP and extensive end-organ damage. Young black men are especially prone to HTN crises with severe renal insufficiency but little obvious prior distress. Even in the elderly, HTN can initially present as an accelerated malignant phase. Left untreated, patients die quickly of brain damage or more gradually from renal damage. Before effective therapy was available, fewer than 25% of patients with malignant HTN survived 1 year, and only 1% survived 5 years [1]. With therapy, including renal dialysis, ≥ 90% survive 1 year and around 80% survive 5 years.

Table 3. Symptoms and signs of hypertensive crises

Blood pressure: Systolic blood pressure usually > 140 mmHg
Fundoscopy: hemorrhages, exudates, papilledema
Neurologic status: headache, confusion, somnolence, stupor, visual loss, focal deficits, seizures, coma
Cardiac status: prominent apical impulse, cardiac enlargement, congestive heart failure, ECG evidence for left ventricular strain or hypertrophy
Renal findings: oliguria, azotemia
Gastrointestinal: nausea, vomiting

Adapted from [1], p. 984

Differential Diagnosis

The presence of HTN encephalopathy or accelerated malignant HTN demands immediate, aggressive therapy to lower BP effectively, often before the specific cause is known [1]. However certain serious diseases, as well as psychogenic problems, can mimic a HTN crisis (Table 4). Management of these conditions usually demands different diagnostic and therapeutic approaches. In particular, BP should not be lowered to abruptly in a patient with a stroke. Specific therapy for a hypertensive crisis is described below.

Table 4. Serious disease and psychogenic problems that can mimic a hypertensive crisis

Acute left ventricular failure
Uremia from any cause, especially from volume overload
Cerebrovascular accident; subarachnoid hemorrhage; brain tumor; head injury
Epilepsy (postictal states); encephalitis
Collagen diseases; especially, lupus erythematosus with cerebral vasculitis
Sympathomimetics: vasopressor overdose; cocaine; amphetamines; some herbals or alternative medicines (see Table 4–2)
Hypercalcemia
Acute anxiety (panic states) with hyperventilation syndrome

Adapted from [1], p. 984

Therapy: Perioperative Settings

When diastolic BP exceeds 140 mm Hg, rapidly progressive damage to the arterial vasculature is demonstrable experimentally, and a surge of CBF may rapidly lead to cerebral encephalopathy [21]. If such high pressures persist or if there are any signs of encephalopathy, the pressure should be lowered using parenteral agents in patients considered to be in immediate danger or oral agents in those who are alert and in no other acute distress [21]. Parenteral anti-HTN drugs are also indicated for perioperative management of true HTN emergencies (Table 2). Recall that HTN emergencies require a stage 2 elevation in systolic BP (160–179 mmHg) and diastolic BP (100–110 mmHg), *associated with* evidence of end-organ damage.

Parenteral drugs used for BP control in HTN emergencies are listed in Table 5 [21-29]. They "target" one or more of the various components that constitute BP:

BP = (SV x HR) x SVR,

where

BP is blood pressure, SV is stroke volume, HR is heart rate, and SVR is systemic vascular resistance.

The product of SV and HR is cardiac output. All parenteral drugs used in HTN emergencies "attack" one or more of these BP components. However, many have shortcomings (Table 5). What, then, would be an "ideal" drug?

- It should have a rapid onset and offset of action.
- Its dose–response relationship should be predictable (little or no cumulative effect).
- It should be easily titrated to the desired amount of BP reduction.
- It should have high efficacy and safety (i.e., minimal or no adverse effects).
- It must not increase intracranial pressure or cause coronary steal.
- There should be an easy transition to oral anti-HTN therapy.

To this the author would add: the "ideal" anti-HTN drug should have little (or, better, "no") effect on "preload," the major determinant of which is venous return. Thus, the "ideal" anti-HTN drug should have no or little effect on venous capacitance (i.e., not be a venodilator). Why?

Patients with HTN are "preload-restricted" (venoconstricted), a compensatory mechanism that helps protect vital organ systems from the chronic adverse effects of HTN. Thus, drugs that are venodilators (e.g., nitroglycerin, sodium nitroprusside) have the potential to do more harm than good. Moreover, SNP is also an equipotent arterial dilator, so it may be difficult to control the amount of BP reduction with sodium nitroprusside: there may be untoward hypotension. Also, an "ideal" anti-HTN drug should be compatible with β-blockers (e.g., esmolol) to control any reflex-mediated increase in

Table 5. Parenteral antihypertensive agents that are commonly used in the treatment of perioperative hypertensive emergencies[a]

Drugs	Dose (onset of action)	Action	Comments
Antiadrenergic			
Esmolol	B: 0.5–1.0 mg/kg (1–2 min) I: 100–300 μg/min (5 min)	Cardioselective β_1-blocker	Hydrolyzed by plasma esterases ($T_{1/2e}$ 9-10 min)
Labetalol	B: 5–12 mg; repeat q. 10–15 min as needed (1–3 min)	Nonselective $\beta_{1,2}$-blocker and competitive α_1-blocker	Titrate to desired heart rate and BP
Metoprolol	B: 2.5–5 mg IV q. 2–5min up to 15 mg (1–3 min)	Cardioselective β_1-blocker	Approved for treating angina and only IV β-blocker approved for use in acute MI
Phentolamine	B: 1–5 mg IM or slowly IV; repeat p.r.n. x 2 (≤ 5 min)	Competitive α_1- and α_2-blocker	Primarily used for short-term HTN control with pheochromocytoma
Diuretics			
Furosemide	B: 20–40 mg over 1–2 min (5–15 min)	Loop diuretic	Volume depletion; potential for hypokalemia
Vasodilators			
Nitroprusside ing;	0.25–10 μg/kg per minute as IV	Direct vascular smooth muscle	Nausea, vomiting, muscle twitching, sweat-
	infusion (immediate)	vasodilator via endogenous	thiocyanate and cyanide toxicity with pro-
longed		NO release	infusions; harbinger of this is tachyphylaxis; protect infusions against light

continue →

Table 5 *continue*

Drugs	Dose (onset of action)	Action	Comments
Nitroglycerine	5–100 μg/min as IV infusion (2–5 min)	Direct venodilator; little effect on arterial bed except at very high doses; dilates epicardial coronary arteries	Methemoglobinuria; headache; vomiting; tolerance with prolonged use
Fenoldopam	0.1–0.6 μg/kg per minute as IV infusion (immediate)	DA_1-receptor agonist	Reflex tachycardia; increased intraocular pressure; headache; recently shown *not* to protect against radiocontrast nephropathy
Nicardipine[b]	B: 1–3 mg IV push (1 min)[c] I: 5–15 mg/h IV (5–10 min)	DHP CCB; arterioselective	eadache; nausea; flushing; tachycardia; local Hphlebitis–give in large peripheral or central vein; reflex tachycardia
Hydralazine	10–20 mg IV (10–20 min) 10–50 mg IM (20–30 min)	Arterioselective dilator; doesn't dilate epicardial coronary arteries	May cause coronary steal: arteriolar dilation ca steel blood away from maximally dilated ischemic region and worsened angina; flushing; headache
Enalaprilat	1.25–5 mg IV q. 6 h (15–30 min)	Angiotensin converting enzyme inhibitor	Precipitous decline in BP in high renin states; long duration of action ($T_{1/2e}$) 11 h; response variable; appears most useful CHF with RAAS activation; avoid in acuteMI; potentially fatal angioedema

continue →

Table 5 *continue*

B, intravenous bolus; BP, blood pressure; IV, intravenous; IM, intramuscular; I, IV infusion; q., every; p.r.n., if necessary; 5-HT, 5-hydroxytryptamine (serotonin); DA_1, dopamine receptor type 1; DHP CCB, dihydropyridine calcium channel blocker; CHF, congestive heart failure; MI, myocardial infarction; RAAS, renin–angiotensin–aldosterone system

[a] These doses may be lower than those used outside of perioperative settings given the effects of anesthetics, sedative-hypnotics, analgesics, central neuraxial blockade, and other drugs with important circulatory effects that my augment those of drugs used to control BP

[b] Intravenous formulations of other dihydropyridine calcium channel blockers are available

[c] Not labeled for intravenous bolus use

Sources: [21, 23–29]

heart rate as BP declines. Finally, it should not cause coronary or cerebral steal, and should have little effect on hepatic or renal function.

References

1. Kaplan NM (2005) Systemic hypertension: mechanisms and diagnosis. In: Zipes DP, Libby P, Bonow RO, Braunwald E (eds) Braunwald's heart disease, 7th edn. Elsevier Saunders, Philadelphia, pp 959–87
2. Domanski M, Mitchell G. Pferffer F, et al (2002) Pulse pressure and cardiovascular disease-related mortality: follow-up study of the Multiple Risk Factor Intervention Trial (MRFIT). JAMA 287:2677–83
3. Joint National Committee (1997) The sixth report of the Joint National Committee on Prevention, Detection, Evaluation, and Treatment of high blood pressure. Arch Intern Med 157:2413–46
4. Joint National Committee (2003) The seventh report of the Joint National Committee on Prevention, Detection, Evaluation, and Trcatmcnt of High Blood Pressure. The JNC 7 Report. JAMA 289:2560–72
5. Zainer CM (2007) Herbals and alternative medicine. In: Atlee JL (ed) Complications in anesthesia, 2nd edition. Elsevier Saunders, Philadelphia, pp 150–8
6. Wong TY, Klein R, Sharrett AR, et al (2002) Retinal arteriolar narrowing and risk of coronary heart disease in men and women: the Atherosclerosis Risk in Communities Study. JAMA 287:1153–9
7. Schussheim AE, Devere RB, de Simone G (1997) Usefulness of subnormal midwall fractional shortening in predicting left ventricular exercise dysfunction in asymptomatic patients with systemic hypertension. Am J Cardiol 79:1070–4
8. Aeschbacher BC, Hutter D, Fuhrer H, et al (2001) Diastolic dysfunction precedes myocardial hypertrophy in the development of hypertension. Am J Hypertens 14:106–13
9. Kozakova M, de Simone G, Morizzo C, Palombo C (2003) Coronary vasodilator capacity and hypertension-induced increase in left ventricular mass. Hypertension 41:224–9
10. Schmieder RE, Messerli FH (2000) Hypertension and the heart. J Hum Hypertens 14:597–604
11. Verdecchia P, Schillaci G, Borgioni C, et al (1998) Prognostic significance of serial changes in left ventricular mass in essential hypertension. Circulation 97:48–54
12. Haider AW, Larson MG, Franklin SS, Levy D (2003) Systolic blood pressure, diastolic blood pressure, and pulse pressure as predictors of risk for congestive heart failure in the Framingham Heart Study. Ann Intern Med 138:10–6
13. Boon D, Piek JJ, van Montfrans GA (2000) Silent ischaemia and hypertension. J Hypertens 18:1355–64
14. Haider AW, Chen L, Larson MG, et al (1997) Antecedent hypertension confers increased risk for adverse outcomes after initial myocardial infarction. Hypertension 30:1020–4
15. Sierra C, de La Sierra A, Mercader J, et al (2002) Silent cerebral white matter lesions in middle-aged essential hypertensive patients. J Hypertens 20:387–9
16. Goldstein IB, Bartzokis G, Guthrie D, Shapiro D (2002) Ambulatory blood pressure and brain atrophy in the healthy elderly. Neurology 59:713–9
17. Reinprecht F, Elmstahl S, Janzon L, Andre-Petersson L (2003] Hypertension and

changes of cognitive function in 81-year-old men: a 13-year follow-up of the population study "Men born in 1914", Sweden. J Hypertens 21:57–66
18. Mansoor GA, Frishman WH (2002) Comprehensive management of hypertensive emergencies and urgencies. Heart Dis 4:358–71
19. Strandgaard S, Paulsen OB (1989) Cerebral blood flow and its pathophysiology in hypertension. Am J Hypertens 2:486–92
20. Preston RA, Jy W, Jinenez JJ, et al (2003) Effects of severe hypertension on endothelial and platelet microparticles. Hypertension 41:211–7
21. Kaplan NM (2005) Systemic hypertension: therapy. In: Zipes DP, Libby P, Bonow RO, Braunwald E (eds) Braunwald's heart disease, 7th edn. Elsevier Saunders, Philadelphia, pp 989–1010
22. Lee TH (2005) Systemic hypertension: guidelines. In: Zipes DP, Libby P, Bonow RO, Braunwald E (eds) Braunwald's heart disease, 7th edn. Elsevier Saunders, Philadelphia, pp 1010–12
23. Moss J, Glick D (2005) The autonomic nervous system. In: Miller RD (ed) Miller's anesthesia, 6th edn. Elsevier Churchill Livingstone, Philadelphia, pp 617–77
24. Hoffman B (2001) Catecholamines, sympathomimetc drugs, and adrenergic receptor antagonists. In: Hardman JG, Limbird LE (eds) Goodman & Gilman's The pharmacological basis of therapeutics, 10th edn. McGraw-Hill, New York, pp 215–68
25. Saunders-Bush E, Mayer SE (2001) 5-Hydroxytryptamine (serotonin): receptor agonists and antagonists. In: Hardman JG, Limbird LE (eds) Goodman & Gilman's The pharmacological basis of therapeutics, 10th edn. McGraw-Hill, New York, pp 269–90
26. Jackson (2001) Diuretics. In, Hardman JG, Limbird LE (2001) Goodman & Gilman's The Pharmacological Basis of Therapeutics, 10th edition. New York, McGraw-Hill, pp 757–87
27. Kerins DM, Robertson RM, Robertson D (2001) Drugs used for treatment of myocardial ischemia. In: Hardman JG, Limbird LE (eds) Goodman & Gilman's The pharmacological basis of therapeutics, 10th edn. McGraw-Hill, New York, pp 843–70
28. Oates LA, Brown NJ (2001) Antihypertensive agents and the drug therapy of hypertension. In: Hardman JG, Limbird LE (eds) Goodman & Gilman's The pharmacological basis of therapeutics, 10th edn. McGraw-Hill, New York, pp 871–900
29. Stone GW, McCullough PA, Tumlin JA, et al (2003) Fenoldopam mesylate for the prevention of contrast-induced nephropathy: a randomized controlled trial. JAMA 290:2284–91

5 Heart Failure, Atrial Fibrillation, and Diabetes Mellitus

A. Aleksova, A. Perkan and G.Sinagra

Diabetes mellitus is a common disease. The worldwide prevalence of diabetes–especially of the predominant type 2 diabetes mellitus which accounts for about 90% of the adult diabetic population–has increased rapidly and continuously during the last several decades. This phenomenon is a direct consequence of negative lifestyle changes in the population, including a reduction of physical activity and the availability of energy-dense food rich in saturated fat, leading to an increased prevalence of obesity. The global prevalence of diabetes mellitus in adults is predicted to increase to 5.4% in the year 2025 [1].

The highest incidence of adult-onset diabetes is to be expected in age groups over 65 years in the developed countries. In the developing countries, the majority of affected individuals are predicted to be among the middle-aged population of 40–65 years [2]. Type 2 diabetes is commonly associated with a whole range of cardiovascular risk factors, such as hypertension, atherogenic dyslipidemia, abdominal obesity, and a procoagulatory state, including platelet dysfunction, impaired fibrinolytic activity, and increased fibrinogen serum concentrations [2–4].

Epidemiology of Heart Failure in Patients with Diabetes Mellitus

Epidemiological evidence in the community shows the prevalence of left ventricular systolic dysfunction in diabetic patients to be twice as high as in nondiabetic patients, with half of the cases being asymptomatic. Diastolic

Cardiovascular Department, "Ospedali Riuniti" and University of Trieste, Trieste, Italy

dysfunction is even more frequent in comparison with nondiabetic persons. This high prevalence has been explained by the frequent coexistence of underlying diabetic cardiomyopathy, hypertension, and ischemic heart disease. In these patients, the diabetic metabolic derangement, together with early activation of the sympathetic nervous system leads to a reduction in myocardial function. Activation of the renin–angiotensin system may also contribute to unfavorable cardiac remodeling. The progression from myocardial damage to overt dysfunction and heart failure is often asymptomatic chronic and frequently undiagnosed and untreated.

The Framingham Study was the first epidemiological study to demonstrate an increased risk for congestive heart failure in patients with diabetes mellitus. Compared with nondiabetic men and women, the estimated increase in the incidences of heart failure for young diabetic men and women were fourfold and eightfold, respectively [3].

A recent Italian cross-sectional study showed a 30% prevalence of diabetes in an elderly population with heart failure. The association with diabetes was independent of age, sex, blood pressure, body mass index, or waist/hip ratio, and also of a family history of diabetes. The incidence of diabetes was 29% during three years of follow-up among heart failure patients initially without this diagnosis, compared with an 18% incidence in a group of matched controls. On the basis of multivariate statistics, congestive heart failure independently predicted the later development of type 2 diabetes. One possible explanation is that increased adrenergic tone associated with heart failure, increases free fatty acid oxidation and insulin resistance, thereby reducing glucose oxidation and precipitating type 2 diabetes [5].

Prevalence of Atrial Fibrillation in Patients with Diabetes Mellitus

With an incidence of 3–6% in patients > 60 years of age, and with significant comorbidities and complications, especially, ischemic cerebrovascular "accidents"(e.g., stroke, thromboembolic events), atrial fibrillation (AF) is the most common sustained arrhythmia in elderly patients managed by cardiologists [6] and constitutes a significant public health problem. Patients with diabetes mellitus constitute 10.7% of all those with AF–a considerable subgroup [7]. The coexistence of these two conditions is associated with a 1.7 relative risk increase for ischemic stroke and thromboembolic events, to which diabetic individuals are especially prone due to their impaired platelet function and decreased spontaneous fibrinolytic capability.

Recently, Maggioni et al. [8] conducted a retrospective analysis of the Val-HeFT database in an attempt to identify independent predictors of AF development, as well as to assess the rate of new-onset AF in patients with chronic symptomatic heart failure. During a follow-up of about two years, they observed new-onset AF in 6.5% of patients with chronic heart failure in sinus rhythm at enrolment. Multivariate analysis showed circulating brain natriuretic peptide level, age over 70 years, diabetes, and heart rate as independent predictors of AF development (Table 1). However, treatment with valsartan reduced the incidence of new-onset AF by 37% compared to placebo.

Table 1. Independent predictors of occurrence of atrial fibrillation (AF) in the Val-HeFT trial (multivariate logistic regression model)

	Odds ratio	95% Confidence interval	*P* value
BNP (≥ 97 vs 97 pg/ml)	2.02	1.56–2.6	<0.001
Age (≥ 70 vs < 70 years)	1.36	1.06–1.76	0.01
Diabetes (yes vs no)	1.31	1.01–1.71	0.04
Heart rate (≥ 72 vs < 72 bpm)	0.77	0.61–0.98	0.04

From [8]. BNP, brain natriuretic peptide

Mechanism of Atrial Fibrillation Development in Patients with Diabetes Mellitus and Heart Failure

Chronic heart failure and AF are closely linked. Heart failure is the strongest risk factor for the development of AF, and about 15–30% of patients with heart failure syndrome have a history of or present with AF [8–11]. In patients with severe heart failure the prevalence of AF may be up to 50% [12]. The pathophysiology of AF is linked to the pathophysiology of heart failure in several ways. Left ventricle diastolic dysfunction and systolic dysfunction lead to left atrial dilatation, which may stimulate stretch-activated cardiac ion channels and increase vulnerability to AF. Blockade of these stretch-activated ion channels increases atrial refractoriness and reduces the propensity to AF despite elevated atrial pressure or volume or both [13]. Sustained atrial overload in chronic heart failure causes atrial enlargement that may facilitate the stability and persistence of AF [14]. Diabetic cardiomyopathy is characterized by predominant impairment of diastolic function of the left ventricle. Diastolic dysfunction, leading to elevated filling pressures and atrial remodeling, predisposes to AF development. Almost 10% of patients with abnormal left ventricle diastolic function have new-onset AF during four years of follow-up [15]. The risk of AF is proportional to the severity of left ventricle diastolic dysfunction as defined by echocardiography [abnormal relaxation (hazard ratio, 3.3), pseudonormal relaxation (hazard ratio, 4.8), and restrictive left ventricle diastolic filling (hazard ratio, 5.3)] [15]. In the latter study [15], both left atrial volume and the extent of diastolic dysfunction had independent predictive value. Another important mechanism that contributes to AF development in diabetic patients with chronic heart failure is neurohumoral modulation with elevated concentrations of catecholamine and angiotensin II. Collectively, elevated catecholamines and angiotensin II may promote and produce changes in atrial fibrosis [16, 17], atrial conduction and refractoriness conducive to AF.

Management of Diabetic Patients with Heart Failure and Atrial Fibrillation

Diabetes mellitus is a diagnosis of considerable and ominous importance in cardiovascular medicine, related to significantly higher mortality and morbidity and causing numerous hospital readmissions. Early activation of the sympathetic nervous system induces a decrease of myocardial function and activation of the renin–angiotensin system results in unfavorable cardiac remodeling. The presence of AF in diabetic patients with heart failure may have an additional deleterious effect. The hemodynamic consequences of AF include inappropriate ventricular rate, loss of atrial contraction, and elevated filling pressures causing atrial dilatation and reductions in stroke volume. AF is also associated with increased risk of stroke. Pharmacological interventions, including meticulous metabolic control of the diabetes, decrease mortality and delay the progression of cardiovascular disease in diabetic patients.

Beta-Blockers

β-blockers are effective in improving outcome in diabetic subjects [2, 12, 18], reducing mortality by 30–40% after myocardial infarction and by 25–30% in congestive heart failure. β-blockers are an important component of pharmacological treatment in diabetic patients for rate control in those with AF. Several mechanisms are proposed to explain the positive effects of β-blockers in preventing AF (Table 2). β-blockers modulating fluctuations in autonomic tone could be beneficial in diabetic patients whose sympathetic overactivity plays a role in the genesis of AF. β-blockers can also contribute by improving autonomic dysfunction and redirecting the myocardial metabolism from free fatty acids towards glucose utilization in diabetic patients. Treatment with carvedilol offers additional benefits compared with metoprolol among patients with AF [19]. In one double-blind multicenter study, carvedilol improved diastolic function in patients with symptomatic heart failure and abnormal diastolic function [20]. In another study in patients with mild chronic heart failure, combination therapy with carvedilol and enalapril reversed left ventricular remodeling to a greater extent than did enalapril monotherapy [21].

Table 2. Mechanisms of AF prevention with β-blockers in chronic heart failure

1) Reduces wall stress
   - Improves LV function and attenuates adverse LV remodeling
   - Reduces atrial intracavitary pressure
   - Decreases mitral regurgitation
2) Favorably modifies sympathetic and RAAS tone
3) Prevents of atrial ischemia
4) Reduces atrial fibrosis
5) Effect on P-wave duration and dispersion

LV, left ventricular; mitral regurgitation; RAAS, renin–angiotensin–aldosterone system

It is known that oxidative stress may have an important role in the genesis of AF [22]. Carvedilol with its antioxidant activity may play an important role in attenuating oxygen radical genesis in patients with hypertension and type 2 diabetes mellitus [23], and thus in preventing new-onset AF. Moreover, in a study by Ohtsuka et al. [24], carvedilol but not metoprolol significantly reduced baseline plasma interleukin-6 (IL-6) levels. It is well known that the amount of C-reactive protein, produced in the liver mainly under control IL-6, correlates with the risk of future development of AF, with increase amounts of IL-6 increasing that risk [25]. Despite these observations, many clinicians are still hesitant to prescribe this life-saving therapy, but historic concerns regarding impaired glucose metabolism and worsening of dyslipidemia should not result in withholding of β-blockers. Another concern could be the possibility for β-blockers to mask symptoms of hypoglycemia, but the low incidence of clinically important hypoglycemia in type 2 diabetes and the substantial mortality benefit of this class of drugs make this concern largely academic. Therefore, β-blockers should be used when tolerated, in diabetic patients with AF and heart failure [26].

Angiotensin-Converting Enzyme Inhibitors and Angiotensin Receptor Blockers

Published data suggest the important benefit of angiotensin-converting enzyme (ACE) inhibitors in diabetic patients with acute coronary syndromes

[27]. A retrospective analysis of the GISSI-3 study [28] has suggested that most if not all of the mortality benefit resulting from treatment with lisinopril versus placebo was found in the diabetic subset of patients. This finding was true at six weeks and at six months of follow-up. ACE inhibitors also contribute to the reduction of microvascular complications (combined endpoint: overt nephropathy, dialysis, or laser therapy) by 16% [29] and improving life expectancy in patients with heart failure [12, 29]. Angiotensin II receptor blockers [30, 31] are also effective in reduction of cardiovascular mortality and morbidity in patients with diabetes, hypertension, and left ventricular hypertrophy.

ACE inhibitors and angiotensin-II receptor blockers also appear to be effective in the prevention of AF. Inhibition of ACE or angiotensin-II receptors not only exerts beneficial effects on ventricular remodeling but also reduces atrial fibrosis and remodeling, factors that predispose AF development. Table 3 shows the different mechanisms proposed to explain the effect of these drugs in AF prevention. One recent animal study showed that angiotensin-II receptor blockade prevented the promotion of AF by reducing atrial structural remodeling [32].

Pedersen et al. [33] investigated the effect of trandolapril on the incidence of AF in patients with reduced left ventricular function. Trandolapril reduced the risk of developing AF by 55%. A subanalysis of the SOLVD study reported that new-onset AF was reduced as much as 78% with enalapril [9].

The effectiveness of ACE inhibitors could be based on their favorable effects on cardiovascular fibrosis and apoptosis [34]. The study by

Table 3. Mechanisms of AF prevention with angiotensin-converting enzyme inhibitors or angiotensin-II receptor blockers in chronic heart failure

Decreases wall stress (improves LV function and attenuates LV remodeling; reduces atrial pressures; decreases MR)
Reduces atrial fibrosis
Modulates and decreases inhomogeneities of ERP; restores rate-dependent adaptation of ERP
Affects atrial action potential duration and intra-atrial conduction velocity (microreentry)
Reduces atrial premature beats
Interferes with ion currents
Modifies sympathetic and RAAS tone
Stabilizes electrolyte concentrations (potassium)

ERP, effective refractory period

Nakashima et al. demonstrated for the first time that angiotensin II contributes to atrial electrical remodeling [35]. In their study, the shortening of the atrial refractory period during rapid pacing was prevented by treatment with candcsartan or captopril but increased by angiotensin II. Val-HeFT [8] demonstrated that the angiotensin-II receptor antagonist valsartan can exert a favorable effect in terms of AF prevention. Another angiotensin-II receptor blocker, candesartan, can prevent the promotion of AF by suppressing the development of structural remodeling [36]. One prospective and randomized study showed that irbesartan combined with amiodarone was more effective than amiodarone alone in the maintenance of sinus rhythm in patients with persistent AF after cardioversion to sinus rhythm [37]. Another study has also demonstrated the ability of losartan to regress fibrosis in hypertensives with biopsy-proven myocardial fibrosis, independently of its antihypertensive efficacy, suggesting that blockade of the angiotensin-II type 1 receptor is associated with inhibition of collagen type I synthesis and regression of myocardial fibrosis [38].

In addition, in the LIFE study [39] losartan was superior to atenolol in reducing the rate of new-onset AF, with similar blood pressure reduction.

Statins

Diabetic patients experience benefits from lipid lowering agents, which accounts for an average 25–29% reduction in risk for adverse cardiovascular events [2,40–45].

Metabolic Control

Several epidemiological surveys have reported a correlation between the degree of elevation of fasting plasma glucose and glycosylated hemoglobin (HbA_{1c}) and clinical outcomes in patients with type 2 diabetes [46–51]. Hyperglycemia and increased turnover of free fatty acids, together with a substantial decrease in the rate of glycolysis and increased oxygen demand, lead to the intracellular accumulation of intermediate oxygenation products. Furthermore, hyperglycemia and increased turnover of free fatty acids interfere with ATP-dependent ion-pumps to cause deleterious calcium overload and impaired myocardial contractile function. In addition to promoting arrhythmias, the foregoing adverse effects of hyperglycemia contribute to contractile dysfunction and attenuate the protective effects of myocardial preconditioning [2]. A growing body of evidence indicates that optimal blood glucose control may counteract the deleterious effects of metabolic abnormalities associated with diabetes [2, 52, 53]. The good glycemic control sustained for five years in a group of diabetics with low cardiovascular risk was associated with a clinical reduction in cardiovascular events by 28% for the first event, and 16% for a myocardial infarction, as shown by the UKPDS study [54]. The meticulous glucose control applied in the DIGAMI study in diabetic patients suffering from an acute myocardial infarction resulted in a 29% reduction in total mortality (after both one year and 3.4 years of follow-up) [55, 56]. In addition, rigorous metabolic control by means of intensive insulin treatment is capable of improving left ventricular diastolic function and myocardial microvasculature reserve [57].

Anticoagulant Therapy

Diabetic patients with AF and left ventricular dysfunction are at increased risk of thromboembolism. In the most recent guidelines for the management of patients with AF, all those with AF and diabetes aged 60 years or older are strongly advised to be given oral anticoagulation (with targeted INR values 2.0–3.0). In addition, 80 to 160 mg aspirin are co-administered daily [58].

Conclusions

Diabetes mellitus is a continuously growing health problem leading to a high rate of cardiovascular events including myocardial infarction, vascular disease, heart failure, and arrhythmias. AF is the type of sustained arrhythmia most commonly observed in cardiology, particularly in heart failure patients with diabetes, and constitutes a significant risk for cardiovascular and cerebrovascular complications. Prevention and treatment of AF in diabetic patients should become a major priority today, and in the years to come, to reduce the risk of cardiovascular complications and adverse outcomes in this patient subset.

References

1. King H, Aubert RE, Herman WH (1998) Global burden of diabetes 1995–2025. Prevalence, numerical estimates and projections. Diabetes Care 21:1414–31
2. Rydén L, Malmberg K (2000) Reducing the impact of diabetic heart's increased vulnerability to cardiovascular disease. Dialogues Cardiovasc Med 5:5–22
3. Kannel WB, McGee DL (1979) Diabetes and cardiovascular disease. JAMA 241:2035–8
4. Clark CM, Perry RC (1999) Type 2 diabetes and macrovascular disease. Epidemiology and etiology. Am Heart J 138:330–3

5. Amato L, Paolisso G, Cacciatore F et al, on behalf of the Osservatorio Geriatrico Regione Campania Group (1997) Congestive heart failure predicts the development of non-insulin dependent diabetes mellitus in the elderly. Diabetes Metab 23:213–8
6. Furberg CD, Psaty BM, Manolio TA et al (1994) Prevalence of atrial fibrillation in elderly subjects (the Cardiovascular Health Study). Am J Cardiol 74:236–41
7. Stratton IM, Adler AJ, Neil HA et al (2000) Association of glycemia with macrovascular and microvascular complicatons of type 2 diabetes (UKPDS 35). BMJ 321:405–12
8. Maggioni AP, Latini R, Carson PE et al (2005) Valsartan reduces the incidence of atrial fibrillation in patients with heart failure: results from the Valsartan Heart Failure Trial (Val-HeFT). Am Heart J 149:548–57
9. Vermes E, Tardif JC, Bourassa MG et al (2003) Enalapril decreases the incidence of atrial fibrillation in patients with left ventricular dysfunction. Insight from the Studies Of Left Ventricular Dysfunction (SOLVD) Trials. Circulation 107:2926–31
10. Poole-Wilson PA, Swedberg K, Cleland JGF et al (2003) Comparison of carvedilol and metoprolol on clinical outcomes in patients with chronic heart failure in the Carvedilol Or Metoprolol European Trial (COMET): randomised controlled trial. Lancet 362:7–13
11. Young JB, Dunlap ME, Pfeffer MA et al (2004) Mortality and morbidity reduction with candesartan in patients with chronic heart failure and left ventricular systolic dysfunction: results of the CHARM Low-Left Ventricular Ejection Fraction Trials. Circulation 110:2618–26
12. The CONSENSUS Trial Study Group (1987) Effect of enalapril on mortality in severe congestive heart failure. N Engl J Med 316:1429–35
13. Bode F, Katchman A, Woosley RL et al (2000) Gadolinium decreases stretch-induced vulnerability to atrial fibrillation. Circulation 101: 2200–5
14. Shinagawa K, Shi YF, Tardif JC et al (2002) Dynamic nature of atrial fibrillation substrate during development and reversal of heart failure in dogs. Circulation 105:2672–8
15. Tsang TS, Gersh BJ, Appleton CP et al (2002) Left ventricular diastolic dysfunction as a predictor of the first diagnosed nonvalvular atrial fibrillation in 840 elderly men and women. J Am Coll Cardiol 40:1636–44
16. Li D, Fareh S, Leung TK et al (1999) Promotion of atrial fibrillation by heart failure in dogs: atrial remodeling of a different sort. Circulation 100:87–95
17. Cha YM, Dzeja PP, Shen WK et al (2003) Failing atrial myocardium: energetic deficits accompany structural remodeling and electrical instability. Am J Physiol Heart Circ Physiol 284:H1313–H1320
18. Wood D, De Backer G, Faergeman O et al (1998) Prevention of coronary heart disease in clinical practice. Summary of recommendations of the Second Joint Task Force of European and other Societies on Coronary prevention. Eur Heart J 19:1434–1503
19. Swedberg K, Olsson L, Charlesworth A et al (2005) Prognostic relevance of atrial fibrillation in patients with chronic heart failure on long-term treatment with beta-blockers: results from COMET. Eur Heart J 26:1303–8
20. Bergstrom A, Andersson B, Edner M et al (2001) Carvedilol improves diastolic function in patients with diastolic heart failure [Abstract 3388]. Circulation 104 (Suppl 2):718
21. Remme WJ, Riegger G, Hildebrandt P et al (2004) The benefits of early combination treatment of carvedilol and an ACE-inhibitor in mild heart failure and left

ventricular systolic dysfunction. The carvedilol and ACE-inhibitor remodelling mild heart failure evaluation trial (CARMEN). Cardiovasc Drugs Ther 18:57–66
22. Mihm MJ, Yu F, Carnes CA et al (2001) Impared myofibrillar energetics and oxydative injury during human atrial fibrillation. Circulation 104:174
23. Giugliano D, Acampora R, Marfella R et al (1997) Metabolic and cardiovascular effects of carvedilol and atenolol in non-insulin dependent diabetes mellitus and hypertension: a randomised, control trial. Ann Intern Med 126:955
24. Ohtsuka T, Hamada M, Saeki H et al (2002) Comparison of effects of carvedilol versus metoprolol on cytokine levels in patients with idopathic dilated cardiomyopathy. Am J Cardiol 89:996
25. Aviles RJ, Martin DO, Apperson-Hansen C et al (2003) Inflammation as a risk factor for atrial fibrillation. Circulation 108:3006–10
26. McGuire DK, Granger CB et al (1999) Diabetes and ischemic heart disease. Am Heart J 138:S366–S375
27. Nesto RW, Zarich S (1998) Acute myocardial infarction in diabetes mellitus: lessons learned from ACE inhibition. Circulation 97:12–5
28. Zuanetti G, Latini R, Maggioni AP et al, for the GISSI-3 investigators (1997) Effect of the ACE inhibitor lisinopril on mortality in diabetic patients with acute myocardial infarction: data from the GISSI-3 study. Circulation 96:4239–45
29. Heart Outcomes Prevention Evaluation (HOPE) Study Investigators (2000) Effects of ramipril on cardiovascular and microvascular outcomes in people with diabetes mellitus: results of the HOPE study and MICRO-HOPE substudy. Lancet 355:253–9
30. Lindholm LH, Ibsen H, Dahlöf B et al, for the LIFE study group (2002) Cardiovascular morbidity and mortality in patients with diabetes in the Losartan Intervention For Endpoint reduction in hypertension study (LIFE): a randomised trial against atenolol. Lancet 359:1004–10
31. Dahlöf B, Devereux RB, Kjeldsen SE et al, for the LIFE study group: cardiovascular morbidity and mortality in the Losartan Intervention For Endpoint reduction in hypertension study (LIFE) (2002): a randomised trial against atenolol. Lancet 359:995–1003
32. Kumagai K, Nakashima H, Urata H et al (2003) Effects of angiotensin II type 1 receptor antagonist on electrical and structural remodeling in atrial fibrillation. J Am Coll Cardiol 41:2197–204
33. Pedersen OD, Bagger H, Køber L et al (1999) Trandolapril reduces the incidence of atrial fibrillation after acute myocardial infarction in patients with left ventricular dysfunction. Circulation 100:376–80
34. Fortuno MA, Ravassa S, Etayo JC et al (1998) Overexpression of Bax protein and enhanced apoptosis in the left ventricle of spontaneously hypertensive rats. Effects of AT1 blockade with losartan. Hypertension 32:280–6
35. Nakashima H, Kumagai K, Urata H et al (2000) Angiotensin II antagonist prevents electrical remodeling in atrial fibrillation. Circulation 101: 2612–7
36. Kumagai K, Nakashima H et al (2003) Effects of angiotensin II type 1 receptor antagonist on electrical and structural remodeling in atrial fibrillation J Am Coll Cardiol 41:2197
37. Madrid AH, Bueno MG, Rebollo JM et al (2002) Use of irbesartan to maintain sinus rhythm in patients with long-lasting persistent atrial fibrillation. A prospective and randomized study. Circulation 106:331–6
38. Lopez B, Querejeta R, Varo N, Gonzalez A et al (2001) Usefulness of serum carboxy-terminal propeptide of procollagen type I in assessment of the cardioreparative ability of antihypertensive treatment in hypertensive patients. Circulation 104:286–91

39. Wachtell K, Lehto M, Gerdts E et al (2005) Angiotensin II receptor blockade reduces new-onset atrial fibrillation and subsequent stroke compared to atenolol: the Losartan Intervention for End Point Reduction in Hypertension (LIFE) study. J Am Coll Cardiol 45:712–9
40. Hansson L, Zanchetti A, Carruthers SG et al (1998) Effects of intensive blood-pressure lowering and low-dose aspirin in patients with hypertension: principial results of the Hypertension Optimal Treatment (HOT) randomised trial. HOT Study Group. Lancet 351:1755–62
41. Opie L (2000) What is the most effective management of hypertension in diabetes? Dialogues Cardiovasc Med 5:23–9
42. Syvanne M, Taskinen MR (1997) Lipids and lipoproteins as coronary risk factors in non insulin dependent diabetes mellitus. Lancet 350(Suppl 1):S120–S123
43. Pyörälä K, Pedersen TR, Kjekshus J et al (1997) Cholesterol lowering with simvastatin improves prognosis of diabetic patients with coronary heart disease. A subgroup analysis of the Scandinavian Simvastatin Survival Study (4S). Diabetes Care 20:614–20
44. Goldberg RB, Mellies MJ, Sacks FM et al (1998) Cardiovascular events and their reduction with pravastatin in diabetic and glucose-intolerant myocardial infarction survivors with average cholesterol levels: subgroup analyses in the cholesterol and recurrent events (CARE) trial. Circulation 98:2513–19
45. The Long-Term Intervention with Pravastatin in Ischaemic Disease (LIPID) Study Group (1998) Prevention of cardiovascular events and death with pravastatin in patients with coronary heart disease and a broad range of initial cholesterol levels. N Engl J Med 339:1349–57
46. Stern MP (1998) The effect of glycemic control on the incidence of macrovascular complications of type 2 diabetes. Arch Fam Med 7:155–62
47. Klein R (1995) Hyperglycemia and microvascular and macrovascular disease in diabetes. Diabetes Care 18:258–68
48. Moss SE, Klein R, Klein BEK et al (1994) The association of glycemia and cause-specific mortality in a diabetic population. Arch Intern Med 154:2473–9
49. Gaster B, Hirsch IB (1998) The effects of improved glycemic control on complications in type 2 diabetes. Arch Intern Med 158:134–40
50. Andersson DKG, Svardsudd K (1995) Long-term glycemic control relates to mortality in type II diabetes. Diabetes Care 18:1534–43
51. Kuusisto J, Mykkanen L, Pyorala K et al (1994) NIDDM and its metabolic control predict coronary heart disease in elderly subjects. Diabetes 43:960–7
52. Mehta S, Yususf S, Peters R et al, for the Clopidogrel in Unstable Angina to Prevent Recurrent Events trial (CURE) Investigators (2001) Effects of pretreatment with clopidogrel and aspirin followed by long-term therapy in patients undergoing percutaneous coronary intervention: the PCI-CURE study. Lancet 358:527–33
53. Rubins HB, Robins SJ, Collins D, Fye CL et al (1999) Gemfibrozil for the secondary prevention of coronary heart disease in men with low levels of high-density lipoprotein cholesterol. Veterans Affairs High-Density Lipoprotein Cholesterol Intervention Trial Study Group. N Engl J Med 34:410–8
54. Clarke PM, Gray AM, Briggs A et al (2004) A model to estimate the lifetime health outcomes of patients with type 2 diabetes: the United Kingdom Prospective Diabetes Study (UKPDS) Outcomes Model (UKPDS no. 68). Diabetologia. 47:1747-1759
55. Malmberg K, Rydén L, Efendic S (1995) A randomized study of insulin-glucose infusion followed by subcutaneous insulin treatment in diabetic patients with acute myocardial infarction: effects on 1-year mortality. J Am Coll Cardiol 26:57–65

56. Malmberg K, Norhammar A, Wedel H et al (1999) Glucometabolic state at admission: important risk marker of mortality in conventionally treated patients with diabetes mellitus and acute myocardial infarction: long term results from the DIGAMI study. Circulation 99:2626–32
57. Von Bibra H, Thrainsdottir IS, Hansen A et al (2004) Augmented metabolic control improves myocardial diastolic function and perfusion in patients with non-insulin dependent diabetes. Heart 9:1483-1484
58. No authors listed (2001) ACC/AHA/ESC guidelines for the management of patients with atrial fibrillation. Task Force Report. Eur Heart J 22:1852–1923

6 Circulatory Failure: Bedside Functional Hemodynamic Monitoring

C. SORBARA, S. ROMAGNOLI, A. ROSSI AND S.M. ROMANO

Introduction

Four basic classes of circulatory shock can be *clinically* defined: hypovolemic, cardiogenic, obstructive, and distributive. Looking at the physiology of cardiac performance, taking a *pathophysiologic* approach we can distinguish between hypovolemic shock, distributive shock, systolic cardiogenic shock, diastolic cardiogenic shock, or a mix of them. All these types evolve, if not treated early and adequately, towards end-organ failure (dysoxia, microcirculatory failure). Multi-organ dysfunction syndrome (MODS) accounts for most deaths in the intensive care unit (ICU). Disturbances in systemic hemodynamics and organ perfusion resulting in tissue hypoxia appear to play a key role in the onset and maintenance of MODS.

In critically ill patients, as well as those with MODS, hemodynamic monitoring is a cornerstone of care, with these *objectives and priorities:* (a) rapid assessment of the determinants of the cardiovascular insufficiency (diagnosis of acute circulatory failure); (b) guidance and titration of cardiopulmonary therapies (treatment algorithm); (c) rapid assessment of regional tissue hypoperfusion, even in a compensated shock patient (i.e, with intrinsic acute and/or chronic circulatory failure); and (d) assessment of the optimization of tissue perfusion. New bedside technologies, more or less invasive, are helping caregivers with increasingly sophisticated and evolving monitoring devices. Nevertheless, despite improvements in resuscitation and supportive care, progression of organ dysfunction occurs in a large proportion of patients with acute, life-threatening illness. Early and aggressive resuscitation of critically ill patients may limit or reverse tissue hypoxia, progression to organ failure,

Anesthesia and Intensive Care Unit, Internal Medicine, Cardiovascular Department, University Hospital Careggi, Florence, Italy and improve outcome [1]. Sometimes, however, although blood pressure, arterial oxygenation, central venous pressure (CVP), and cardiac output (CO) may be in the "normal range," the patient may continue to suffer from inadequate microcirculatory perfusion not reflected by "classic" hemodynamic parameters. Consequently, simultaneous monitoring of global and regional tissue oxygenation is needed, because tissue hypoxia plays a crucial role in the pathogenesis of MODS.

Using a functional approach–because no monitoring device, no matter how simple or how complex, invasive or noninvasive, measuring variables directly or indirectly by signal processing, will improve outcome unless coupled with correct diagnosis and a treatment algorithm – we examine hemodynamic data/indices from 'unstable' patients for dynamic measures of preload *reserve*, afterload *reserve*, cardiac *reserve*, and perfusion *reserve*, that could guide and titrate the four major therapeutic options: fluid challenge; vasopressor/vasodilator; inotropic/inodilator; and oxygen/hemoglobin ther apy.

Preload Reserve: Preload and Preload Responsiveness

Fluid therapy is often the first-line approach to the critically ill patient with circulatory failure. However, only half of such patients have been shown to respond to volume expansion with a significant improvement in hemodynamics, as indicated by an increase in cardiac output, stroke volume, or mean arterial pressure [2]. Nonresponders may suffer deleterious effects from volume expansion such as worsening of gas exchange, longer ventilation time, or cor pulmonale. An inotropic agent and/or vasopressor support should be preferentially used in these patients. Bearing in mind the high risk of volume overload, before giving fluid the clinician should be able to predict, by continuous hemodynamic monitoring, the response of individual patients to volume expansion instead of inotropic/vasoactive agents. Several clinical factors (detected at physical examination) and biological measured variables have been proposed as markers of fluid requirement, although they have limited sensitivity and specificity [3].

Neither cardiac filling pressures, such as CVP and pulmonary artery occlusion pressure (PAOP), nor their changes in response to fluid challenge are sufficiently reliable for predicting response to fluid load [4]. Since the introduction of the pulmonary artery catheter (PAC), many studies have shown that PAOP alone poorly reflects left ventricular (LV) preload, unless LV volume is measured as well [5]. Further, PAOP is a poor predictor of the LV preload responsiveness due to its high dependence on LV compliance. The latter is frequently reduced in critically ill patients, and can change over a period of hours to days. Moreover, importantly, values for PAOP may be misinterpreted, especially with extrinsic or intrinsic positive end-expiratory pressure [6].

Since echocardiography can provide accurate information on LV dimensions (diameters, areas, and volumes), its use has been proposed to assess LV preload and to guide fluid therapy in critically ill patients. LV end-diastolic area (LVEDA)–one of the parameters measured most often in echocardiographic hemodynamic evaluation of the critically ill–can be easily measured by both transthoracic (TTE) and transesophageal echocardiography (TEE) in the midpapillary short axis view. However, many studies have demonstrated that, while this index is valid in the hypovolemic patient with normal right and left cardiac function (low LVEDA), a given LVEDA, like a given LV end-diastolic volume (LVEDV), has poor validity in discriminating between potential responders and nonresponders before a fluid challenge, both in normal patients (high LVEDA) and in patients with right and/or left cardiac dysfunction [7, 8]. As for the filling pressures (CVP, PAOP), even the filling volumes (EDA, EDV) are inadequate to predict the compliance (the "stretching point") of the cardiac chamber unless the corresponding ventricular pressure is measured as well. Moreover, LVEDA cannot reflect end-diastolic volume in the presence of acute or chronic myocardial ischemia with regional wall motion abnormalities.

From this analysis, it is striking that in physiologic as much as in pathophysiologic clinical conditions, no "cut-off" high values of the most frequently used "static" indicators of cardiac preload (pressure–CVP, PAOP, and volume–LVEDA, LVEDV) can forecast preload responsiveness. The latter relies more on the *slope of the Frank-Starling curve* than on the absolute values of cardiac preload (Fig. 1). "Dynamic" parameters, derived from the heart–lung interaction, have been more recently proposed as an alternative.

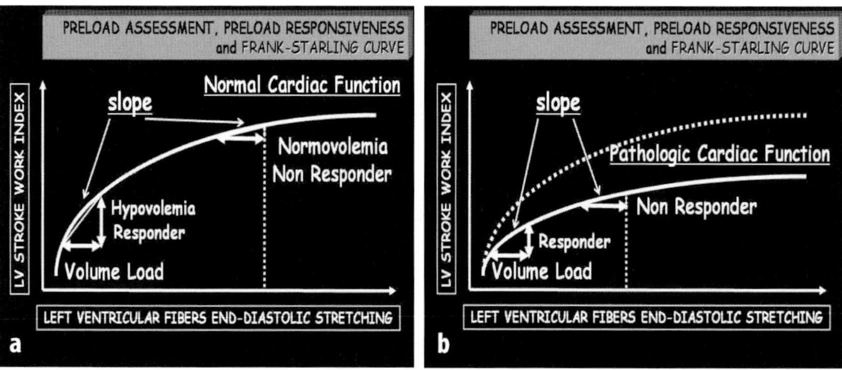

Fig. 1. Preload assessment, preload responsiveness, and Frank–Starling Curve in normal (**a**) and pathologic (**b**) cardiac function. LV, left ventricular

Preload Responsiveness and Dynamic Parameters

The development of pulse contour analysis (arterial pressure waveform analysis), first described in the early 1940s, led to a growing interest in the clinical significance of the analysis of variations in blood pressure and stroke volume that result from the heart–lung interactions during mechanical ventilation. Pulse contour analysis is a minimally invasive method that analyzes the systolic and diastolic portions under the arterial pressure waveform in order to determine LV stroke volume, thus providing beat-to-beat measurement of CO.

The calculation of LV stroke volume (beat-to-beat) from arterial pressure is based on the principle that the magnitude of the arterial pulse pressure and pressure decay profile describe a unique LV stroke volume for a given arterial input impedance (resistance, compliance, inertness of the arterial tree and blood). How the pressure profile is analyzed compared with the strength given to spectral power analysis, the weight given to resistive versus compliant elements, and mean arterial pressure vary among published proprietary algorithms [the PiCCO TM monitor (Pulsion Medical System, Hessen, Germany), the LiDCO plus System (LiDCO Ltd., Cambridge, UK), the PRAM TM monitor (Pressure Recording Analytic Method) (Mostcare TM, BIOSI, Italy), and the Flow Trac technology and Vigileo monitor (Edwards Lifesciences, Irvine CA, USA)].

During intermittent positive pressure ventilation (IPPV), the oscillations of respiratory changes in LV stroke volume can be used as indicators of preload responsiveness. The loading conditions of both ventricles are cyclically modified by modification of intrathoracic pressures during mechanical ventilation (Fig. 2).

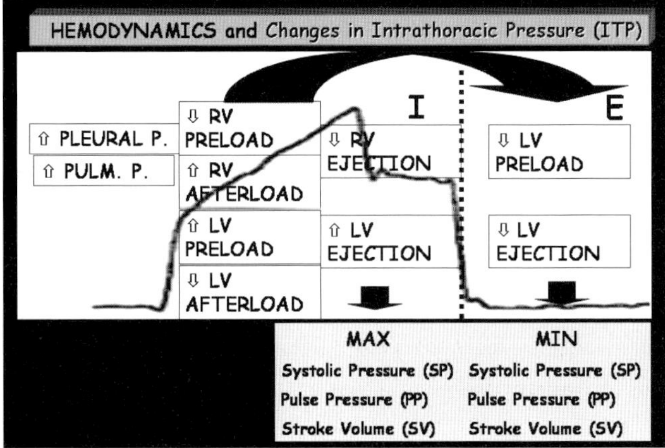

Fig. 2. Changes in intrathoracic pressure and cardiac hemodynamics

During the inspiratory phase of IPPV, a rise in arterial stroke volume can be observed due to an increase in LVEDV as a consequence of increased drainage from the pulmonary veins and left atrium. In addition, improved LVEDV as a consequence of reduced right ventricular (RV) end-diastolic volume (ventricular interdependence) and a decrease in systemic afterload due to a reduction in transmural pressure contribute to the systolic enhancement.

However, experimental and clinical data suggest that the major determinant of cyclic changes in the loading conditions is reduced venous return to the right heart as a consequence of increased pleural pressure and transpulmonary pressure during the inspiratory phase [9, 10]. Moreover, the increase in pulmonary vascular resistances occurring during inflation creates an obstacle to RV ejection (RV afterload enhancement). Consequently, during the early expiratory phase in IPPV, systemic blood pressure begins to fall as a consequence of the reduced RV output (due to decreased venous return and increased RV afterload). If the expiratory phase is extended, the level of pressure will rise again to baseline [11–13].

IPPV-induced oscillations in RV preload lead to cyclic oscillations in RV stroke volume and consequently in LV stroke volume. The magnitude of these changes is greater when the ventricles operate on the *steep* rather than on the *flat* portion of the Frank-Starling curve, as in both normal and pathologic cardiac function [14]. Thus, the respiratory changes in LV stroke volume induced by IPPV could be considered an indicator of biventricular preload dependence. Beat-to-beat changes in LV stroke volume can be easily monitored as beat-to-beat changes in arterial pulse pressure, since the only other determinants of pulse pressure, arterial compliance and resistance, cannot change enough to alter pulse pressure during a single breath (Fig. 3).

Stroke volume variation (SVV) can be defined as the percentage of change between the maximum and minimum stroke volumes divided by the average of the minimum and the maximum [SVmax – SVmin/(SVmax + SVmin)/2]. Pulse contour analysis registers the SV in real time and measures the SVV. Benkerstadt et al. [15] demonstrated that it was possible on the basis of SVV to predict fluid responsiveness in patients undergoing brain surgery. According to the receiver operating characteristic (ROC) curve analysis, a cut-off value of 9.5% distinguished between responders (increase in cardiac index, CI > 15%) and nonresponders to fluid infusion with a sensitivity of 79% and a specificity of 93%. Recent confirmations that SVV predicts fluid responsiveness also come from studies in cardiac surgery [16, 17].

Pulse pressure variation (PPV) can be defined as the maximum difference in pulse pressure observed over a respiratory cycle, where pulse pressure equals systolic blood pressure minus diastolic blood pressure divided by the average of the minimum and the maximum [PPmax – PPmin/(PPmax +

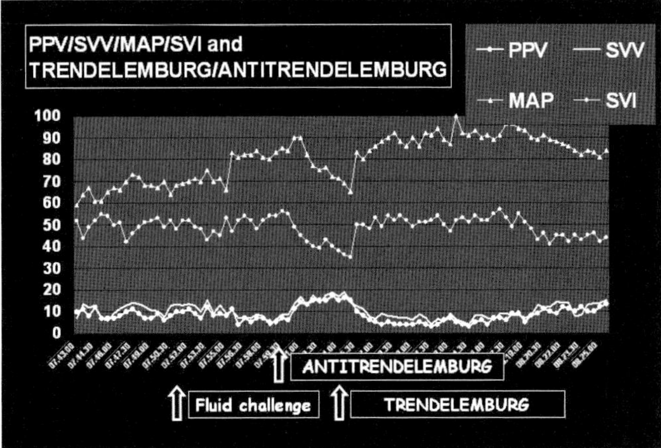

Fig. 3. Hemodynamic monitoring by the PRAM monitor (Mostcare, BIOSI) of mean arterial pressure (MAP), stroke volume index (SVI), pulse pressure variation (PPV), and stroke volume variation (SVV) during Trendelemburg/ anti-Trendelemburg testing in one patient

PPmin)/2]. Michard and coworkers [18] demonstrated that PPV accurately predicts the hemodynamic effects of volume expansion with a threshold value of 13% that discriminates between responders and nonresponders with a sensitivity of 94% and a specificity of 96%. Indeed, if PPV is less than 13%, volume expansion can generate deleterious effects (e.g., worsening of gas exchange) and inotropic or vasoactive therapy can be chosen to improve hemodynamics; on the other hand, if PPV is over 13%, an improvement in CI can be observed in response to fluid infusion.

Aortic blood flow variation (AFV). Since the primary determinant of arterial pulse pressure (P = CO x R) is the phasic aortic flow (SV) generated by the heart's contraction with each heart beat–as arterial resistance and compliance cannot change enough during a single breath–AFV, as measured by pulsed wave Doppler (PWD) TEE at the LV outflow tract (LVOT) or by esophageal Doppler imaging at the thoracic descending aorta, can also be used to determine preload responsiveness and the subsequent change in CO in response to fluid treatment.

Esophageal Doppler ultrasonography measures blood flow velocity in the descending aorta by means of a transducer (4 MHz continuous-wave, or 5 MHz pulsed-wave, according to manufacturer) placed at the tip of a flexible probe. The cross-sectional area of the aorta can be estimated from a nomogram based on age, height, and weight [19] (CardioQ, Deltex Medical Ltd, Sussex, UK) or measured from a second echo beam originating from a second transducer (10 MHz) placed on the probe (Hemosonic 100, Arrow, International Reading, PA, USA).

The Doppler beam allows calculation of the aortic blood flow beat-to-beat from the velocity of red blood cells and the diameter of the aorta. Moreover, since the blood flow in the descending aorta represents around 70% of the blood ejected by the left ventricle, the instrument can calculate CO [20]. Slama and coworkers demonstrated, in mechanically ventilated rabbits subjected to hemorrhage, that the respiratory variation of aortic blood velocity increased progressively during incremental blood withdrawal [21]. More recently, Monnet and coworkers also demonstrated, in patients with acute circulatory failure, that an aortic blood flow inspiratory variation greater than 18% predicted volume responsiveness with a sensitivity of 90% and a specificity of 94% [22].

Echocardiography is the least invasive (TEE) or noninvasive technique (TTE) that can be useful in detecting fluid responsiveness in critically ill patients. It measures the aortic velocity time integral (VTI) and peak velocity of aortic blood flow (V_{peak}) (Fig. 4). Respiratory changes in VTI (ΔVTI) and V_{peak} (ΔV_{peak}), measured at the aortic annulus level, reflect the fluctuations of stroke volume induced by modifications of loading conditions during IPPV. In this regard, Feissel and coworkers demonstrated, in sedated and ventilated patients with septic shock who underwent TEE, that a threshold value of 12% discriminated between responders and nonresponders, with a positive predictive value of 91% and a negative predictive value of 100% [23].

A further method that allows prediction of fluid responsiveness is measurement of *inferior vena cava (IVC) diameter respiratory changes.*

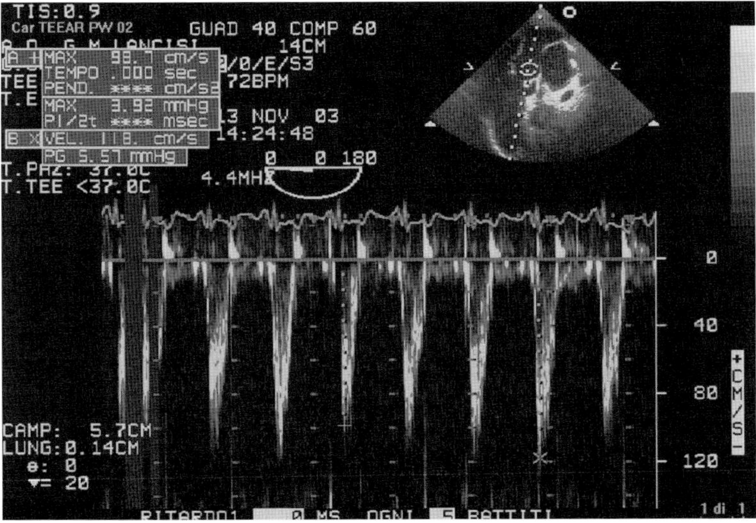

Fig. 4. Echocardiography and preload responsiveness during mechanical ventilation: aortic flow variation

Intrathoracic and intra-abdominal pressures may influence the diameter of IVC that can be visualized by TTE (short-axis or long-axis subcostal view). In self-breathing patients, the collapsibility index (inspiratory percentage decrease in IVC diameter) have been shown to be a good indicator of right atrial pressure (collapsibility index > 50% indicates a right atrial pressure < 10 mmHg) [24]. However, as is known, right atrial pressure is a weak predictor of fluid responsiveness. Instead, the respiratory changes in the IVC diameter induced by mechanical ventilation have been proposed as indicator of fluid responsiveness. A threshold value of 12% was found to be able to discriminate between responders and nonresponders, with a positive predictive value of 93% and a negative predictive value of 92% [25].

In addition, Vieillard-Baron et al. [26, 27] also proposed *superior vena cava (SVC) inspiratory collapse* (visualized by TEE) as a predictor of fluid responsiveness. They found that a marked inspiratory collapse in the SVC was associated with a major inspiratory drop in right ventricular outflow.

Limitations and Pitfalls

Cardiorespiratory interactions are of clinical interest and useful in detecting preload sensitivity, but several important considerations must be pointed out.

Rhythm

A “rhythmical sinus rhythm” is recommended during measurements, because the beat-to-beat changes in LV stroke volume cannot reflect the effect of mechanical insufflations when different diastolic times are present.

Ventricular Function

PPV and SVV are valid methods for fluid responsiveness identification if biventricular preload dependence is present, but incorrect interpretation of preload dependency could be made when the RV is dysfunctional. In the presence of severe RV dysfunction, an inspiratory decrease in RV output is mainly due to an increase in pulmonary resistance (RV afterload). In such a situation, a volume load will not correct the PPV because the RV is not able to fill the pulmonary circulation and enhance LVEDV (false-positive response) [28].

As mentioned above, during the inspiratory phase of IPPV, the rise in arterial blood pressure is the consequence of an increase in LVEDV due to squeezing of the blood from the pulmonary veins and capillaries into the left heart. Therefore, this phenomenon, which suggests a potential benefit from a volume load, is frequently observed in conditions of congestive heart failure where fluid removal therapy is one of the main aims.

Tidal Volume

PPV is the consequence of cyclic changes in intrathoracic and transpulmonary pressures. Therefore, the higher the tidal volume, the greater the LV SVV and PPV. Tidal volume significantly influences these indices [29]. In adult respiratory distress syndrome (ARDS), the tidal volume is low because lung compliance is significantly impaired, but for the same reason, high airway pressure is still present during ventilation [30]. Tavernier and Michard [7, 18] ventilating patients with a large range of tidal volumes (8–12 ml kg^{-1}) and plateau pressures (11–34 cmH_2O) confirmed the accuracy of PPV as a predictor of fluid responsiveness. Moreover, Vieillard-Baron [27] also reported the accuracy of PPV as a predictor of fluid responsiveness with lower tidal volume (8 ml kg^{-1}). In contrast, De Backer et al. recently found that PPV was inaccurate if a tidal volume below 8 ml kg^{-1} was used [31]. Looking at these data, no final conclusions can be drawn; however, the role of tidal volume during IPPV must always be considered when PPV is used in a fluid therapy decision-making process.

These dynamic parameters have been validated in deeply sedated patients. Whether they also predict fluid responsiveness in nonsedated, self-ventilating patients remains to be determined.

Afterload Reserve and Dynamic Parameters

Systemic hypotension, even with a "supranormal" CO, is always pathologic, as physiologic mechanisms normally keep central arterial pressure constant to maintain coronary, cerebral, and end-organ perfusion despite a widely varying CO. Moreover, the relationship between arterial pressure and regional blood flow is both nonlinear and different among vascular beds: a primary condition of vasoplegia may induce blood flow redistribution and/or frank ischemia in specific organs (brain, heart, gut, kidney), even with a normal or supranormal value of CO [32]. On the other hand, the presence of peripheral vasoconstriction with systemic normotension does not imply a stable cardiovascular state and represent compensation for unrecognized underlying cardiac failure.

Thus, knowledge of the level of vasomotor tone and its change in response to changes in CO and vasoactive therapy is relevant in the decision-making process on specific therapies and their titration. The evaluation of arterial tone, as studied by Pinsky [33], can be performed by analyzing the relationship between pulse pressure and stroke volume.

As CO = mean arterial pressure (MAP)/systemic vascular resistance, the arterial tone, or arterial elastance (E_a) [34], can be defined by the ratio between MAP and LV stroke volume and the slope of the line drawn from the variations between the two values. If so, and assuming that arterial impedance remains constant throughout the respiratory cycle, then variations of MAP during mechanical ventilation are a reliable reflection of variations in LV stroke volume. However, MAP also depends on arterial compliance or arterial tone: the more compliant the artery, the lower the MAP for a given LV stroke volume; the less compliant the artery, the higher the MAP for a given LV stroke volume. If, instead of MAP, one uses arterial pulse pressure, then one can estimate *the SVV to PPV ratio, and the ratio of change of the ratio* as a direct measure of large vessel arterial tone. Small respiratory changes in LV stroke volume in a preload-unresponsive patient might be able to induce significant PPV in the case of high arterial tone. On the other hand, large changes in LV stroke volume might be able to induce only small PPV in a preload-responsive patient with very compliant arteries and a low arterial tone. Arterial tone may differ from one patient to another or in the same patient depending on the time of measurement, the disease, and the continuous infusion of the vasoactive drug at the moment of the measurement (Fig. 5).

The primary limitation to the application of arterial elastance analysis is not its scientific validity, but the difficulties in measuring beat-to-beat changes in LV stroke volume at the patient's bedside. Today, thanks to pulse contour analysis, transesophageal PWD echocardiography, and esophageal pulsed Doppler techniques, the physician has the capability to easily measure beat-to-beat changes in LV stroke volume (SVV) simultaneously with beat-to-beat changes in pulse pressure (PPV) at the patient's bedside.

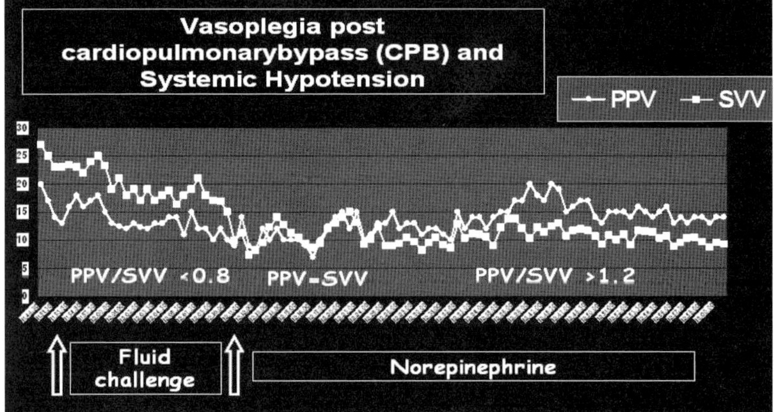

Fig. 5. Hemodynamic monitoring by the PRAM monitor (Mostcare, BIOSI) of pulse pressure variation to stroke volume variation ratio (PPV/SVV) after cardiopulmonary bypass in one patient: PPV/SVV<1 (low arterial tone) during a fluid challenge, followed by a PPV/SVV ≈ 1, and PPV/SVV >1 (high arterial tone) during infusion of norepinephrine

Cardiac Reserve: Contractility and Efficiency

Cardiac Power

CO is the primary determinant of global oxygen transport; unfortunately, many studies have shown that neither absolute values for CO nor its change in response to therapy reflect the "normality" or the "adequacy" of local blood flow or the outcome of critical illness. Detrimental values of CO can be considered only in critically ill patients who are unable to sustain a cardiac index in excess of 2 l min^{-1} m^{-2}, despite aggressive therapy [35]. Moreover the strong load dependency of stroke volume, CO, and ejection fraction preclude the capability of these hemodynamic parameters to aid in evaluating *myocardial contractile performance* in daily clinical practice. This is in practical terms the capability of the heart to maintain an "effective" blood flow with an acceptable perfusion pressure in the presence of variable arterial impedance, without going into failure, without high filling pressure, and without overly expensive myocardial energy expenditure (oxygen consumption).

Ideally, measurement of ventricular performance as an independent parameter of cardiovascular function couples CO with a beat-to-beat assessment of systolic pump function, independent of loading conditions. Such a measurement is useful both as an index of contractility and as an index of ventricular functional reserve. Why? Because knowing the amount of contractile reserve is important for prevention of complications from fluid overload and in assessing a patient's response to hemodynamic stress (e.g., weaning from mechanical ventilation, surgery, sepsis, etc.).

The slope of the LV end-systolic pressure–volume (P-V) relation (E_{es} = *end-systolic ventricular elastance*) has been used in experimental medicine for assessment of cardiac contractility [36–38]. Its clinical application, however, is limited by technical difficulties associated with instantaneous volume measurements, by the necessity of complicated off-line analysis, and by medical and ethical limitations related to the required episodes of load alterations.

If the cardiovascular system is thought of as a hydraulic system, then the heart works as a pump to circulate blood to both the pulmonary and systemic circulations. The effort performed by the ventricle to pump blood against gravity and to overcome both the inertia and viscosity of blood is "ventricular work". If so, cardiac power (PWR) is ventricular work per unit of time; namely, the product of cardiac output and the pressure generated in the arterial system [39, 40]. In clinical practice, PWR is calculated on a beat-to-beat basis as a clinical index of contractility by matching arterial pressure tracing and Doppler echocardiographic flow velocity across the aortic valve [41].

In the absence of mitral regurgitation, beat-to-beat basis cardiac flow during systole equals aortic flow. Hence, PWR can be described as the product of instantaneous aortic pressure and instantaneous aortic flow, where the maximal value (*PWRmax*) is obtained by the analysis of instantaneous data for pressure and flow, and by their product during ventricular ejection (PWRmax = P_{ao} x V_{ao}max x AVA x 1.333 x 10^{-4}), where P_{ao} is instantaneous aortic pressure, V_{ao}max is instantaneous maximum aortic blood flow velocity, and AVA is time-averaged aortic valve area; thus, PWRmax is the maximum PWR (in watts) [42]. Unfortunately, although this index (PWRmax) is highly dependent on contractility, showing great stability concerning changes in afterload, it is otherwise highly dependent on preload. For this reason, several authors have proposed decreasing this load dependency dividing the PWRmax by the square of the end-diastolic volume (EDV), with the resulting preload-adjusted maximal power index of contractility (PAMP = PWR/EDV^2), which is independent of load status and available by beat-to-beat measurements [43, 44]. In clinical conditions, instantaneous aortic pressure is *arterial blood pressure* at the time point at which the product of pressure and flow is *at maximum.* Although PAMP has appealing characteristics (PAMP is cardiac load-independent index), an important limitation to its clinical use is a series of off-line, time-consuming analyses required to obtain it.

To overcome this clinical limitation, Amà et al. [45] validated a more practical measure of contractility: the *preload adjusted peak power (PAPP).* PAPP represents the estimated ventricular power from the *peak* systolic pressure (invasive radial artery) and flow (continuous-wave Doppler echocardiography at the level of the aortic valve), normalized for preload ($LVEDV^2$)(2D transesophageal echocardiography at two-chamber view of the left ventricle) (Fig. 6). The authors found an excellent correlation between the PAMP and PAPP (r = 0.99; y = 1.0168x + 0.0796; P < 0.0001). The study also confirmed the independence of this hemodynamic parameter on loading conditions, and, most importantly, the practical bedside and on-line assessment from a single beat steady-state condition.

PAPP has been also used to measure the cardiac *contractile reserve* as a reliable marker of progression and worsening of heart failure. Marmor et al. [46] measured PAPP with a validated noninvasive device consisting of a sphygmomanometric arm cuff, a Doppler transducer, and an electrocardiographic monitoring system, while aortic velocities and diameter were measured by TEE. Interestingly, the study results showed that the best discriminator among New York Heart Association (NYHA) functional classes was the contractile reserve.

During β_{1-2}-adrenergic stimulation achieved by infusion of dobutamine, CO measured in patients affected by different degrees of heart failure

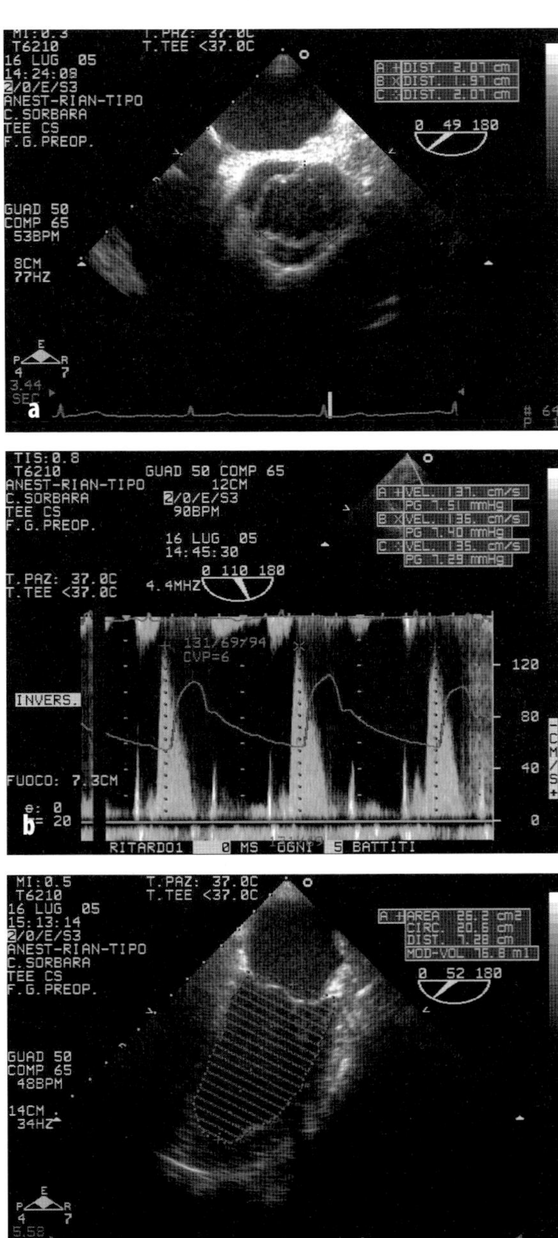

Fig. 6. Transesophageal echocardiography recordings from a sample patient. **a** Short-axis image of the aortic valve. The aortic opening appears as an equilateral triangle. **b** Continuous-wave Doppler echocardiography at the level of the aortic valve. The blood flow velocity is given in centimeters per second. **c** Two-chamber view of the left ventricle in a longitudinal plane. Semiautomatic calculation of left ventricular volume according to Simpson's rule

(NYHA classes 1–3) was remarkably similar, because of the simultaneous and opposite actions of the drug on contractility (increased), on systemic vascular resistance (decreased), and on heart rate (increased). In contrast, PAPP was significantly enhanced in healthy patients and those in lower NYHA classes compared with patients with higher degrees of heart failure, demonstrating that the contractility reserve, as measured with PAPP, decreases with the progression of heart failure.

Cardiac Cycle Efficiency (CCE)

Sunagawa and coworkers, in experimental studies on optimal left ventriculoarterial coupling [47- 49] demonstrated that for any given ventricular elastance (E_{es}) and end-diastolic volume, the cardiovascular system will operate optimally in term of maximum stroke work only in presence of a restricted range of values of arterial elastance (E_a).

This condition corresponds with the concept of maximal efficiency, defined as the "best" ratio of stroke work (mechanical, external work: the work accomplished by the ventricle that contributes to ejection) to total work (pressure–volume area, i.e., the potential energy still stored in the myocardium at end-systole). This ratio is maximized when E_{es} is equal to twice the E_a (Fig. 7).

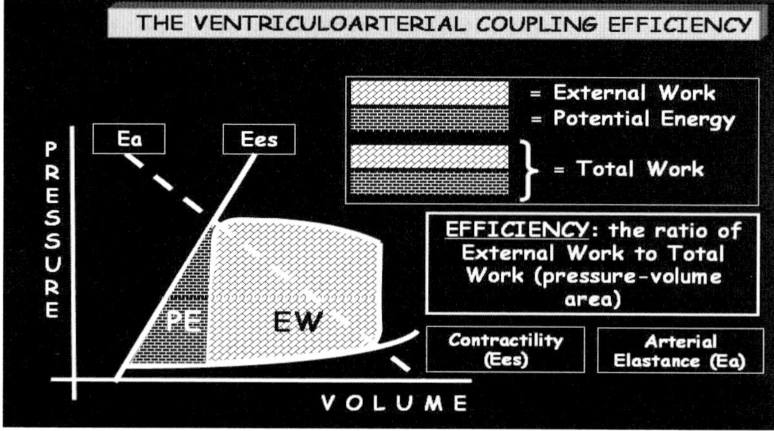

Fig. 7. Stroke work area versus pressure volume area. The *shaded* region represents pressure volume area (the total work performed by the ventricle). The *lighter shaded* region is stroke work (external work). The *darker shaded* region represents potential energy (still stored in the myocardium at end-systole)

In physiological terms, for any given hemodynamic state (inotropy, end-diastolic volume, and heart rate), there is a unique combination of arterial properties and afterload values (aortic impedance Z_c, total arterial resistance R, and total arterial compliance C) which will allow stroke work to be maximized. Likewise, at any given afterload, there is a unique combination of ventricular properties that will fulfil the demands of the systemic circulation with minimal energy expenditure (oxygen consumption).

Romano et al. [50-52] used the PRAM arterial waveform analysis (Mostcare, BIOSI) to measure CO and developed another parameter for continuous hemodynamic monitoring - *cardiac cycle efficiency (CCE). CCE is similar to maximal ventriculoarterial coupling efficency, just discussed. It is the hemodynamic work performed by the heart divided by the energy expenditure ratio. Thus, CCE reflects the energetic cost for the cardiovascular system to maintain some degree of hemodynamic balance.*

Technically, PRAM acquires the arterial pressure waveform signal at frequency of 1000 Hz. It uses a proprietary algorithm to analyze this signal and to calculate aortic input impedance (Z_{im}). Z_{im} relates pressure (the forces acting on blood) to flow (the resultant motion of blood) at the aortic root. Thus Z_{im} relates ventricular mechanical properties to systemic arterial mechanics. Such high-frequency signal acquisition and analysis allows accurate calculation of the three determinants of aortic input impedance (Z_{im}): 1) aortic impedance (Z_c), 2) total arterial resistance (R), and 3) total arterial compliance (C) - the Windkessel model. At the same time, it accounts for the variable effects of the wave reflection phenomenon, a hydraulic impedance mismatch caused by branching vessels of the arterial tree. Thus, some forward ventriculo-arterial energy is reflected back toward the heart. Intuitively, it might be expected that the morphology of the pressure waveform should be similar to that of the flow waveform. In fact, if the forward component is separated from the reflected component, the waveforms should be identical. However, since the reflected waveform adds to the pressure waveform, but subtracts from the flow waveform, the net result is a unique or "individual" relation between pressure and flow waveforms. The timing of waveform reflections during the cardiac cycle (systole or diastole) depends on both the anatomical characteristics of the cardiovascolar system and on the patient's clinical condition. Further, such timing determines positive or negative effects on cardiac performance in terms of the efficiency of the arterial tree in accepting pulsatile flow from the heart [53]. Thus, for all intents and purposes, CCE is the ratio between the ideal shape (derived by a mathematical formula) of the pressure waveform that the patient should have and that detected during examination of one cardiac cycle in any given patient. Too, CCE provides continuous and on-line bedside assessing of the result/cost ratio for cardiac performance; namely, the correlation between different values of CO (result) and energy expenditure (cost). Lastly, it expresses the ability of cardiovascular system to maintain homeostasis at different degrees of energy expenditure, and thus has potential prognostic value (Figs. 8,9).

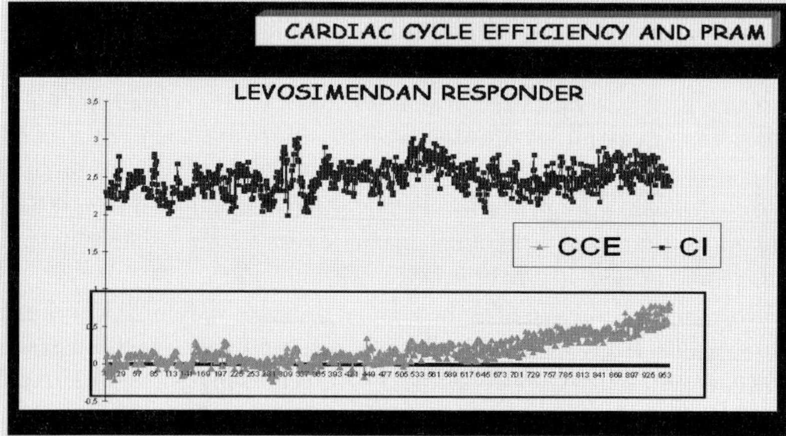

Fig. 8. Cardiac cycle efficiency (CCE) and cardiac index (CI) recorded by the PRAM monitor from the radial artery of a patient with low CO syndrome and being treated with levosimendan. The CI has not changed significantly from the beginning to the end of the recordings, but this result was obtained with increasing efficiency of energy expenditure (CCE), and the patient had a positive outcome

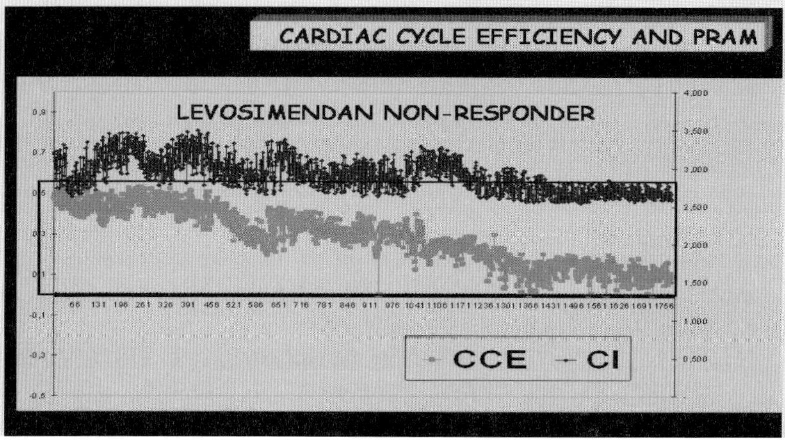

Fig. 9. CCE and CI recorded by the PRAM monitor from the radial artery in another patient with low-output syndrome and treated with levosimendan. The CI has not changed significantly from the beginning to the end of the recordings, but this result was obtained with decreasing efficiency of energey expenditure (CCE), and the patient had a negative outcome

Conclusions

The cardiovascular system in critically ill patients has a moment-to-moment continuous variable arrangement of its determinants, i.e., ventricular compliance, ventricular elastance, right *versus* left ventricular failure, and arterial elastance. This process involves both physiologic and pathophysiologic adaptive mechanisms that interact with each other, many times in a patient with low functional cardiovascular reserve.

In the last 30 years, many tools, more or less sophisticated, have been proposed to physicians for hemodynamic monitoring of critically ill patients with widely questioned impact on patient outcome. Recently, minimally invasive monitoring systems, such as arterial pulse contour analysis and transesophageal echocardiography, have provided promising advances in the approach to hemodynamic assessment of patients. We can now distinguish, on a beat-to-beat basis, real-time cardiac performance, including such parameters as preload and preload responsiveness, high and low arterial tone, and load-dependent (CO, ejection fraction, cardiac cycle efficiency) and load-independent (cardiac power) cardiac performance indices.

Nevertheless, *"all"* hemodynamic monitoring technologies (i.e., pulmonary artery catheter, echocardiography, pulse contour analysis), invasive or non-invasive, simple or complex, measuring variables directly or indirectly by signal processing, are associated with caveats and limitations (which can be pathophysiologic [end-diastolic pressure and end-diastolic volume as single expression of preload and/or preload responsiveness] and/or technical [pulse pressure variation and stroke volume variation, until now validated only in a steady-state sedated patient with sinus rhythm and controlled ventilation]). These caveats, if not known, may cause inappropriate and/or delayed treatment of unstable, critically ill patients.

Due to these considerations, a "gold standard" hemodynamic monitoring system and/or parameter doesn't exist at the moment. An isolated value of CO could be appropriate or not for a critically ill patient although "in normal range". But the same value, and overall its trend, when read contemporary with the indices of organs perfusion (i.e. SvO2, blood lactate, tonometry, or artero-venous gradient of PCO2) can offer precious information on hemodynamic status and on the adequacy of therapy.

So, for a correct hemodynamic assessment, changes in static parameters for pressure, volume and flow must be considered *together with* those in dynamic, functional parameters, interpreted for different clinical scenarios, and with as much attention given to *trends* as to absolute values.

We speculate that *future* bedside hemodynamic assessment will be directed towards quick and specific diagnosis, with articulated, simultaneous treatment for multiple aspects of cardiovascular reserve, such as preload responsiveness, arterial capacitor tone, cardiac cycle reserve and ventriculo-arterial coupling efficiency.

References

1. Rivers E, Nguyen B, Havstad S et al (2001) Early goal-directed therapy in the treatment of severe sepsis and septic shock. N Engl J Med 345:1368–1377
2. Michard F, Teboul JL (2000) Using heart-lung interactions to assess fluid responsiveness during mechanical ventilation. Crit Care 4:282–289
3. Vincent JL, Weil MH (2006) Fluid challenge revisited. Crit Care Med 34:1333–1337
4. Kumar A, Anel R, Bunnel E et al (2004) Pulmonary artery occlusion pressure and central venous pressure fail to predict ventricular filling volume, cardiac performance, or the response to volume infusion in normal subjects. Crit Care Med 32:691–699
5. Raper R, Sibald WJ (1984) Misled by the wedge? The Swan-Ganz catheter and left ventricular preload Chest 89:427–434
6. Teboul JL, Pinsky MR, Mercat A et al (2000) Estimating cardiac filling pressure in mechanically ventilated patients with hyperinflation. Crit Care Med 28:3631–3636
7. Tavernier B, Makhotine O, Lebuffe G et al (1998) Systolic pressure variation as a guide to fluid therapy in patients with sepsis induced hypotension. Anesthesiology 89:1313–1321
8. Tousignant CP, Walsh F, Mazer CD (2000) The use of transesophageal echocardiography for preload assessment in critically ill patients. Anesth Analg 90:351–355
9. Pizov R, Ya'ari Y, Perel A (1989) The arterial pressure waveform during acute ventricular failure and synchronized external chest compression. Anesth Analg 68:150–156
10. Szold A, Pizov R, Segal E et al (1989) The effect of tidal volume and intravascular volume state on systolic pressure variation in ventilated dogs. Intensive Care Med 15:368–371
11. Jardin F, Farcot JC, Gueret P et al (1983) Cyclic changes in arterial pulse during respiratory support. Circulation 68:266–274
12. Theres H, Binkau J, Laule M et al (1999) Phase-related changes in right ventricular cardiac output under volume-controlled mechanical ventilation with positive end expiratory pressure. Crit Care Med 27:953–958
13. Brower R, Wise RA, Hassapoyannes C et al (1985) Effect of lung inflation on lung blood volume and pulmonary venous flow. J Appl Physiol 58:954–963
14. Michard F, Teboul JL (2000) Respiratory changes in arterial pressure in mechanically ventilated patients. In: Vincent J-L (ed) Yearbook of intensive care and emergency medicine. Springer, Berlin, pp 696–704
15. Berkenstadt H, Margalit N, Hadani M et al (2001) Stroke volume variation as a predictor of fluid responsiveness in patients undergoing brain surgery. Anesth Analg 92:984–989
16. Hofer CK, Müller SM, Furre L et al (2005) Stroke volume and pulse pressure variation for prediction of fluid responsiveness in patients undergoing off-pump coronary artery bypass grafting. Chest 128:848–854
17. Reuter DA, Goepfert MSG, Goresch T et al (2005) Assessing fluid responsiveness during open chest conditions. Br J Anaesth 94:318–323
18. Michard F, Boussat S, Chemla D et al (2000) Relationship between respiratory

changes in arterial pulse pressure and fluid responsiveness in septic patients with acute circulatory failure. Am J Resp Crit Care Med 162:134–138
19. Singer M, Clark J, Bennet ED (1989) Continuous hemodynamic monitoring by esophageal Doppler. Crit Care Med 17:447–452
20. Boulnois JL, Pechoux T (2000) Non-invasive cardic output monitoring by aortic blood flow measurement with the Dynemo 3000. J Clin Monit Comput 16:127–140
21. Slama M, Masson H, Teboul JL et al (2004) Monitoring of respiratory variations of aortic blood flow velocity using esophageal Doppler. Intensive Care Med 30:1182–1187
22. Monnet X, Rienzo M, Osman D et al (2005) Esophageal Doppler monitoring predicts fluid responsiveness in critically ill ventilated patients. Intensive Care Med 31:1195–1201
23. Feissel M, Michard F, Mangin I et al (2001) Respiratory changes in aortic blood velocity as an indicator of fluid responsiveness in ventilated patients with septic shock. Chest 119:867–873
24. Kircher BJ, Himelman RB, Schiller NB (1990) Noninvasive estimation of right atrial pressure from the inspiratory collapse of the inferior vena cava. Am J Cardiol 66:493–496
25. Feissel M, Michard F, Mangin I et al (2002) Respiratory changes in inferior vena cava diameter predict fluid responsiveness in septic shock (abstract). Am J Resp Crit Care Med 165(Suppl):A712
26. Vieillard-Baron A, Augarde R, Prin S et al (2001) Influence of superior vena caval zone condition on cyclic change in right ventricular outflow during respiratory support. Anesthesiology 95:1083–1088
27. Vieillard-Baron A, Chergui K, Rabiller A et al (2004) Superior vena cava collapsibility as a gauge of volume status in ventilated septic patients. Intensive Care Med 30:1734–1739
28. Vieillard-Baron A (2006) Pulse pressure variations in managing fluid requirement: beware the pitfalls! In: Vincent J-L (ed) Yearbook of intensive care and emergency medicine. Springer, Berlin, pp 185–191
29. Reuter D, Felbinger T, Schmidt C et al (2002) Stroke volume variations for assessment of cardiac responsiveness to volume loading in mechanically ventilated patients after cardiac surgery. Intensive Care Med 28:392–398
30. Gattinoni L, Pelosi P, Suter P et al (1998) Acute respiratory distress syndrome caused by pulmonary and extra-pulmonary disease. Different syndromes? Am J Resp Crit Care Med 156: 3–11
31. De Backer D, Heenen S, Piagnerelli M et al (2005) Pulse pressure variations to predict fluid responsiveness: influence of tidal volume. Intensive Care Med 31:517–523
32. Schlichtig R, Kramer D, Pinsky MR (1991) Flow redistribution during progressive hemorrhage is a determinant of critical O2 delivery. J Appl Physiol 70:169–178
33. Pinsky MR (2002) Functional hemodynamic monitoring: applied physiology at the bedside. Springer, Berlin, pp 537–552
34. Sunagawa K, Maughn WL, Burkoff (1983) Left ventricular interaction with arterial load studied in the isolated canine ventricle. Am J Physiol 245:H733-H788
35. Tuchschmidt J, Fired J, Astiz M et al (1992) Elevation of cardiac output and oxygen delivery improves outcome in septic shock. Chest 102:216–220
36. Sagawa K (1981) The end-systolic pressure-volume relation of the ventricle: definition, modification, and clinical use. Circulation 63:1223–1227
37. Suga H, Sagawa K (1974) Instantaneous pressure-volume relationships and their ratio in the excised, supported canine left ventricle. Circ Res 35:117–126

38. Suga H, Sagawa K, Shoukas AA (1973) Load independence of the instantaneous pressure-volume ratio of the canine left ventricle and effects of epinephrine and heart rate on the ratio. Circ Res 32:314–322
39. Snell R, Luchsinger P (1965) Determination of the external work and power of the left ventricle in intact man. Am Heart J 69:529–537
40. Stein P, Sabbah H (1976) Rate of change of ventricular power: an indicator of ventricular performance during ejection. Am Heart J 91:219–227
41. Cotter G, Williams SG, Vered Z (2003) Role of cardiac power in heart failure. Curr Opin Cardiol 18:215–222
42. Schmidt C, Roosens C,Struys M et al (1999) Contractility in humans after coronary artery surgery: echocardiographic assessment with preload-adjusted maximal power. Anaesthesiology 91:58–70
43. Kass D, Beyar R (1991) Evaluation of contractile state by maximal ventricular power divided by the square of end-diastolic volume. Circulation 84:1698–1708
44. Nakayama M, Chen CH, Nevo E et al (1998) Optimal pre-load adjustment of maximal ventricular power index varies with cardiac chamber size. Am Heart J 136:281–288
45. Amà R, Claessens T, Roosens C et al (2005) A comparative study of preload adjustment maximal and peak power: assessment of ventricular performance in clinical practice. Anaesthesia 60:35–40
46. Marmor A, Raphael T, Marmor M et al. (1996) Evaluation of contractile reserve by dobutamine echocardiography: non-invasive estimation of the severity of heart failure. Am Heart J 132:1195–1201
47. Sunagawa K, Sugimachi M, Todako K et al. (1993) Optimal coupling of the left ventricle with the arterial system. Basic Res Cardiol 88:75–90
48. Sunagawa K, Sagawa K, Maughan WL (1984) Ventricular interaction with the loading system. Ann Biomed Eng 12:163–189
49. Sunagawa K, Maughan WL, Sagawa K (1985) Optimal arterial resistance for the maximal stroke work studied in isolated canine left ventricle. Circ Res 56:586–595
50. Romano SM, Pistolesi M (2002) Assessment of cardiac output from systemic arterial pressure in humans. Crit Care Med 30:1834–1841
51. Giomarelli P, Biagioli B, Scolletta S (2004) Cardiac output monitoring by pressure recording analytical method in cardiac surgery. Eur J Cardiothorac Surg 26:515–520
52. Scolletta S, Romano SM, Biagioli B et al. (2005) Pressure recording analytical method (PRAM) for measurement of cardiac output during various haemodynamic states. Br J Anaesth 95:159–65
53. O'Rourke MF (1982) Vascular impedance in studies of arterial and cardiac function. Physiol Rev 62:570–623

7 Perioperative Cardiac Risk Stratification

F.R.B.G. Galas[1], L.A. Hajjar[1] and J.O.C. Auler jr.[2]

Introduction

Cardiovascular events are considered the main cause of death in the perioperative period. The most important events are acute myocardial infarction (MI), unstable angina, cardiac failure, severe arrhythmias, nonfatal cardiac arrest, and death. Patients experiencing an MI after noncardiac surgery have a hospital mortality rate of 15–25% [1, 2], and nonfatal perioperative MI is an independent risk factor for cardiovascular death and nonfatal MI during the 6 months following surgery. Patients who have a cardiac arrest after noncardiac surgery have a hospital mortality rate of 65%, and nonfatal perioperative cardiac arrest is a risk factor for cardiac death during the 5 years following surgery [3, 4]. The objectives of preoperative evaluation are: (a) performing an evaluation of the patient's current medical status; (b) making recommendations concerning the evaluation, management, and risk of cardiac problems over the entire perioperative period; and (c) providing a clinical risk profile that the patient, primary physician, anesthesiologist, and surgeon can use in making treatment decisions that may influence short- and long-term outcomes. No test should be performed unless it is likely to influence patient treatment [5]. The cost of risk stratification cannot be ignored. Accurate estimation of a patient's risk for postoperative cardiac events (MI, unstable angina, ventricular tachycardia, pulmonary edema, and death) after surgery can guide allocation of clinical resources, use of preventive therapies, and priorities for future research.

[1]Surgical Intensive Care Unit and Department of Anesthesiology, Hospital das Clínicas, InCor (Heart Institute), University of São Paulo Medical School, São Paulo, Brazil; [2]Surgical Intensive Care Unit Department and InCor (Heart Institute), University of São Paulo Medical School, São Paulo, Brazil

The prevalence of cardiovascular disease increases with age, and it is estimated that the number of persons older than 65 years in the United States will increase 25–35% over the next 30 years [6]. Unfortunately, this is the same age group in which the largest number of surgical procedures is performed [7].

If successful, cardiac risk stratification classifies patients into various risk categories so that their management can be tailored to their needs. The goal of risk stratification is to reduce overall mortality and morbidity. Clarification of risk status allows the clinicians to provide better information as the basis for informed consent. From a societal perspective, reducing perioperative complications and avoiding unnecessary testing could result in substantial cost savings. The major harms of stratification arise from the use of potentially unnecessary preoperative exams and the consequent possibility of ineffective or harmful interventions. Harm may also result from delay of the planned noncardiac surgery [6]. Therefore, the goal of the consultation is the rational use of testing in an era of cost containment and optimal care of the patient [8]. The need for better methods of objectively measuring cardiovascular risk has led to the development of multiple noninvasive techniques in addition to established invasive procedures [9].

The consultant must also bear in mind that the perioperative evaluation may be the ideal opportunity to affect long-term treatment of a patient with significant cardiac disease or risk of such disease. The referring physician and patient should be informed of the results of the evaluation and implications for the patient's prognosis. The consultant can also assist in planning for follow-up [10].

Clinical Predictors of Risk

There are three clinical predictor groups of surgical risk: the type of surgery, the patient's functional status, and comorbid diseases (the assessment of which is based on clinical data).

Type of Surgery

The clinician should analyze whether the surgery is emergency or not, and the nature of the surgical procedure. Emergency surgery is associated with a large number of perioperative cardiac events. Mangano [1] determined that cardiac complications are two to five times more likely to occur in emergency surgical procedures than in elective operations. This finding is not surprising, because the necessity for immediate surgical intervention may make it impossible to evaluate and treat such patients optimally. For example, patients undergoing repair of ruptured abdominal aortic aneurysms have a mortality rate more than ten times higher than those undergoing an elective surgery for asymptotic aneurysms [11, 12]. For elective surgery, cardiac risk can be stratified according to a number of factors, including the magnitude of the surgical procedure. A large-scale study supported low morbidity and mortality rates in superficial procedures performed on an ambulatory basis [13]. Several large surveys have demonstrated that perioperative cardiac morbidity is particularly concentrated among patients undergoing major thoracic, abdominal, or vascular surgery, especially when aged 70 years or older [14]. Major surgery is related to procedural stress, which depends on anesthetic–surgery time, loss of fluids and blood, and hemodynamic instability (Table 1) [15]. Patients who require vascular surgery appear to have an increased risk of cardiac complications, because many of the risk factors contributing to peripheral vascular disease are also risk factors for coronary artery disease (CAD). This is because the usual symptomatic presentation for CAD in these patients may be obscured by exercise limitations imposed by advanced age and/or intermittent claudication. It is also because major arterial operations are often time-consuming and may be associated with substantial fluctuations in intravascular fluid volumes, cardiac filling pressures, systemic blood pressure, heart rate, and thrombogenicity [16]. Some studies [17, 18] suggest that clinical evidence of CAD in a patient who has peripheral vascular disease appears to be a better predictor of subsequent cardiac events than the particular type of peripheral vascular operation to be performed. In addition, some situations do not lend themselves to comprehensive cardiac evaluation, although surgical care may be qualified as semi-elective. In some patients, the impeding danger of the disease is greater than the anticipated perioperative risk. Examples include patients who require arterial bypass for limb salvage or mesenteric revascularization to prevent intestinal gangrene. Although CAD is the overwhelming risk factor for perioperative morbidity, procedures with different levels of stress are associated with different levels of morbidity and mortality [16] . Superficial and ophthalmologic procedures represent the lowest risk and are rarely associated with excess morbidity and mortality. Major vascular procedures represent the highest-risk procedures. Within the intermediate risk category, morbidity and mortality vary, depending on the surgical location, and extent of the procedure. Some procedures may be short, with minimal fluid shifts, while others may be associated with prolonged duration, large fluid shifts, and greater potential for postoperative myocardial ischemia and respiratory depression. Therefore the physician must exercise judgment to correctly assess perioperative surgical risks and the need for further evaluation [3].

Table 1. AHA cardiac risk[a] stratification for noncardiac surgical procedures

Risk	Surgery
High (reported cardiac risk often greater than 5%)	Emergent major operations, particularly in the elderly Aortic and other major vascular surgery Peripheral vascular surgery Anticipated prolonged surgical procedures associated with large fluid shifts and/or blood loss
Intermediate (reported cardiac risk generally less than 5%)	Carotid endarterectomy Head and neck surgery Intraperitoneal and intrathoracic surgery Orthopedic surgery Prostate surgery
Low[b] (reported cardiac risk generally less than 1%)	Endoscopic procedures Superficial procedure Cataract surgery Breast surgery

[a] Combined incidence of cardiac death and nonfatal myocardial infarction
[b] Patients do not generally require further preoperative cardiac testing

Patient's Functional Status

Functional status scales have been shown to be good predictors of future cardiac events in the general population. The most important scales are described in detail elsewhere: Duke Activity Status Index [15], Canadian Cardiovascular Society's (CCS) classification of angina [16], New York Heart Association (NYHA), classification of congestive heart failure (CHF) [17], and the Specific Activity Scale [18]. These scales try to correlate clinical data with patients' functional status without carrying out supplemental tests. The Duke Activity Status Index was developed to assess functional capacity in a manner that correlates with oxygen uptake by weighting questions according to the known metabolic cost of each activity [15]. The clinician should also observe the limitations of these scales. The Duke Activity Status Index was not studied as a predictor of cardiac events in the perioperative period of noncardiac surgery [6], neither was the Specific Activity Scale (the application of which is very difficult). Physician and patient subjectivity is difficult to control for when applying these scales; and the NYHA and CCS scales are appropriate for specific groups of patients, and therefore cannot be generalized to all patients. Studies of patients undergoing major noncardiac surgery have shown that severe limitation of activity [19] or inability to reach a target heart rate on bicycle ergometry [20] predicts postoperative cardiac risk.

Comorbid Diseases and Risk Factors

The consultant must evaluate the cardiovascular system and analyze comorbid diseases within the framework of the patient's overall health. Associated conditions often heighten the risk of anesthesia and may complicate cardiac management. In a recent analysis, Lee and colleagues [21] revisited the cardiac risk index to identify patients at high risk and identified the following as predictors: history of ischemic heart disease, history of heart failure, history of stroke or transient ischemic attack, preoperative insulin treatment, renal failure and high risk procedure. The presence of two or more of these risk variables conferred an event rate as high as 11% in a group of 1422 patients, whereas the event rate was under 1% in the presence of one or none of these variables. In most of the studies of comorbidity and risk factors, conditions which impose greater risk are:

- Age > 70 years
- Coronary artery disease (history of myocardial infarction, angina pectoris, ischemic ST-segment changes on the electrocardiogram)
- Heart failure (HF) (evidence of ventricular dysfunction is the best predictor)
- Arterial hypertension
- *Diabetes mellitus* (greater incidence of acute MI and silent myocardial ischemia) as well as peripheral vascular disease
- Renal impairment
- Pulmonary disease

Table 2 lists clinical predictors of increased perioperative risk of MI, HF, and death established by multivariate analysis. Clinical factors should be placed into the following three categories:

1. Major predictors: when present, mandate intensive management, which may result in delay or cancellation of surgery unless it is emergent.
2. Intermediate predictors: well-validated markers of increased risk of perioperative cardiac complications; justify careful assessment of the patient's status.
3. Minor predictors: recognized markers of cardiovascular disease that have not been proven to independently increase perioperative risk.

Cardiac Risk Indices and Algorithms in Noncardiac Surgery

During the past 20 years or so, a number of risk indices have been developed. The American Society of Anesthesiologists (ASA) score was the first clinical index developed to predict risk for potential adverse otucomes related to anesthesia and surgery, and was based solely on the patient's age, body

Table 2. Clinical predictors of increased perioperative cardiovascular risk (myocardial infarction, heart failure, death)

Major
Unstable coronary syndromes
Acute or recent MI[a] with evidence of important ischemic risk by clinical symptoms or noninvasive study
Unstable or severe[b] angina (Canadian class III or IV)
Decompensated heart failure
Significant arrhythmias
High-grade atrioventricular block
Symptomatic ventricular arrhythmias in the presence of underlying heart disease
Supraventricular arrhythmias with uncontrolled ventricular rate
Severe valvular disease

Intermediate
Mild angina pectoris (Canadian class I or II)
Previous MI by history or pathological Q waves
Compensated or prior heart failure
Diabetes mellitus (particularly insulin-dependent)
Renal insufficiency

Minor
Advanced age
Abnormal ECG (left ventricular hypertrophy, left bundle-branch block, ST-T abnormalities)
Rhythm other than sinus (e.g., atrial fibrillation)
Low functional capacity (e.g., inability to climb one flight of stairs with a bag of groceries)
History of stroke
Uncontrolled systemic hypertension
ECG, electrocardiogram; MI, myocardial infarction

[a]The American College of Cardiology National Database Library defines 'recent' MI as occurring more than 7 days but less than or equal to 1 month (30 days) previously; 'acute' MI is within the preceding 7 days;
[b]May include "stable" angina in patients who are unusually sedentary

habitus, comorbidities, etc...[22]. Although it is subjective, it has been found to be a sensitive predictor of death in very large numbers of patients (> 100 000) and of major nonfatal complications [23–24]. The ASA score performs less well than other clinical risk indices in predicting cardiac complications [20, 25].

In 1977, Goldman et al. developed the original Cardiac Risk Index (Table 3). It was the first validated multivariate model developed to predict cardiac complications in a general surgical population [25]. Scores were assigned to each variable according to its weight in the model, and a risk index for car-

Table 3. Cardiac Risk Index and modified Cardiac Risk Index

Multivariate cardiac risk indicator variables	Goldman Index		Detsky Index	
	Variable	**Points (0–53)**	**Variable**	**Points (0–110)**
Age	> 70 years	5	> 70 years	5
History of MI or Q-wave on ECG	Within 6 months	10	Within 6 months More than 6 months previously	10 5
History of angina	Not independently predictive		CCS class III CCS class IV	10 20
Left ventricular dysfunction or CHF	S3 or jugular venous distention	11	Pulmonary edema within 1 week Any previous pulmonary edema	10 5
Arrhythmia	Any rhythm other than sinus > 5 PVCs	7 7	Any rhythm other than sinus > 5 PVCs	5 5
Other heart disease	Important aortic stenosis	3	Critical aortic stenosis	20
Other medical problems	Any of the following: $PO_2 < 60$ mmHg, $PCO_2 > 50$ mmHg, K^+ concentration < 3 mmol/l, BUN level > 50 mmol/l, creatinine concentration > 260 _mol/l, bedridden	3	Any of the following: $PO_2 < 60$ mmHg, $PCO_2 > 50$ mmHg, K^+ concentration < 3 mmol/l, BUN level > 50 mmol/l, creatinine concentration > 260 _mol/l, bedridden	5

continue →

continue **Table 3**

Multivariate cardiac risk indicator variables	Goldman Index		Detsky Index	
	Variable	**Points (0–53)**	**Variable**	**Points (0–110)**
Findings for ischemia on ECG	Not independently predictive		Not independently predictive	
Type of surgery	Emergency Intrathoracic or abdominal	4 3	Emergency	10
Scores	Class I Class II Class III Class IV	0—5 6—12 13–25 > 25	Class I Class II Class III	0—15 20–30 > 30

From [27]
MI, myocardial infarction; ECG, electrocardiogram; CCS, Canadian Cardiovascular Society; CHF, congestive heart failure; PVCs, premature ventricular contractions; BUN, blood urea nitrogen

diac death and life-threatening complications was developed. The higher the score, the higher the predicted risk; scores range from class I (low risk) to class IV (high risk). Patients with angina were excluded from this index. This is a good index for low-risk and high-risk patients, however it may fail in intermediate-risk patients. Nine years later, Detsky et al. [26] modified the original Cardiac Risk Index, added the variables of significant angina and remote myocardial infarction, and simplified the scoring system into three classes of risk (class I, 0–15 points; class II, 20–30 points; class III >30 points) (Table 3). It improved predictive accuracy among higher-risk patients. Classes II and III predict a high risk of perioperative cardiac events (10–15%). Low Cardiac Risk Index scores (class I) still do not reliably identify patients who are at low risk of perioperative cardiac events. Information on "low-risk" variables should be collected for these patients [16]. In summary, based on American College of Physicians (ACP) guidelines, patients should initially be assessed by using the modified Cardiac Risk Index so that patients at high risk of postoperative cardiac events can be detected. For the remaining patients, obtaining information about "low-risk" variables will allow further clinical classification into low-risk and intermediate-risk groups [6].

Algorithms are used in the assessment of cardiac risk in the perioperative period as an assistant in the judgment as to whether the clinician should perform supplementary evaluation or not. The most commonly used algorithms are from the American College of Cardiology (ACC)/American Heart Association (AHA) and from the ACP. The ACP uses the modified Cardiac Risk Index for initial cardiac risk arrangement, and then, in Detsky class I patients, assesses risk variables (Table 4) for greater precision (Figs. 1, 2). The ACC/AHA algorithm does not use a specific Cardiac Risk Index (Fig. 3). It determines risk of cardiac events through variables. It ranks patients as low-, intermediate-, or high-risk for cardiac events, and uses noninvasive

Table 4. Low-risk variables (Detsky Class I patients) that require further assessment to allow clinical classification into low-risk and intermediate-risk groups

Age > 70 years	Heart failure history
History of angina	Hypertension with severe left ventricular hypertrophy
Diabetes mellitus	Ischemic ST abnormalities on resting ECG
Q-waves on ECG	History of ventricular ectopy
History of AMI	

Adapted from ACP guidelines[17]
ECG, electrocardiogram; AMI, acute myocardial infarction

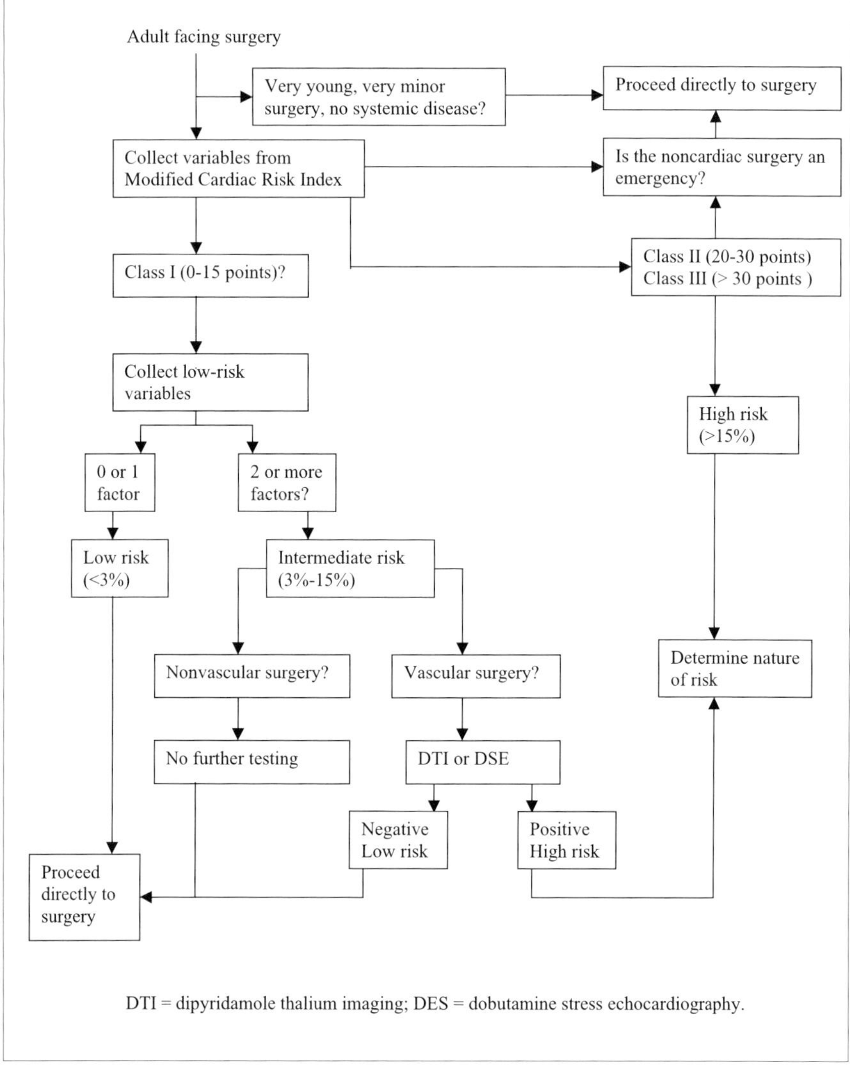

Fig. 1. Adaptation of American College of Physicians (ACP) algorithm for the risk assessment and management of patients at low or intermediate risk of perioperative cardiac events. Illustrated is application of ACP algorithm for further risk stratification in Detsky Class I (Table 3). DTI, dipyridamole thallium imaging; DES, dobutamine stress echocardiography

tests, based on metabolic equivalents and type of surgery, for the diagnosis of perioperative ischemia. However, only a few prospective or randomized studies have been performed to evaluate these guidelines.

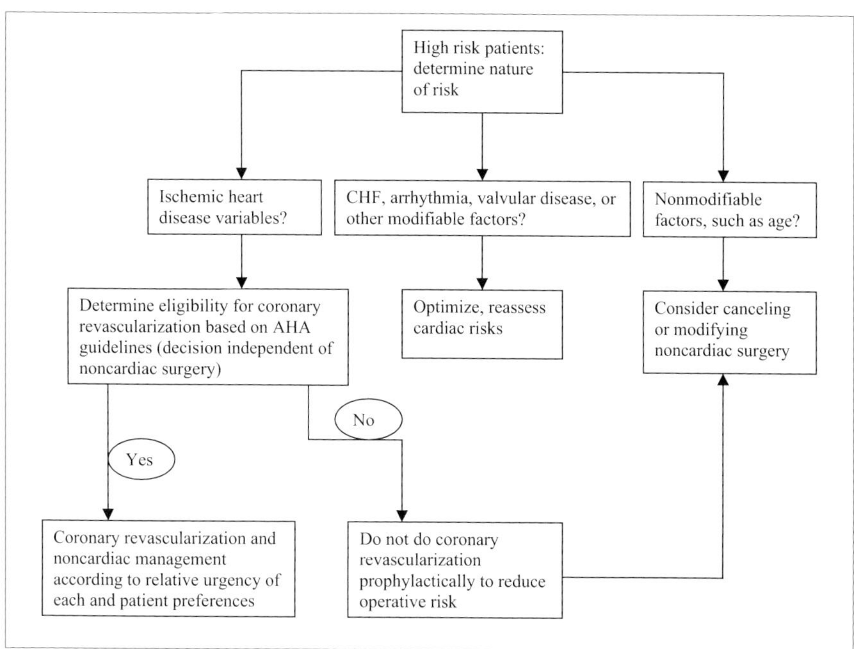

Fig. 2. Adaptation of ACP algorithm for the management of patients at high risk of perioperative cardiac events

Supplemental Preoperative Evaluation

When assessing a patient's risk of major cardiac events during or after a noncardiac operation, the clinician uses clinical evaluation to determine the risk of fatal and nonfatal cardiac events and may refine the risk assessment of intermediate-risk patients through noninvasive testing [16].

Noninvasive tests available for further risk stratification include those that assess left ventricular function (radionuclide angiography, echocardiography, and contrast ventriculography), cardiac ischemia (exercise or pharmacological stress testing and ambulatory electrocardiography monitoring), or both (dobutamine stress echocardiography) [16]. Identification of high-risk patients whose long-term outcome would be improved with medical therapy or coronary revascularization procedures is a major goal of preoperative noninvasive testing [3].

Postoperative events probably have multifactorial causes, and therefore noninvasive testing may never be able to stratify patient risk fully. Tests done before surgery cannot account for every intra- and postoperative factor. For example, the perioperative period is a time of hypercoagulability, cate-

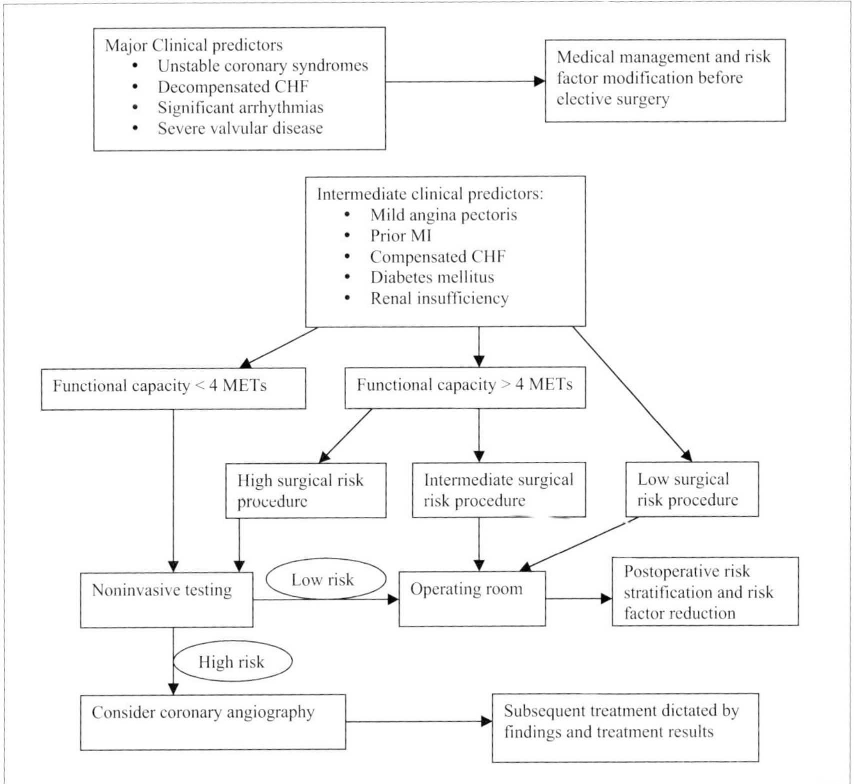

Fig. 3. Adaptation of ACC/AHA algorithm for preoperative cardiac assessment. CHF, congestive heart failure; MI, myocardial infarction; METs, metabolic equivalents; ECG, electrocardiogram

cholamine surges, pain, and operative stresses, all of which may influence oxygen demand, and factors other than coronary stenosis that may influence oxygen supply, leading to myocardial ischemia [6].

The perioperative guidelines from the ACC/AHA recommend testing before surgery when two of three factors are present, which are intermediate clinical predictors (Canadian class 1 or 2 angina, prior MI based on history or pathologic Q waves, compensated or prior heart failure, or diabetes), poor functional capacity (less than 4 METs - metabolic equivalents), and high surgical risk procedure (aortic repair or peripheral vascular surgery, prolonged surgical procedures with large fluid shifts or blood loss, and emergency major operations). Emergency major operations may require immediate proceeding to surgery without sufficient time for noninvasive testing or preoperative interventions [3].

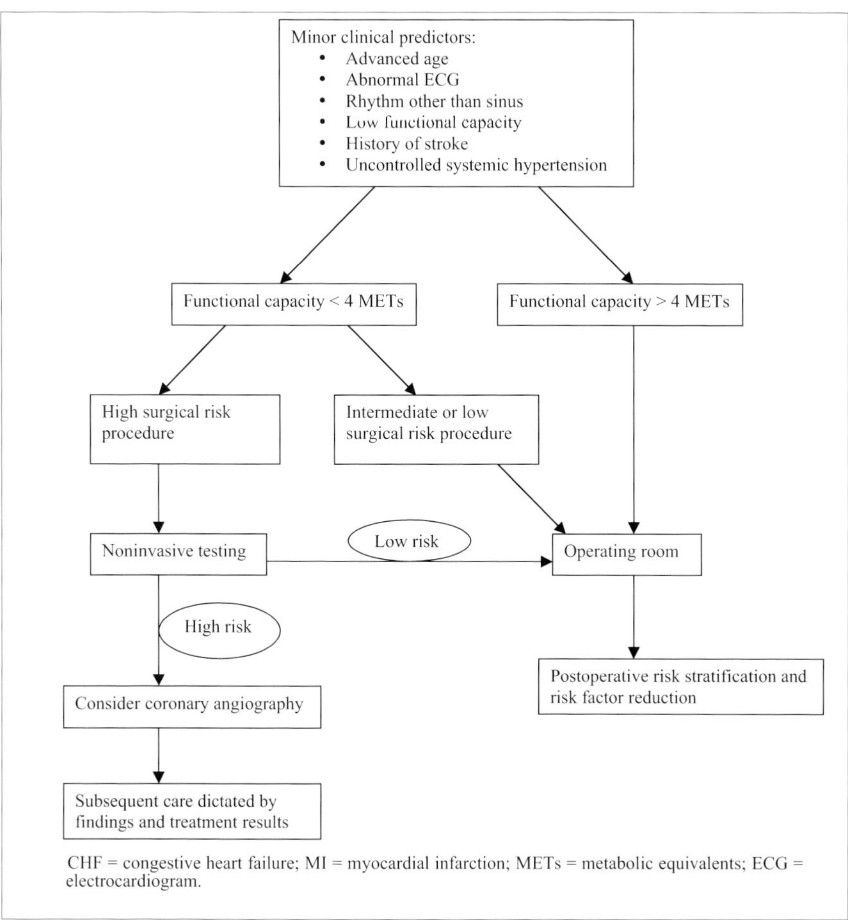

CHF = congestive heart failure; MI = myocardial infarction; METs = metabolic equivalents; ECG = electrocardiogram.

Resting Left Ventricular Function

Studies have demonstrated a greater risk of complications in patients with a left ventricular ejection fraction (LVEF) of less than 35% [27–33]. Poor left ventricular systolic or diastolic function is mainly predictive of postoperative heart failure and, in critically ill patients, death. However, left ventricular function was not found to be a consistent predictor of perioperative ischemic events [3].

Recommendations for preoperative noninvasive evaluation of left ventricular function:

Class I: Patients with current or poorly controlled heart failure (HF)

Class IIa: Patients with prior HF, and patients with dyspnea of unknown origin

Class III: As a routine test of left ventricular function in patients without prior HF

Assessment of Risk for CAD and Functional Capacity

The 12-Lead Electrocardiogram

The 12-lead rest electrocardiogram (ECG) contains important prognostic information that relates to long-term morbidity and mortality [3].

Recommendations for preoperative ECG:

Class I Recent episode of chest pain or ischemic equivalent in clinically intermediate or high-risk patients scheduled for an intermediate or high-risk operative procedure

Class IIa Asymptomatic persons with diabetes mellitus

Class IIb Patients with prior coronary revascularization
Asymptomatic men more than 45 years old or women more than 55 years old with two or more atherosclerotic risk factors
Patients with prior admission for cardiac causes

Class III As a routine test in asymptomatic subjects undergoing low-risk operative procedures

Exercise Stress Testing for Myocardial Ischemia and Functional Capacity

The aim of supplemental preoperative testing is to provide an objective measure of functional capacity, to identify the presence of important preoperative myocardial ischemia or cardiac arrhythmias, and to estimate perioperative cardiac risk and long-term prognosis [31–34]. According to the ACC/AHA guidelines, preoperative noninvasive testing should be considered in patients identified to be at increased risk of cardiac complications based on clinical risk profile, functional capacity, and type of surgery [3]. An exercise or pharmacological stress test is recommended in patients with intermediate pretest probability of CAD [33–35];

- to establish prognostic assessment of patients undergoing initial evaluation for suspected or proven CAD;
- to give an evaluation of subjects with a significant change in their clinical status;
- to demonstrate myocardial ischemia before coronary revascularization;
- to evaluate the adequacy of medical therapy;
- and for prognostic assessment after an acute coronary syndrome.

Exercise electrocardiography, which can be safely performed in an outpatient setting, is considered the least expensive noninvasive test for the detection of myocardial ischemia. Pooled data from seven studies indicate that exercise electrocardiography has a sensitivity of 74% and a specificity of

69% for the prediction of cardiac death and myocardial infarction in patients undergoing major vascular surgery [7]. However, patients are often unable to exercise because of claudication, peripheral neuropathy, or as a consequence of a prior cerebrovascular event. Up to 40% of vascular patients also have preexisting electrocardiographic abnormalities that may preclude reliable ST-segment analysis. For this reason, pharmacological rather than exercise testing is often required in patients undergoing surgery. In this respect, dipyridamole myocardial perfusion scintigraphy combined with clinical risk assessment is the most extensively studied noninvasive approach [34–37]. Meta-analysis of 24 studies performed in patients undergoing major vascular surgery showed that dipyridamole myocardial perfusion scintigraphy has a sensitivity of 83% and a specificity of 49% for prediction of cardiac death and myocardial infarction [7].

Recently, pharmacological stress echocardiography with dobutamine has also been proposed for risk stratification. This method may also provide information about the presence and severity of coexisting valvular heart disease and to evaluate ventricular function [35–37]. A recent review of 6595 stress tests revealed that the incidence of side effects such as cardiac arrhythmias (8%) and hypotension (3%) was low [7].

Recommendations for exercise or pharmacological stress testing:

Class I Diagnosis of adult patients with intermediate pretest probability of CAD

Prognostic assessment of patients undergoing initial evaluation for suspected or proven CAD; evaluation of subjects with significant chance in clinical status

Demonstration of proof of myocardial ischemia before coronary revascularization

Evaluation of adequacy of medical therapy; prognostic assessment after an acute coronary syndrome

Class IIa Evaluation of exercise capacity when subjective assessment is unreliable

Class IIb Diagnosis of CAD patients with high or low pretest probability; those with resting ST depression less than 1 mm; those undergoing digitalis therapy; and those with ECG criteria for left ventricular hypertrophy

Detection of restenosis in high-risk asymptomatic subjects in the initial months after angioplasty

Class III For exercise stress testing, diagnosis of patients with resting ECG abnormalities that preclude adequate assessment

Severe comorbidity likely to limit life expectancy or candidacy for revascularization

Routine screening of asymptomatic men or women without evi-

dence of CAD
Investigation of isolated ectopic beats in young patients

Preoperative Testing: Which Test to Use?

There are only a few studies comparing the prognostic accuracy of various noninvasive tests used for preoperative cardiac risk assessment. In a meta-analysis of 20 studies, different noninvasive tests were compared according to the predictive value [7]. With the exception of dobutamine stress echocardiography, each of the tests demonstrated a bias for better predictive value in earlier studies. Although dobutamine stress echocardiography appeared to be the best among these tests and ambulatory electrocardiography seemed to have the least predictive value, the data analyzed were not sufficient to determine the optimal test. Meta-analysis of 15 studies showed that the prognostic value of both noninvasive stresses tests had a similar predictive accuracy but the summed odds ratios for cardiac death and myocardial infarction were greater for dobutamine stress echocardiography than for dipyridamole perfusion scintigraphy [7].

Therefore, dobutamine stress echocardiography or perfusion myocardial scintigraphy can be considered. Because stress echocardiography has a higher specificity and adds additional information about valvular and left ventricular dysfunction, it could be considered the favored test. However, the physician's choice of preoperative cardiac testing should also take into account factors such as local expertise and experience, availability, and costs.

Coronary Angiography

For certain patients at high risk, it may be appropriate to proceed with coronary angiography rather than perform a noninvasive test [38]. The following recommendations provide a summary of indications for preoperative coronary angiography in patients before surgery [3].

Class I Patients with suspected or known CAD
Evidence for high risk of adverse outcome based on noninvasive test results
Angina unresponsive to appropriate medical therapy
Unstable angina
Equivocal noninvasive test results in patients at high clinical risk undergoing high-risk surgery

Class IIa Multiple markers of intermediate clinical risk and planned vascular surgery
Moderate to large region of ischemia on noninvasive test
Nondiagnostic noninvasive test results in patients of intermediate clinical risk undergoing high risk noncardiac surgery
Urgent noncardiac surgery while convalescing from acute MI

Class IIb Perioperative MI
Medically stabilized class III or IV angina and planned low-risk or minor surgery

Class III Low-risk noncardiac surgery with known CAD and no high-risk results on noninvasive testing
Asymptomatic after coronary revascularization with excellent exercise capacity
Mild stable angina with good left ventricular function and no high-risk noninvasive test results
Noncandidate for coronary revascularizations owing to concomitant medical illness, severe left ventricular dysfunction, or refusal to consider revascularization
Candidate for liver, lung, or renal transplant more than 40 years old as part of evaluation

Assessing and Reducing the Cardiac Risk of Noncardiac Surgery: Evidence Base

Auerbach and Goldman recently published a review emphasizing available evidence in cardiac risk, after the ACC/AHA and ACP guidelines [39].

Preoperative Clinical Assessment: Developing Initial Estimates of Risk

Consensus-derived algorithms such as those suggested by the AHA/ACC [39] approximate clinical decision making and incorporate specific recommendations. However, differences among algorithms may lead to conflicting advice. Implementation of the AHA/ACC algorithm may reduce length of stay and resource use and improve outcomes. Risk indices, which are derived in hundreds or thousands of patients through the use of rigorous statistical methods and then tested in thousands of patients, require clinicians to sum weights assigned to risk factors and do not automatically provide guidance as to how to act after a score is calculated. In three studies that have prospectively compared risk indices head to head, the Revised Cardiac Risk Index (RCRI) performed best; the original index was the second best in two studies and equivalent to the modified index in the third.

Evidence Limitations

The ACC/AHA and ACP algorithms and risk indices were developed in patients seen a decade or more ago, when perioperative care was quite different.

Summary

The AHA/ACC guidelines and the RCRI are useful, although different, approaches to documenting cardiac risk. The RCRI has been tested extensively and provides accurate estimates of risk that can be used to direct subsequent steps in care.

Use of Exercise Capacity as a Preoperative Screening Tool

Patient report of poor exercise tolerance (e.g., inability to walk at least four blocks) is associated with two-fold-higher odds for postoperative complications and a nearly five-fold increase in odds for myocardial ischemia after adjustment for clinical risk. In the larger RCRI study, however, functional status was not independently associated with risk.

Evidence Limitations

The positive predictive value of poor exercise capacity in the perioperative setting is only 10%, with a negative predictive value of 95%. If patients reduce exertion because of cardiac symptoms but still meet a 4-MET threshold, clinicians will underestimate risk. Conversely, noncardiac functional limitations (e.g., knee or back pain) may overestimate cardiac risk.

Summary

Exercise capacity is most informative when patients report exercise-induced cardiopulmonary symptoms; the ability to exercise to at least 4 METs reduces risk somewhat. Inability to exercise, especially if limitations may not be due to cardiopulmonary symptoms, has a poor positive predictive power and often requires further evaluation.

Valvular Heart Disease

Aortic stenosis carries a strong risk for perioperative complications, with an independent relative risk (RR) of 5.2 for gradients 25–50 mmHg and 6.8 for gradients above 50 mmHg.

Mitral stenosis, seen predominantly in patients who spent their childhoods in developing countries, may be underappreciated clinically and increases the risk of perioperative atrial arrhythmias. Except for risks associated with anticoagulation and a higher risk of endocarditis, no reliable data suggest that patients with prosthetic heart valves have different risks than patients with similar degrees of native valvular disease and heart failure. Other valvular diseases are important primarily because of their association with heart failure or arrhythmias.

Evidence Limitations

Patients with aortic stenosis who are referred for noncardiac surgery are probably healthier than the overall population of patients with aortic stenosis. The true risks are unknown because, in the absence of routine screening echocardiography, some patients go to surgery with undiagnosed aortic stenosis.

Summary

Patients undergoing noncardiac surgery should be assessed by careful cardiac auscultation, with echocardiography in patients with findings suspicious for aortic stenosis. For native valvular lesions other than aortic stenosis and for patients with prosthetic mitral valves, the degree of heart failure is the best indication of risk.

Heart Failure

Heart failure is a well-described risk for postoperative cardiac complications, equivalent to or perhaps even greater than ischemic heart disease.

Evidence Limitations

No data document an optimal approach to managing heart failure before, during, or after noncardiac surgery.

Summary

A general recommendation is to control heart failure optimally preoperatively while avoiding overdiuresis that may exacerbate intraoperative hypotension. β-blockade may not be an appropriate acute therapy because it should be begun and titrated carefully in the outpatient setting.

Arrhythmias

Ventricular and atrial arrhythmias were initially identified as important predictors of perioperative cardiac complications, but subsequent data indicate that this link is explained by the severity of underlying ischemic heart disease and heart failure.

Evidence Limitations

Other than trials to prevent postoperative atrial fibrillation, the evidence base is slim.

Summary

Arrhythmias reflect the severity of coronary disease or heart failure, so preoperative assessment should focus on these possibilities, unless the arrhythmia would warrant treatment independent of the planned surgery. Indications for implantation of pacemakers and cardioverter–defibrillators should follow guidelines used in nonoperative settings.

Systemic Hypertension

Except in one study, hypertension has not been an independent risk factor for perioperative cardiac events unless it is very marked (i.e., systolic blood pressure > 180 mmHg or diastolic pressure > 110 mmHg). In one small randomized trial, patients with a history of hypertension without other cardiac disease and who had a diastolic blood pressure of 110– 130 mmHg on preoperative evaluations were randomized to postponement of surgery until blood pressure was controlled or to proceeding with surgery after intranasal administration of 10 mg nifedipine; neither group had any postoperative cardiac complications or strokes.

Evidence Limitations

Large-scale trials might identify benefits of interventions to address hypertension.

Summary

Patients should continue antihypertensive medications up to the morning of surgery and resume them as soon as possible postoperatively. In patients with underlying cardiovascular disease, limited data support delaying surgery if diastolic pressure exceeds 110 mm Hg.

Pulmonary Hypertension and Congenital Heart Disease

Limited data are available on the risk of perioperative myocardial infarction in patients with pulmonary hypertension, but the mortality rate in these patients is very high (7% in patients with pulmonary artery systolic pressures of 68 mmHg), as are rates of respiratory failure. Adverse outcomes are associated with severity of right ventricular strain, worse functional status, and a history of pulmonary embolism. Data are insufficient to recommend perioperative use of prostacyclin, inhaled nitrous oxide, or sildenafil. Patients with congenital heart disease have a 3.5-fold-increased risk of perioperative complications with noncardiac surgery, with risks depending on the extent of surgery and severity of the underlying abnormality, cyanosis, and heart failure.

Evidence Limitations

No large studies guide perioperative care of pulmonary hypertension or congenital heart disease specifically.

Summary

It is unclear what interventions, except antibiotic prophylaxis, may reduce operative risk in patients with pulmonary hypertension or congenital heart disease.

Refining Initial Risk Estimates: Risk Stratification Tests

Noninvasive Stress Testing

Patients at higher risk after initial evaluation are often referred for noninvasive testing, and three general conclusions are reasonable. First, exercise and pharmacological stress testing have excellent negative predictive values (between 90% and 100%) but poor positive predictive values (between 6% and 67%), making them more useful for reducing risk estimates when negative (or normal) than for identifying very high risk when positive. Second, compared with exercise testing, pharmacological stress tests have superior discriminative power and can be used in patients with functional limitations—the majority of patients referred for noninvasive testing. Third, dobutamine echocardiography may be preferable because of higher specificity, because it assesses ventricular and valvular function as well as pulmonary pressures, and because its findings may be more independent of clinical risk.

Evidence Limitations

Extensive evidence supports the ability of stress testing to provide reassurance when "negative." Clinicians, however, tend to rely too much on "positive" tests. Additionally, most studies enrolled patients at higher risk (e.g., with known coronary disease or undergoing vascular surgery), potentially inflating estimates of positive predictive value and making the sensitivity and specificity of testing in lower risk subgroups less certain.

Summary

Pharmacological stress tests markedly reduce clinical risk estimates in all but the highest-risk patients, in whom additional testing may be appropriate. Whether judicious use of noninvasive tests improves outcomes remains unproved. Dobutamine echocardiography may have superior test characteristics and can provide additional information, but these advantages have yet to be shown to be clinically important. As a result, choices among noninvasive tests should be based on the need to assess valvular or ventricular function and on which test is most reliable and available locally.

Echocardiography

Echocardiograms assess several conditions (e.g., left ventricular dysfunction, aortic stenosis) that pose risks for surgery, but routine echocardiographic screening is not helpful. Preoperative echocardiography is appropriate in patients who meet AHA/ACC clinical guidelines and who would require echocardiography even if no surgery was planned, as well as in patients with a systolic murmur with characteristics (e.g., peaks late, obscures the second heart sound, or is associated with delayed carotid upstroke) suggestive of aortic stenosis, especially in symptomatic patients.

Evidence Limitations

Other than to detect aortic stenosis, evidence to support preoperative echocardiograms is indirect.

Summary

Patients in whom echocardiography would be indicated in the absence of planned surgery and patients with signs or symptoms suggestive of aortic stenosis should have a preoperative echocardiogram.

Approaches to Reducing Risk

Approaches for preventing cardiac complications include practices that are under the purview of the anesthesiologist and surgeon but of which the cardiology consultant should be aware, as well as interventions that are properly recommended or managed by cardiologists.

Risk Stratification in Cardiac Surgery

In cardiac surgery, it has long been accepted that operative or hospital mortality is an indicator of quality of care. This is true to a large extent: death following heart surgery is often due to failure to achieve a satisfactory cardiac outcome; it is itself the cause of major early morbidity as well as poor long-term results. For operative mortality to remain a valid measure of quality of care, it must be related to the risk profile of the patients receiving surgery, hence the need for a reliable risk stratification model [40]. Another reason for the regular use of risk stratification in the assessment of cardiac surgical results is to avoid surgeons and hospitals who treat high-risk patients seeming to have worse results than others [40, 41].

For risk stratification in cardiac surgery we have two scales: the EuroSCORE [40] and the Bedside Estimation of Risk (Bernstein and Parsonnet) [41].

The EuroSCORE has three groups of risk factors with respective weights:

1. *Patient-related factors:* age over 60 (1 per 5 years or part thereof), female gender (1), chronic pulmonary disease (1), extracardiac arteriopathy (2), neurological dysfunction (2), previous cardiac surgery (3), serum creatinine > 200 μmol/l (2), active endocarditis (3), and critical preoperative state (3).
2. *Cardiac factors:* unstable angina on intravenous nitrates (2), reduced left ventricular ejection fraction (30–50%: 1; < pulmonary systolic pressure > 60 mmHg (2).
3. *Operation-related factors:* emergency (2), other than isolated coronary surgery (2), thoracic aorta surgery (3), and surgery for postinfarct septal rupture (4).

In a study of 14 799 patients, the mortality rates per group were: low-risk group (EuroSCORE 1–2): 0.8%, medium-risk group (EuroSCORE 3–5): 3%, and high-risk group (EuroSCORE 6 plus): 11.2% [40]. This is a simple, objective, and up-to-date system for assessing risk in heart surgery.

In 2000, Bernstein and Parsonnet reported the Bedside Estimation of Risk in cardiac surgery through a logistic regression model in which 47 potential risk factors were considered, and a method requiring only simple addition and graphic interpretation was designed for approximating the estimated risk easily and quickly [41].

The risk factors and respective points analyzed by this score system are: female gender (6), age (70–75 years: 2.5, 76–79 years: 7, > 80 years: 11), congestive failure (2.5), severe chronic obstructive pulmonary disease (6), diabetes (3), ejection fraction (30–49%: 6.5, < 30%: 8), hypertension (3), left-mainstem stenosis > 50% (2.5), morbid obesity (1), preoperative intraaortic balloon pump (4), first operation (10), second or subsequent reoperation (20), aortic valve procedure (0), mitral valve procedure (4.5), combination valve procedure and aortocoronary bypass (6). The graphic allows determination of the estimated risk from the total score obtained by summing the individual scores for the risk factors present. It allows an estimate of the risk of surgical mortality faced by an individual patient, as an aid to patients and physicians contemplating cardiac surgery [36].

Implications of Risk Assessment Strategies and Costs

The decision to recommend preoperative evaluation for the individual patient being considered for noncardiac surgery ultimately becomes a balancing act between the estimated probabilities of effectiveness versus risk. The proposed benefit is the possibility of identifying risk factors and comorbidities that might result in significant cardiac morbidity or mortality in the perioperative period or in the long term. In the process of further screening and treatment, the risks from the tests and treatments may offset the potential benefit of evaluation. In addition, cost-effectiveness analyses should be considered.

Successful perioperative evaluation and management of patients undergoing surgery requires careful teamwork and communication between the surgeon, the anesthesiologist, the patient's primary care physician, and the consultant. Evidence-based medicine added to clinical judgment should help the physician get better results. Future research should be directed at determining the real value of more extensive diagnostic testing and interventions.

References

1. Mangano DT (1990) Perioperative cardiac morbidity. Anesthesiology 7:153–184
2. Fleisher LA, Eagle KA (2001) Lowering cardiac risk in noncardiac surgery. N Engl J Med 345:1677–1682
3. Eagle KA, Berger PB, Calkins H et al (2002) ACC/AHA guideline update for perioperative cardiovascular evaluation for noncardiac surgery: a report of the American College of Cardiology/American Heart Association Task Force on Practice Guidelines (Committee to Update the 1996 Guidelines on Perioperative Cardiovascular Evaluation for Noncardiac Surgery). Circulation 105:1257–1267
4. Wong T, Detsky AS (1992) Preoperative cardiac risk assessment for patients having peripheral vascular surgery. Ann Intern Med 116:743–753
5. Wenger NK (1990) A 50-year-old useful report on coronary risk for noncardiac surgery [Editorial]. Am J Cardiol 66:1375–1376
6. Palda VA, Detsky AS (1997) Perioperative assessment and management of risk from coronary artery disease. Ann Intern Med 127:313–3328
7. Devereaux PJ, Goldman L, Cook DJ et al (2005) Perioperative cardiac events in patients undergoing noncardiac surgery: a review of the magnitude of the problem, the pathophysiology of the events and methods to estimate and communicate risk. CMAJ 173:627–634
8. Taylor LM Jr, Porter JM (1987) Basic data related to clinical decision-making in abdominal aortic aneurysms. Ann Vasc Surg 1:502–504
9. Warner MA, Shields SE, Chute CG (1993) Major morbidity and mortality within 1 month of ambulatory surgery and anesthesia. JAMA 270:1437–1441
10. Backer CL, Tinker JH, Robertson DM et al (1980) Myocardial reinfarction following local anesthesia for ophthalmic surgery. Anesth Analg 59:257–262
11. Greenburg AG, Saik RP, Pridham D (1985) Influence of age on mortality of colon

surgery. Am J Surg 150:65–70
12. Plecha FR, Bertin VJ, Plecha EJ et al (1985) The early results of vascular surgery in patients 75 years of age and older: an analysis of 3259 cases. J Vasc Surg 2:769–774
13. Goldman L (1983) Cardiac risks and complications of noncardiac surgery. Ann Intern Med 98:504–513
14. Roger VL, Ballard DJ, Hallett JW Jr et al (1989) Influence of coronary artery disease on morbidity and mortality after abdominal aortic aneurysmectomy: a population-based study. J Am Coll Cardiol 14:1245–1552
15. L'Italien GJ, Cambria RP, Cutler BS et al (1995) Comparative early and late cardiac morbidity among patients requiring different vascular surgery procedures. J Vasc Surg 21:935–944
16. Hlatky MA, Boineau RE, Higginbotham MB et al (1989) A brief self administered questionnaire to determine functional capacity (The Duke Activity Status Index). Am J Cardiol 64:651–654
17. Palda VA, Detsky AS (1997) Guidelines for assessing and managing the perioperative risk from coronary artery disease associates with major noncardiac surgery. Report of the American College of Physicians. Ann Intern Med 127:309–328
18. Eagle KA, Brundage BH, Chaitman BR et al (1996) Guidelines for perioperative cardiovascular evaluation for noncardiac surgery. Report of the American College of Cardiology/American Heart Association Task Force on Guidelines (Committee) On Perioperative Cardiovascular Evaluation for Noncardiac Surgery. Circulation 93:1280–1316
19. Goldman L, Hashimoto B, Cook F et al (1981) Comparative reproducibility and validity of systems for assessing cardiovascular functional class: advantages of a new specific activity scale. Circulation 64:1227–1234
20. Browner WS, Li J, Mangano DT (1992) In-hospital and long-term mortality in male veterans following noncardiac surgery. The Study of Perioperative Ischemia Research Group. JAMA 268:228–32
21. Lee TH, Marcantonio CM et al (1999) Derivation and prospective validation of a simple index for prediction of cardiac risk of major noncardiac surgery. Circulation 100: 1043–1049
22. Gerson MC, Ilurst JM, Ilertzberg VS et al (1985) Cardiac prognosis in noncardiac geriatric surgery. Ann Intern Med 103:832–7
23. Drips RD, Lamont A, Eckenhoff JE (1961) The role of anesthesia on surgical mortality. JAMA 178:261–266
24. Cohen MM, Duncan PG (1988) Physical status score and trends in anesthetic complications. J Clin Epidemiol 41:83–90
25. Owend WD, Dykes MI, Gilbert JP et al (1975) Development of two indices of postoperative morbidity. Surgery 77:586–592
26. Menke IL, Klein A, John KD et al (1993) Predictive value of ASA classification for the assessment of perioperative risk. Int Surg 78:266–270
27. Goldman L, Caldera DL, Nussbaum SR et al (1977) Multifactorial index of cardiac risk in noncardiac surgical procedures. N Engl J Med 297:845–850
28. Detsky AS, Abrams HB, McLaughlin JR et al (1986) Predicting cardiac complications in patients undergoing non-cardiac surgery. J Gen Intern Med 1:211–219
29. Fletcher JP, Antico VF, Gruenewald S et al (1989) Risk of aortic aneurysm surgery as assessed by preoperative gated heart pool scan. Br J Surg 76:26–28
30. Pedersen T, Kelbaek H, Munck O (1990) Cardiopulmonary complications in high-risk surgical patients: the value of preoperative radionuclide cardiography. Acta Anaesthesiol Scand 34:183–189

31. Lazor L, Russel JC, DaSilva J et al (1988) Use of the multiple uptake gated acquisition scan for the preoperative assessment of cardiac risk. Surg Gynecol Obstet 167:234–238
32. Pasternack PF, Imparato AM, Bear G et al (1984) The value of radionuclide angiography as a predictor of perioperative myocardial infarction in patients undergoing abdominal aortic aneurysms resection. J Vasc Surg 1:320–325
33. Mosley JG, Clarke JM, Ell PJ, Marston A (1985) Assessment of myocardial function before aortic surgery by radionuclide angiocardiography. Br J Surg 72:886–887
34. Fiser WP, Thompson BW, Thompson AR et al (1983) Nuclear cardiac ejection fraction and cardiac index in abdominal aortic surgery. Surgery 94:736–739
35. Halm EA, Browner WS, Tubau JF et al (1996) Echocardiography for assessing cardiac risk in patients having noncardiac surgery. Ann Intern Med 125:433–441
36. Kertai MD, Klein J, Bax JJ et al (2005) Predicting perioperative cardiac risk. Prog Cardiovasc Dis 47:240–257
37. Scanlon PJ, Faxon DP, Audet AM et al (1999) ACC/AHA guidelines for coronary angiography: a report of the American College of Cardiology/American Heart Association Task Force on practice guidelines (Committee on Coronary Angiography). Developed in collaboration with the Society for Cardiac Angiography and Interventions. J Am Coll Cardiol 33:1756–1824
38. Karthikeyan G, Bhargava B (2006) Managing patients undergoing non-cardiac surgery: need to shift emphasis from risk stratification to risk modification. Heart 92:17–20
39. Auerbach A, Goldman L (2006) Assessing and reducing the cardiac risk of noncardiac surgery. Circulation 113:1361–1376
40. Nashef SAM, Roques F, Michel P et al (1999) European system for cardiac operative risk evaluation (EuroSCORE). Eur J Cardiothorac Surg 16:9–13
41. Bernstein AD, Parsonnet V (2000) Bedside estimation of risk as an aid for decision-making in cardiac surgery. Ann Thorac Surg 69:823–828

8 Hemodynamic Monitoring in Patients with Acute Heart Failure

J.-L. Vincent and R. Holsten

Introduction

Acute heart failure has been defined simply as "the rapid onset of symptoms and signs secondary to abnormal cardiac function" [1]. Acute heart failure can present de novo with no prior history of heart disease (although asymptomatic cardiac disease may well have been present), or on a background of decompensated chronic cardiac failure. Acute heart failure is, therefore, a syndrome with varying etiologies and ranging in severity from relatively mild dyspnea, through severe pulmonary edema with acute respiratory distress, to full-blown cardiogenic shock, where tissue perfusion is compromised. Whatever the etiology, the result is an inability of the heart to maintain cardiac output, and hence oxygen supply, sufficient to meet the needs of the peripheral tissues.

Ischemic heart disease is the underlying cause of acute heart failure in 60–70% of patients [2, 3], particularly in the elderly. In younger patients, cardiomyopathy, myocarditis, and arrhythmias present relatively more commonly. In-hospital mortality rates from acute heart failure have been reported to be between 2% and 7% [2, 4, 5], but these can rise to as high as 80% in patients with cardiogenic shock [6]. Many patients with acute heart failure will be admitted to an intensive care unit (ICU) [4], and many of these patients will have severe disease or cardiogenic shock. In such patients, close hemodynamic monitoring—the collection and analysis of qualitative and quantitative data of cardiopulmonary function—is essential to ensure that adequate organ blood flow and oxygenation are maintained. Hemodynamic monitoring includes clinical observation, and various noninvasive and inva-

Department of Intensive Care, Erasme University Hospital, Free University of Brussels, Belgium

sive measures, which will be discussed briefly below. In addition to categorizing each patient's clinical condition, hemodynamic data can help to determine appropriate therapy. Importantly, monitoring is of little value in itself: it is the interpretation and application of the data obtained which is crucial.

Hemodynamic Monitoring in Acute Heart Failure

The hemodynamic monitoring of the patient with acute heart failure should be initiated as soon as a diagnosis is made, but the precise nature of the monitoring will depend on the severity of the heart failure and on the patient's response to therapy. Monitoring of electrocardiogram, blood pressure, and heart rate must be conducted routinely in all patients with heart failure. Central hemodynamic monitoring should be considered in all patients with acute heart failure, and many patients admitted to the ICU with heart failure will require invasive hemodynamic monitoring. Guidelines have been developed, largely based on expert opinion [1].

Invasive Monitoring

Arterial Line

Noninvasive measurement of blood pressure is one of the most widely used procedures in clinical medicine, but in patients in intensive care, accuracy of measurement is critical, particularly in patients with low blood pressure. Intra-arterial monitoring of pressure is more precise in such patients, may be more comfortable for the patient, and has the additional benefit of being continuous [7]. It is also essential to monitor closely the effects of vasodilating therapies. Many such patients also require multiple arterial blood analyses, which can be done through the same line. The complication rate for the insertion of a radial or femoral artery catheter is low [8].

Central Venous Line

Central venous lines provide access to the central venous circulation and are therefore useful for the delivery of fluids and drugs. These lines are usually inserted via the subclavian or internal jugular veins. They can also be used to monitor the central venous pressure (CVP), which provides a measure of circulatory filling and cardiac preload, and central venous oxygen saturation ($ScvO_2$), which provides an indication of the adequacy of oxygen utilization.

$ScvO_2$ monitoring has seen a surge in interest since the study by Rivers et al. demonstrated improved outcomes in patients with sepsis managed by early goal-directed therapy in which one of the targets was an $ScvO_2 > 70\%$

[9]. Of course, the goal should not be to reach a normal $ScvO_2$ in patients with heart failure. There has been considerable debate regarding whether $ScvO_2$ can be used as a surrogate for mixed venous oxygen saturation (SvO_2). Although $ScvO_2$ is physiologically lower than SvO_2, it is approximately 10% higher than SvO_2 in stable acutely ill patients, and this difference may vary even more under septic conditions [10, 11]. Nevertheless, several studies have demonstrated a good correlation between $ScvO_2$ and SvO_2 [12], particularly when changes over time are considered [10, 13], and if a pulmonary artery catheter (PAC), allowing measurement of SvO_2, is not required for other reasons, it would seem reasonable to use $ScvO_2$ as an indicator of the adequacy of tissue oxygenation.

The CVP is measured at the junction of the superior vena cava and the right atrium, and provides an estimate of right atrial pressure. The typical CVP waveform is complex with three ascending waves (a, c, and v) and two descents (x and y). This typical waveform is altered in certain diseases, such as atrial fibrillation, tricuspid regurgitation, and pericardial disease. In addition, the CVP is influenced by changes in thoracic pressure, including during respiration, and by the application of positive end-expiratory pressure (PEEP). The CVP is monitored by a pressure transducer, situated at the level of the right atrium, linked to a monitor that can show the pressure wave continuously. Ideally, the CVP is measured at the onset of the c wave, the start of ventricular systole, this indicating right ventricular end-diastolic pressure. However, most monitoring systems measure a mean CVP value over the whole cardiac cycle, and average this value over several cycles. The CVP is often used as a measure of preload, and hence as an indicator of likely response to fluid infusion, although the effectiveness of CVP in this role has not been convincingly demonstrated. Nevertheless, many ICU patients will require a central venous line for other reasons (large fluid infusions, drugs, etc.) and CVP measurement can therefore be performed without additional risk to the patient. The normal CVP range is 3–8 cmH_2O. A low CVP can certainly indicate a low intravascular volume, but normal or high values do not necessarily exclude this. The limitations of CVP measurements must be stressed, including that they may be misleading in patients with significant tricuspid regurgitation, pulmonary hypertension, or tension pneumothorax. PEEP ventilation can also affect the CVP waveform. Risks of central venous line insertion include hematoma, subclavian or superior vena caval thrombosis, pulmonary embolization, pneumothorax, hemothorax, ventricular arrhythmia, cardiac perforation, and infection.

The central venous line, with an arterial line, may also be used to measure cardiac output. The pulse contour cardiac output (e.g., PiCCO, Pulsion Medical Systems, Munich, Germany) system monitors temperature changes in the arterial system after injection of a cold saline bolus intravenously. The cardiac output is then calculated by analysis of the thermodilution curve using the Stewart–Hamilton algorithm. The lithium dilution cardiac output (e.g., LiDCOplus, LiDCO, Cambridge, UK) uses the measurement of the arterial lithium concentration after a small intravenous bolus injection of lithium and development of a concentration–time curve to calculate the cardiac output [14]. This technique cannot be used in patients being treated with lithium and nondepolarizing muscle relaxants interfere with calibration. Using either technique, other parameters can also be estimated including pulse pressure variation and stroke volume variation, which can indicate fluid responsiveness [15]. Measurement of cardiac output with these techniques has been validated against standard PAC thermodilution cardiac output [16–19], and they may be of use in patients who do not require a PAC.

Pulmonary Artery Catheter

The PAC possesses at its tip an inflatable balloon that allows it to move with the blood by flotation. Introduced intravenously, usually via the subclavian or internal jugular veins, the PAC progresses through the right atrium and ventricle to the pulmonary artery. The PAC was initially developed to measure the pulmonary artery occlusion pressure (PAOP), measured from the distal end of the catheter but with the balloon briefly inflated. The inflated balloon is carried by the flow of blood and wedges in a branch of the PA, occluding blood flow distal to this point. The pressure measured at this time thus represents the pressure that exists beyond the pulmonary capillaries, i.e., the pressure present in the left atrium, which, in the absence of any abnormality of the mitral valve, is itself equal to the filling pressure in the left ventricle, thus providing an indication of left ventricular preload. However, the PAC also provides measurement of right atrial pressure (equivalent to the CVP), right ventricular pressure, and pulmonary artery pressures. The PAC can be equipped with a thermistor, which can measure the blood temperature several centimeters from the distal end of the catheter, allowing calculation of the cardiac output by the so-called thermodilution technique. The rapid injection of cold fluid into the right atrium (through the proximal lumen of the PAC) causes a transient reduction in the temperature of the blood in the pulmonary artery. Computerized analysis of the thermodilution curve produced by this technique allows reliable calculation of the cardiac output. PACs can also be equipped with a system of intraventricular thermistors, which enable almost continuous measurement of cardiac output without need for injection of cold water (e.g., Vigilance, Edwards, Life Sciences, Irvine, CA, USA). The PAC can also be used to measure the SvO_2 as venous blood from all parts of the body is collected and mixed in the right heart chambers before passing through the pulmonary capillaries. SvO_2 can be measured either intermittently by repeated blood withdrawal, or continuously if the PAC is equipped with fiberoptic fibers that transmit light at different wavelengths, allowing measurement of oxygen saturation by reflectance oximetry.

There has been considerable debate in recent years over the need for PA catheterization in ICU patients. Several studies have suggested that the use of the PAC in critically ill patients may result in worse outcomes [20–22], although others have not confirmed these findings [23–29]. In a randomized controlled trial of patients with severe symptomatic and recurrent heart failure, the ESCAPE study, Binanay et al. reported that management guided by clinical assessment and PAC-derived data was not superior to management guided by clinical assessment alone [30]. This study [30] was terminated early because of the significant number of excess adverse events noted in the PAC group (4.2%), and the lack of any likely benefit of PAC on the primary end point of days alive out of the hospital at 6 months.

The results from ESCAPE and other studies suggest that a PAC should probably not be used routinely in all patients with acute heart failure, but PAC use is recommended in hemodynamically unstable patients who are not responding in a predictable fashion to traditional treatments, and in patients with a combination of congestion and hypoperfusion [1]. The acquisition of PAC-derived data in such patients can allow for a comprehensive evaluation of hemodynamic status and be of value in guiding therapy. Interpretation of PAC-derived data must take into account the presence of conditions such as mitral stenosis or aortic regurgitation, pulmonary occlusion, ventricular interdependence, and high airway pressures, in which PAOP values may be inaccurate. Severe tricuspid regurgitation, frequently found in patients with acute heart failure, can lead to overestimation or underestimation of the cardiac output value measured by thermodilution.

The risks associated with PA catheterization are similar to those seen with insertion of a central line and are listed in Table 1. Importantly, the PAC should be removed as soon as it is no longer necessary (with the patient hemodynamically stable and therapy optimized).

Less-Invasive Hemodynamic Monitoring

With many raising concerns about the benefits, or lack thereof, of invasive monitoring systems, many researchers have focused on the development of reliable alternatives, particularly for the monitoring of cardiac output and related hemodynamic parameters.

Table 1. Potential complications of pulmonary artery catheterization

Problems due to difficult insertion:
- Pneumothorax
- Hematoma at the site of puncture (particularly if the carotid artery is used)
- Air embolus
- Damage to local structures including nerves

Arrhythmias:
- Extrasystoles, supraventricular and ventricular, by irritation of the endocardium (particularly as the catheter passes through the right ventricle)
- Right bundle branch block; carries the risk of complete atrioventricular block if there is preexisting left bundle branch block

Catheter knotting
Endocardial and valvular damage
Thrombosis and pulmonary infarction
Pulmonary artery rupture
Infection

Echocardiography

Echocardiography is an essential tool for evaluating the underlying etiology of acute heart failure, particularly in terms of structural cardiac abnormalities, but is increasingly also being used to monitor cardiac output and ventricular volumes. Echo-Doppler studies are very useful in the initial evaluation of the patient with acute heart failure, to evaluate left and right heart functions and valvular function. Echo-Doppler can guide initial fluid and vasoactive drug therapy. Various hemodynamic variables can be estimated using different echocardiography techniques, including cardiac output, pulmonary artery pressure, PAOP, left atrial pressure, pulmonary vascular resistance, and transvalvular pressures [31, 32]. Transesophageal echocardiography can be used to calculate cardiac output using Doppler beams across a cardiac valve or by measuring Doppler flow velocity in the descending aorta [33]. However, both techniques require considerable operator skill, and studies have demonstrated inconsistent results in terms of correlation with PAC thermodilution cardiac output [34, 35]. These techniques may be more suitable for monitoring changes in cardiac output over time.

Bioimpedance

This is a noninvasive technique that uses variation in the impedance to flow of a high-frequency, low-magnitude alternating current across the thorax or the whole body to generate a measured waveform from which cardiac output can be calculated by a modification of the pulse contour method. Some [36, 37], but not all [38], studies have shown fair to moderate agreement between bioimpedance- and thermodilution-derived cardiac output. Cotter et al.

reported a correlation of 0.851 between whole body bioimpedance and thermodilution cardiac output in patients with acute heart failure [39], and Albert et al. similarly reported a correlation coefficient of 0.89 between thoracic impedance and thermodilution in patients with acutely decompensated complex heart failure [40]. However, bioimpedance can be unreliable in patients with pronounced aortic disease, significant edema or pleural effusion, and increased PEEP [33]. Movement artifacts can also be problematic.

Partial CO_2 Rebreathing

With the partial CO_2 rebreathing method, changes in CO_2 elimination and end-tidal CO_2 in response to a brief rebreathing period are used to estimate cardiac output. In patients undergoing cardiac or vascular surgery, several studies have reported good agreement between the partial CO_2 rebreathing technique and thermodilution cardiac output [41, 42], although others have reported poor agreement [43]. This technique is quite unreliable in patients with respiratory failure [33].

Integration into Clinical Practice

Effective hemodynamic monitoring of the patient with acute heart failure can help diagnosis of the underlying etiology and monitor changes in condition over time in response to therapeutic interventions. Critically, however, attaching a patient to one or multiple hemodynamic monitoring devices will not on its own improve that patient's outcome—hemodynamic monitoring can only be effective when the data it supplies are correctly interpreted and applied.

In the patient with acute heart failure, the traditional hemodynamic targets for therapy have been to reduce PAOP and/or increase cardiac output. Additional targets may include control of blood pressure, preservation of renal function, and myocardial protection [44]. Results from hemodynamic monitoring must be taken in conjunction with a full and repeated clinical examination, including signs and symptoms of pulmonary congestion, such as dyspnea, orthopnea, abdominal discomfort, and rales. Noninvasive monitoring can provide information on a variety of hemodynamic parameters including blood pressure, heart rate, cardiac output, PAOP, right atrial pressure, and pulmonary artery pressures. Insertion of an arterial line and a central line are frequently necessary in patients with severe acute heart failure and can be used to assess CVP and $ScvO_2$. In patients with continuing hemodynamic instability who fail to respond to standard therapy, insertion of a PAC can provide additional, semicontinuous information on filling pressures and SvO_2. The PAC can be of particular use in evaluating complex clinical scenarios where heart failure is just one component in a patient with multiple pathologies, and in the evaluation of elevated right-sided pressures in a patient with concomitant pulmonary and cardiac disease.

References

1. Nieminen MS, Bohm M, Cowie MR et al (2005) Executive summary of the guidelines on the diagnosis and treatment of acute heart failure: the Task Force on Acute Heart Failure of the European Society of Cardiology. Eur Heart J 26:384–416
2. Rudiger A, Harjola VP, Muller A et al (2005) Acute heart failure: clinical presentation, one-year mortality and prognostic factors. Eur J Heart Fail 7:662–670
3. Zannad F, Mebazaa A, Juilliere Y et al (2006) Clinical profile, contemporary management and one-year mortality in patients with severe acute heart failure syndromes: The EFICA study. Eur J Heart Fail Mar 2 [Epub ahead of print]
4. Fonarow GC (2003) The Acute Decompensated Heart Failure National Registry (ADHERE): opportunities to improve care of patients hospitalized with acute decompensated heart failure. Rev Cardiovasc Med 4(Suppl7):S21-S30
5. Tavazzi L, Maggioni AP, Lucci D et al (2006) Nationwide survey on acute heart failure in cardiology ward services in Italy. Eur Heart J 27:1207–1215
6. Tayara W, Starling RC, Yamani MH, Wazni O, Jubran F, Smedira N (2006) Improved survival after acute myocardial infarction complicated by cardiogenic shock with circulatory support and transplantation: comparing aggressive intervention with conservative treatment. J Heart Lung Transplant 25:504–509
7. Bennett D (2005) Arterial pressure: a personal view. In: Pinskly MR et al (eds) Functional hemodynamic monitoring. Springer, Berlin Heidelberg New York, pp 89–97
8. Frezza EE, Mezghebe H (1998) Indications and complications of arterial catheter use in surgical or medical intensive care units: analysis of 4932 patients. Am Surg 64:127–131
9. Rivers E, Nguyen B, Havstad S et al (2001) Early goal-directed therapy in the treatment of severe sepsis and septic shock. N Engl J Med 345:1368–1377
10. Reinhart K, Kuhn HJ, Hartog C, Bredle DL (2004) Continuous central venous and pulmonary artery oxygen saturation monitoring in the critically ill. Intensive Care Med 30:1572–1578
11. Edwards JD, Mayall RM (1998) Importance of the sampling site for measurement of mixed venous oxygen saturation in shock. Crit Care Med 26:1356–1360
12. Ladakis C, Myrianthefs P, Karabinis A et al (2001) Central venous and mixed venous oxygen saturation in critically ill patients. Respiration 68:279–285
13. Dueck MH, Klimek M, Appenrodt S et al (2005) Trends but not individual values of central venous oxygen saturation agree with mixed venous oxygen saturation during varying hemodynamic conditions. Anesthesiology 103:249–257
14. Pearse RM, Ikram K, Barry J (2004) Equipment review: an appraisal of the LiDCO plus method of measuring cardiac output. Crit Care 8:190–195
15. De Backer D, Heenen S, Piagnerelli M et al (2005) Pulse pressure variations to predict fluid responsiveness: influence of tidal volume. Intensive Care Med 31:517–523
16. Goedje O, Hoeke K, Lichtwarck-Aschoff M et al (1999) Continuous cardiac output by femoral arterial thermodilution calibrated pulse contour analysis: comparison

with pulmonary arterial thermodilution. Crit Care Med 27:2407–2412

17. Sakka SG, Reinhart K, Wegscheider K, Meier-Hellmann A (2000) Is the placement of a pulmonary artery catheter still justified solely for the measurement of cardiac output? J Cardiothorac Vasc Anesth 14:119–124
18. Linton R, Band D, O'Brien T et al (1997) Lithium dilution cardiac output measurement: a comparison with thermodilution. Crit Care Med 25:1796–1800
19. Kurita T, Morita K, Kato S et al (1997) Comparison of the accuracy of the lithium dilution technique with the thermodilution technique for measurement of cardiac output. Br J Anaesth 79:770–775
20. Connors AF, Speroff T, Dawson NV et al (1996) The effectiveness of right heart catheterization in the initial care of critically ill patients. JAMA 276:889–897
21. Polanczyk CA, Rohde LE, Goldman L et al (2001) Right heart catheterization and cardiac complications in patients undergoing noncardiac surgery: an observational study. JAMA 286:309–314
22. Peters SG, Afessa B, Decker PA et al (2003) Increased risk associated with pulmonary artery catheterization in the medical intensive care unit. J Crit Care 18:166–171
23. Murdoch SD, Cohen AT, Bellamy MC (2000) Pulmonary artery catheterization and mortality in critically ill patients. Br J Anaesth 85:611–615
24. Afessa B, Spencer S, Khan W et al (2001) Association of pulmonary artery catheter use with in-hospital mortality. Crit Care Med 29:1145–1148
25. Yu DT, Platt R, Lanken PN et al (2003) Relationship of pulmonary artery catheter use to mortality and resource utilization in patients with severe sepsis. Crit Care Med 31:2734–2741
26. Rhodes A, Cusack RJ, Newman PJ et al (2002) A randomised, controlled trial of the pulmonary artery catheter in critically ill patients. Intensive Care Med 28:256–264
27. Sandham JD, Hull RD, Brant RF et al (2003) A randomized, controlled trial of the use of pulmonary-artery catheters in high-risk surgical patients. N Engl J Med 348:5–14
28. Chittock DR, Dhingra VK, Ronco JJ et al (2004) Severity of illness and risk of death associated with pulmonary artery catheter use. Crit Care Med 32:911–915
29. Sakr Y, Vincent JL, Reinhart K et al (2005) Use of the pulmonary artery catheter is not associated with worse outcome in the intensive care unit. Chest 128:2722–2731
30. Binanay C, Califf RM, Hasselblad V et al (2005) Evaluation study of congestive heart failure and pulmonary artery catheterization effectiveness: the ESCAPE trial. JAMA 294:1625–1633
31. Nohria A, Mielniczuk LM, Stevenson LW (2005) Evaluation and monitoring of patients with acute heart failure syndromes. Am J Cardiol 96:32G-40G
32. McLean AS , Huang SJ (2006) Intensive care echocardiogrphy. In: Vincent JL (ed) Yearbook of intensive care and emergency medicine. Springer, Berlin Heidelberg New York, pp 131–141
33. Hofer CK, Zollinger A (2006) Less invasive cardiac output monitoring: characteristics and limitations. In: Vincent JL (ed) Yearbook of intensive care and emergency medicine. Springer, Berlin Heidelberg New York, pp 162–175
34. Bettex DA, Hinselmann V, Hellermann JP et al (2004) Transoesophageal echocardiography is unreliable for cardiac output assessment after cardiac surgery compared with thermodilution. Anaesthesia 59:1184–1192
35. Dark PM, Singer M (2004) The validity of trans-esophageal Doppler ultrasonography as a measure of cardiac output in critically ill adults. Intensive Care Med 30:2060–2066

36. Sageman WS, Riffenburgh RH, Spiess BD (2002) Equivalence of bioimpedance and thermodilution in measuring cardiac index after cardiac surgery. J Cardiothorac Vasc Anesth 16:8–14
37. Spiess BD, Patel MA, Soltow LO, Wright IH (2001) Comparison of bioimpedance versus thermodilution cardiac output during cardiac surgery: evaluation of a second-generation bioimpedance device. J Cardiothorac Vasc Anesth 15:567–573
38. Hirschl MM, Kittler H, Woisetschlager C et al (2000) Simultaneous comparison of thoracic bioimpedance and arterial pulse waveform-derived cardiac output with thermodilution measurement. Crit Care Med 28:1798–1802
39. Cotter G, Moshkovitz Y, Kaluski E et al (2004) Accurate, noninvasive continuous monitoring of cardiac output by whole-body electrical bioimpedance. Chest 125:1431–1440
40. Albert NM, Hail MD, Li J, Young JB (2004) Equivalence of the bioimpedance and thermodilution methods in measuring cardiac output in hospitalized patients with advanced, decompensated chronic heart failure. Am J Crit Care 13:469–479
41. Botero M, Kirby D, Lobato EB et al (2004) Measurement of cardiac output before and after cardiopulmonary bypass: comparison among aortic transit-time ultrasound, thermodilution, and noninvasive partial CO2 rebreathing. J Cardiothorac Vasc Anesth 18:563–572
42. Kotake Y, Moriyama K, Innami Y et al (2003) Performance of noninvasive partial CO2 rebreathing cardiac output and continuous thermodilution cardiac output in patients undergoing aortic reconstruction surgery. Anesthesiology 99:283–288
43. Mielck F, Buhre W, Hanekop G et al (2003) Comparison of continuous cardiac output measurements in patients after cardiac surgery. J Cardiothorac Vasc Anesth 17:211–216
44. Gheorghiade M, Zannad F, Sopko G et al (2005) Acute heart failure syndromes: current state and framework for future research. Circulation 112:3958–3968

9 Electrocardiography of Heart Failure: Features and Arrhythmias

J. L. Atlee

While this chapter addresses the electrocardiographic (ECG) features of heart failure (HF) and physiologically significant arrhythmias in patients with HF, neither ECG findings nor specific arrhythmias establish the diagnosis of HF, regardless of its origin. The diagnosis of HF is established by the patient's symptoms and physical signs, along with confirmatory evidence of mechanical heart dysfunction (e.g., by echocardiography or cardiac catheterization). HF can be due to systolic and/or diastolic dysfunction affecting one or both ventricles. Regardless of which, because of ventricular interdependence, HF ultimately leads to compromise of both systemic and pulmonary hemodynamics. Unchecked, the end result is multiorgan system failure and death, whether HF results from congenital or acquired heart disease. This chapter highlights the ECG features of HF and arrhythmias in patients with HF.

Heart Failure: Definitions and Perspectives

Heart failure is a complex clinical syndrome that results from structural or functional disorders that impair the ability of the ventricle(s) to fill with blood (diastolic HF) or eject blood (systolic HF) [1]. The primary symptoms of HF are dyspnea and fatigue, which may limit exercise tolerance and lead to fluid retention as pulmonary congestion (left-sided HF) and/or peripheral edema (right-sided HF). Either can impair the functional capacity and quality of life in affected individuals, but they do not necessarily dominate the

Department of Anesthesiology, Medical College of Wisconsin, Milwaukee, WI 53226, USA

clinical picture at the same time. Since not all patients have volume overload ("congestion" as pulmonary or peripheral edema at the time of initial or subsequent evaluation), "HF" is now preferred to the older term "congestive HF" [2]. The term "myocardial failure" denotes abnormal systolic or diastolic function. It may be asymptomatic or may become symptomatic. Further, myocardial failure is not synonymous with "circulatory failure." The latter may be caused by a variety of noncardiac conditions (e.g., hemorrhagic or septic shock) in patients with preserved myocardial function. Finally, "cardiomyopathy" and "left ventricular dysfunction" are more general terms that describe abnormalities of cardiac structure or function, either or both of which may lead to HF.

The clinical manifestations of HF vary and depend on many factors, including the patient's age, the extent to which and rate at which cardiac performance becomes impaired, and the ventricular chamber first involved in the process. The clinical stages of HF include a broad spectrum of severity of impaired cardiac function, from mild (manifest only during stress) to advanced forms in which the heart requires pharmacologic or mechanical support to sustain life (Table 1).

Table 1. Clinical stages of heart failure (HF) as defined by the American College of Cardiology and American Heart Association

Stage	Description	Examples
A	At high risk for developing HF due to existing conditions that are strongly associated with its development No identified structural or functional abnormalities of the pericardium, myocardium, or cardiac valves No history or symptoms or signs of HF	Systemic hypertension Coronary artery disease Diabetes mellitus History of cardiotoxic drug therapy History of alcohol abuse Family history of cardiomyopathy
B	Presence of structural heart disease that is strongly associated with the development of HF No history or signs or symptoms of HF	Left ventricular hypertrophy or fibrosis Left ventricular dilatation or dysfunction Asymptomatic valvular heart disease Previous myocardial dysfunction
C	Current or prior symptoms of HF associated with underlying structural heart disease	Dyspnea or fatigue due to left ventricular systolic dysfunction
		Asymptomatic patients on therapy for prior symptoms of HF

continue →

Table 1 *continue*

Stage	Description	Examples
D	Advanced structural heart disease and marked symptoms of HF despite maximal medical therapy	Frequent HF hospitalizations and cannot be discharged In the hospital awaiting heart transplant
	HF that requires specialized interventions	At home with continuous inotropic or mechanical circulatory support In hospice setting for the management of HF

Adapted from [2]

Finally, in one study of patients admitted nonelectively to an urban university hospital with the diagnosis of HF, precipitating factors for HF could be identified in 66% of 435 patients [3]. Perhaps the most common cause of decompensation in a previously compensated patient with HF is inappropriate reduction in the intensity of treatment, be it dietary sodium and fluid restriction, drug therapy, or both [1]. Sodium and fluid retention may be the result of dietary excesses incurred by vacations and travel or patient noncompliance with or removal by the physician of effective pharmacotherapy.

Electrocardiographic Features of Heart Failure

There are no ECG features that are specific to HF. Rather, there are ECG findings in patients with structural heart disease, whether congenital or acquired, that reflect myocardial remodeling or specific chamber enlargement or dilation. Discussed are: right and left atrial abnormalities (or enlargement), and ventricular hypertrophy and enlargement [4, 5]. Not discussed are ECG changes associated with other processes (e.g., coronary artery disease, cardiomyopathies, infectious processes, drug-induced or environmental toxicities) that adversely affect the heart and may ultimately lead to HF. Unless otherwise stated, all discussion below applies to adults.[1]

[1] In the neonate, the right ventricle is more hypertrophied than the left because there is greater resistance in the pulmonary than in the systemic circulation during fetal development [5]. Right-sided resistance is greatly diminished when the lungs fill with air. Left-sided resistance becomes greatly increased when the placenta is removed. From this time on, the ECG evidence of right-sided ventricular predominance is gradually lost as the left ventricle becomes "hypertrophied" in relation to the right ventricle.

Left and Right Atrial Abnormalities (Enlargement)

Various pathological and pathophysiological events can affect the normal sequence of atrial activation and produce abnormal P waves in the surface ECG. These are best appreciated with full 12-lead ECG. Abnormal P waves are also seen with non-sinus-origin P waves generated by subsidiary or latent atrial pacemakers found along the sulcus terminalis, or in Bachmann's bundle, the coronary sinus ostia, or the tricuspid annulus [6]. Most commonly, the ECG with subsidiary atrial pacemaker rhythms (e.g., wandering atrial pacemaker; ectopic atrial rhythm) records bifid, negative, or nearly isoelectric P waves in leads with normally upright P waves (i.e., I, II, aVF, and V_4 through V_6) [4-6]. Also, a negative P wave in lead I suggests left atrial rhythm [4]. Apparent left atrial rhythms can arise in the pulmonary vein orifices and may play a role in the generation of atrial fibrillation [4, 7]. However, because of the uncertainties of localizing the origin of atrial rhythms with such unusual P waves, collectively, these rhythms or tachycardias (with atrial rates > 120 beats/min–adults) are referred to as ectopic atrial rhythms or tachycardias.

Left Atrial Abnormality (Enlargement)

Anatomical or functional abnormalities of the left atrium can alter the morphology, duration, and amplitude of the P waves in the clinical ECG [4, 5]. Specific ECG findings with left atrial abnormalities (a term preferred to "left atrial enlargement" [4]) include increased amplitude and duration of the P waves in the limb leads, as well as an increase in the amplitude of the terminal negative portion of the P wave in lead V_1 (and leads II, III, and aVF if extreme [5]). Such abnormal patterns reflect increased left atrial mass or chamber size, or conduction delays within the atria. Increased P wave amplitudes are due to increased atrial mass. Because the left atrium is usually activated late during the inscription of the P wave, the effects of increased left atrial mass and electrical force increase P wave duration and augment the P terminal force in the right precordial leads. In addition, these patterns correlate with delayed interatrial conduction, which prolongs the P wave and shortens the P-R interval. It also reduces the overlap between right and left atrial activation, so that the ECG patterns generated by each atrium may be separated as two humps in lead II (*P mitrale*). Common criteria for diagnosing left atrial abnormality (enlargement) are listed in Table 2. However, the diagnostic accuracy of these criteria is limited. For example, one report discussed by Mirvus and Goldberger[2] [4] showed that various P wave mor-

[2] The cited report (Hazen MS, Marwick TH, Underwood DA (1991) Diagnostic accuracy of the resting electrocardiogram in detection and estimation of left atrial enlargement: an echocardiographic correlation in 551 patients. Am Heart J 122:823-828

Table 2. Electrocardiographic diagnostic criteria suggestive of left and right atrial abnormalities (enlargement)

Left atrial abnormality (enlargement)	Right atrial abnormality (enlargement)[a]
1. P wave duration >120 ms (lead V_1 or II)	1. Does not affect the duration of the P wave
2. Conspicuous notching ("humping"; " M-like") of P waves (V_1 or II), with an interval between notches ≥ 0.04 s (*P mitrale*)	2. Peaked ("A-like") appearance to P waves (amplitudes > 0.2 mV) in leads II and aVF, and > 0.1 mV in V_1 and V_2 (*P pulmonale*)
3. Ratio between the duration of the P wave (lead II) and the P–R interval > 1.6	3. Possible *rightward shift* of mean P wave axis to > 75°
4. Increased duration and deepening of the terminal negative portion of the P wave in V_1 causing the area subtended by the P wave to exceed 0.04 s. Usually, does not increase overall amplitude of the P wave, unless extreme. If it does, the terminal portion of P wave may become negative in leads II, III and aVF as well	4. Increased area under initial positive portion of P wave in lead V_1 to > 0.06 millimeter seconds
5 Possible *leftward shift* of the mean P wave axis to between –30° and +45°	

Adapted from criteria given in [4], p 120, and [5], p 75

[a] In addition to criteria based on P-wave morphologies, right atrial abnormalities (enlargement) are suggested by QRS changes: (1) Q waves (especially, qR patterns) in the right precordial leads without evidence of myocardial infarction, and (2) low amplitude (< 600 μV) QRS complexes in lead V_1 with a ≥ 3-fold increase in their amplitude in lead V_2

phologies (e.g., *P mitrale*) (in body surface ECG) were found to be poorly sensitive (20%), but highly specific (98%), for detecting echocardiographically enlarged left atria.

Combinations of P wave morphologies did not improve sensitivity or specificity of surface ECG. Surface ECG features did give an estimate of the magnitude of LA enlargement. When PTFVl (P wave terminal forces in ECG lead V_1) were ≥ 0.040 sec.mm, 95% of patients had a left atrial size of ≥ 40 mm. Further, when when PTFVl was ≥ 0.060 sec.mm, 75% had a left atrial size ≥ 60 mm. Thus, these PTFVl criteria for LA enlargement in the surface ECG are specific and highly predictive of the degree of LA enlargement as measured by surface echocardiography with two-dimensional guidance. Finally, the ECG findings of left atrial abnormality are associated with more severe left ventricular dysfunction in patients with ischemic heart disease and more severe valve damage in patients with aortic or mitral valve disease [4]. In addition, with these ECG findings, patients have a higher than normal incidence of paroxysmal atrial tachyarrhythmias.

Right Atrial Abnormality (Enlargement)

ECG features of right atrial abnormality include abnormally high P wave amplitudes in the limb and right precordial leads. Criteria commonly used to diagnose right atrial abnormality are listed in Table 2 [4, 5]. Such abnormal patterns reflect an increase in right atrial mass and the generation of greater electrical forces early during atrial activation. In patients with chronic pulmonary disease, these abnormalities may more reflect the vertical position of the heart within the chest secondary to pulmonary hyperinflation as opposed to heart disease per se. The QRS changes commonly associated with right atrial abnormalities are those of the underlying pathophysiology that is producing right atrial hemodynamic changes–often right ventricular hypertrophy secondary to chronic obstructive pulmonary disease.

Ventricular Hypertrophy and Enlargement

The thick-walled ventricles dilate in response to receiving excess volume during diastole, and become hypertrophied in response to ejecting blood against chronically increased pulmonary or systemic vascular resistance during systole. Enlargement of the right or left ventricle commonly is accompanied by enlargement of its corresponding atrium. ECG features that meet the criteria for atrial abnormality (LA enlargement -P wave terminal forces in ECG lead $V_1 \geq 0.040$ sec. mm) should be considered suggestive of enlargement of the corresponding ventricle [5].

Left Ventricular Hypertrophy and Enlargement

Left ventricular (LV) hypertrophy (LVH) or LV chamber enlargement produces changes in the QRS complex, ST segment, and the T wave [4, 5]. The most characteristic of these is increased amplitude of the QRS complex and R waves in leads facing the LV: namely, I, aVL, V_5, and V_6. These are taller than normal, whereas S waves in leads overlying the right ventricle (V_1 and V_2) are deeper than normal. ST segment and T wave patterns can vary widely in patients with LV enlargement and hypertrophy. ST segment and T wave amplitudes are normal or increased in leads with tall R waves [4]. However, in many patients, the ST segment is depressed and followed by an inverted T wave. Most often, the ST segment slopes downward from a depressed J point and T waves are asymmetrically inverted. These repolarization changes most commonly occur in patients with QRS changes, but can occur alone. Especially prominent inverted T waves (i.e., "giant negative T waves") are characteristic of hypertrophic cardiomyopathy with predominant apical thickening. Other ECG changes in LVH include widening (QRS > 0.11 s) and notching of the QRS complex and a delay in the intrinsicoid deflection.[3] These may reflect the longer duration of activation of the thickened LV wall or damage to its conducting system. Finally, these ECG changes are most typical of LVH consequent to pressure (systolic) overload. Volume (diastolic) overload can produce a somewhat different pattern, including tall, upright T waves and sometimes narrow (< 25 s) but deep (= 0.2 mV) Q waves in leads facing the left side of the ventricular septum (II, III, aVF, V_4, V_5, and V_6). However, the diagnostic value of these changes in predicting the underlying hemodynamics is very limited.

Diagnostic Criteria for Left Ventricular Hypertrophy

Many sets of diagnostic criteria for LVH have been developed on the basis of the aforementioned ECG attributes. Common criteria are: the Sokolow–Lyon index; Romhilt–Estes point score system; Cornell voltage criteria; Cornell regression equation; Cornell voltage–duration measurement; Novacode criterion (for men) [4]. Diagnostic criteria for each of these are detailed in Table 3 [4]. Commonly, these methods assess the presence or absence of LVH as a binary function based on empirically determined criteria. For example, the Sokolow–Lyon and Cornell voltage criteria require that voltages in specific leads exceed certain values. The Romhilt–Estes point score system assigns point values to amplitude and other criteria. "Definite" or "probable" LVH are diagnosed if scores of 5 or 4 are computed, respectively. The Cornell voltage–duration method includes measurement of QRS duration as well as amplitude. The other two methods (Cornell regression equation; Novacode system) seek to quantify LV mass as a continuum. The diagnosis of LVH is based on a computed mass that exceeds an independently determined threshold. Also, as with atrial enlargement, the relative diagnostic accuracy of these ECG methods for diagnosing LVH or chamber enlargement is compared to echocardiographic with radiographic or autopsy measurements of LV size as "gold standards." In general, as for atrial enlargement, these studies have reported low sensitivity (10–50%: lowest for Sokolow–Lyon and

[3] An electrode overlying the LV free wall records a rising R wave as transmural activation of the underlying LV free wall proceeds [4]. Once the activation front reaches the epicardium, the full thickness of LV free wall under the electrode will be in an activated state, with no propagating electrical activity. At that moment, the electrode will register a sudden reversal of potential to record a negative potential from remote areas of myocardium still undergoing activation. This sudden reversal of potential with a sharp downslope is the "intrinsicoid deflection", and marks the timing of activation of the epicardium under the electrode.

Table 3. Electrocardiographic measurements and diagnostic criteria for left ventricular hypertrophy (enlargement) (LVH)

Electrocardiographic measurement	Diagnostic criteria
1. Sokolow–Lyon index	1. $S_{V1} + (R_{V5}$ or $R_{V6}) > 3.5$ mV 2. $R_{aVl} > 1.1$ mV
2. Romhilt–Estes point score system[a]	1. Any limb lead R wave or S wave ≥ 2.0 mV; *or* S_{V1} or $S_{V2} \geq 3.0$ mV; *or* R_{V5} to $R_{V6} \geq 3.0$ mV (3 points for each of these) 2. ST–T wave abnormality (in absence of digitalis (3 points) 3. ST–T wave abnormality with digitalis (1 point) 4. Left atrial abnormality—e.g., P mitrale (3 points) 5. Left axis deviation ≥ 30° (2 points) 6. QRS duration ≥ 90 ms (1 point) 7. Intrinsicoid deflection in V_5 or V_6 ≥ 50 ms (1 point)
Cornell voltage criteria	$S_{V3} + S_{aVl} \geq 2.8$ mV (for men) $S_{V3} + S_{aVl} \geq 2.0$ mV (for women)
Cornell regression equation[b]	Risk of LVH = $1/(+ e^{-exp})$, where exp = $4.558 - 0.092(R_{aVl} + S_{V3}) - 0.212$ (QRS) $- 0.278$ $PTF_{V1} - 0.859$ (sex)
Cornell voltage-duration measurement	1. QRS duration (ms) ? Cornell voltage < 2436 2. QRS duration x sum of voltages in all leads > 17 472
Novacode criteria (for men)[c]	LVMI (g/m²) = $-36.4 + 0.182\ R_{V5} + 0.20\ S_{V1} + 0.28\ S_m{}^c + 0.0.182\ T_{(neg)}V_6 - 0.148\ T_{(pos)}aVr + 1.049\ QRS_{duration}$

From criteria given in [4], p 122. S_{V1}, R_{V6}, R_{aVl}, etc. are the S wave in unipolar lead V_1, the R wave in unipolar lead V_6, the R wave unipolar lead aV_l, etc., respectively, [a] For the Romhilt-Estes point score system, probable LVH is diagnosed with 4 points, and definite LVH with ≥ 5 points, [b] For the Cornell regression equation, voltages are in millivolts, QRS is the QRS duration in milliseconds, PTF is the area under the P terminal force in V_1 (in millimeter seconds), and sex = 1 for men and 2 for women; LVH is present if exp is < −1.55, [c] For the Novocode criteria, "neg" and "pos" refer to the amplitudes of the negative and positive portions of the T waves, respectively; $S_m{}^c$ indicates the amplitude of S, Q, and QS wave, whichever is larger

Romhilt–Estes criteria, but higher for all Cornell and the Novacode criteria) and high specificity (85–95%) for all measures. The accuracy of these criteria can also vary with demographic and related features of the populations studied. For example, the precordial QRS voltages are often higher in blacks of African descent (especially males) than in white persons. This leads to a higher prevalence of false-positive ECG diagnoses of LVH in blacks of African descent with hypertension.

Clinical Significance of Left Ventricular Hypertrophy 4 liv

The presence of ECG criteria for LVH identifies a subset of the general population at significantly increased risk of cardiovascular morbidity and mortality [4]. This increased risk is especially apparent in women and in persons in whom ST-T wave abnormalities are present. The relative risk of cardiovascular events for patients with LVH voltage criteria alone is approximately 2.8, whereas the relative risk increases to > 5.0 if ST segment depression is also present [8]. Interestingly, the positive diagnoses of LVH by Sokolow–Lyon criteria and Cornell criteria (see [4]) have independent prognostic value [9].

Finally, the ECG finding of LVH correlates with more severe heart disease, including higher blood pressure in patients with hypertension (HTN), and greater ventricular dysfunction in those with HTN or coronary artery disease [4]. Effective HTN treatment reduces the ECG evidence of LVH and reduces the associated risk of cardiovascular mortality [4] (see also Chapter 4).

Right Ventricular Hypertrophy and Enlargement

The right ventricle (RV) is considerably smaller than the LV. It produces electrical forces that are largely canceled by those generated by the larger LV mass. Thus, for RV hypertrophy (RVH) to be manifested on the ECG, it must be severe enough to overcome the concealing forces of the larger LV electromotive forces [4, 5].

Normally, the final third of the QRS complex is produced solely by activation of the thicker-walled LV and interventricular septum [5]. As the RV hypertrophies, it provides increasing contribution to the early portion of the QRS complex, and also begins to contribute to the later portion of this complex. Lead V_1, with its left–right orientation, provides the optimal view of the competition between the two ventricles for electrical predominance. In normal adults, the QRS complex in V_1 is predominantly negative, with a small R wave ("r") followed by a large S ("S") wave. When the RV hypertrophies in response to pressure overload, this negative predominance may be lost, producing a prominent R wave and small or absent S wave in V_1. In mild RVH, the LV retains predominance, and there is either no ECG change or the QRS axis moves rightward. With moderate RVH, the initial QRS electromotive forces are predominantly anterior (with an increased R wave in V_1), and the terminal forces may or may not be predominantly rightward.

With severe concentric RVH, the QRS complex typically becomes predominantly negative in lead I, and positive in V_1. Delayed repolarization of the RV myocardium may produce negativity of the ST segment, and a T wave pattern (negative in V_1 to V_3) indicative of "RV strain."

Biventricular Hypertrophy and Enlargement

Hypertrophy or enlargement of both ventricles produces complex ECG patterns [4, 5, 10]. In contrast to biatrial enlargement, the result is not simply the sum of two sets of abnormalities. Thus, the effects of enlargement of one ventricular chamber may cancel the effects of enlargement of the other chamber. For example, enhanced posterior forces generated by LVH may cancel anterior forces produced by RVH. Furthermore, the greater LV forces generated by LVH increase the degree of RVH needed to overcome the dominance of LVH. Therefore biventricular enlargement is suggested when any of the following combinations of ECG changes is present [4, 5]:

1. High-voltage RS complexes in the midprecordial leads; seen in many congenital lesions, and perhaps most common with ventricular septal defect.
2. Voltage criteria for LVH in the precordial leads with combined vertical heart position or right-axis deviation in the limb leads.
3. A low-amplitude S wave in V_1, combined with a very deep S wave in lead V_2, or deep S waves in the left precordial leads in the presence of ECG criteria for LVH.
4. Criteria for LVH in the left precordial leads, combined with prominent R waves in the right precordial leads (i.e., tall R waves in both the left and right precordial leads).
5. Left atrial enlargement as the sole criterion for LVH, with any criterion suggestive of RVH.

Finally, prominent left atrial abnormality (or atrial fibrillation) along with evidence of RV or biventricular enlargement (e.g., LVH with vertical or rightward QRS axis deviation) should suggest chronic rheumatic valvular heart disease [4].

Conduction Disturbances and Arrhythmias in Patients with Heart Failure

Cardiac arrhythmias and atrioventricular (AV) conduction disturbances are common in patients with underlying structural heart disease and commonly precipitate or worsen HF [1]. Indeed, some arrhythmias and conduction disturbances may be the immediate cause of sudden death, which has led to the emergence of implanted pacemaker (PM) and cardioverter-defibrillator (ICD) therapies (with or without cardiac resynchronization therapy [11]) as preventive and therapeutic modalities in patients with HF or predisposed to HF (see also Chapter 12). The development of arrhythmias or conduction disturbances may precipitate HF through several mechanisms [4]:

1. *Tachyarrhythmias.* The most common tachyarrhythmia in patients with HF is atrial fibrillation. This and other fast atrial rhythms (sinus, ectopic or reentry tachycardias) reduce the time available for ventricular filling. If there is already impaired ventricular filling (e.g., mitral stenosis) or reduced ventricular compliance (e.g., LVH), tachycardia raises atrial pressure and further reduces cardiac output by shortening ventricular filling time. Also, tachyarrhythmias increase myocardial O_2 demand and utilization, which may trigger or worsen myocardial ischemia in patients with fixed occlusive coronary artery disease, thereby raising left atrial pressure and causing pulmonary congestion. Finally, tachycardia may also directly impair contractility in failing myocardium, in part owing to a negative force-frequency relationship [12].
2. *Bradycardia (pronounced/severe).* This usually decreases cardiac output in patients with underlying structural heart disease, because stroke volume may already be maximal and cannot rise further to maintain cardiac output. The effects of bradycardia will be augmented greatly if there is concurrent loss of atrial transport function (e.g., with AV junctional or ventricular escape rhythms).
3. *Dissociation between atrial and ventricular contractions.* This occurs with AV junctional and idioventricular escape rhythms or tachycardia, and advanced second-degree and third-degree AV heart block. In addition, atrial contractions are ineffective in atrial fibrillation, and may be greatly impaired with fast supraventricular tachycardias and preexcitation syndromes. The mechanism is impairment of or loss of atrial transport function, which leads to impaired ventricular filling, reduced cardiac output, and increased atrial pressure. Impairment of or the loss of atrial transport function is especially disadvantageous in patients with reduced ventricular compliance due to aging or hypertrophic cardiomyopathy (e.g., secondary to systemic HTN or aortic stenosis), or restrictive conditions (e.g., pericarditis, large pericardial effusions, hemorrhagic tamponade).
4. *Abnormal intraventricular conduction.* This occurs with many tachyarrhythmias (e.g., ventricular tachycardias and supraventricular tachycardias) associated with aberrant ventricular conduction. It impairs myocardial performance due to the loss of normally (mechanically) synchronized RV and LV contractions (i.e., ventricular interdependence). In addition to triggering HF, tachyarrhythmias associated with abnormal intraventricular conduction may be the early manifestations of acute HF.

Death in patients with severe HF occurs with progressive mechanical ("pump") failure; or, in as many as one-half of all patients, suddenly and unexpectedly from primary "electrical failure" [1]. This could be attributed to a tachyarrhythmia (e.g., preexcited atrial fibrillation or flutter, rapid ventricular tachycardia, or ventricular fibrillation), asystole or pulseless electrical activity (PEA), or the failure of AV conduction (i.e., advanced or complete AV heart block with ineffective or absent ventricular contractions) [1, 6]. When present, a variety of arrhythmias, especially frequent ventricular extrasystoles, ventricular tachycardia, left bundle branch block, and atrial fibrillation, are predictors of mortality and sudden death [1]. What remains unclear is whether these electrical disturbances are simply indicators of the severity of left ventricular dysfunction or whether they are responsible for and trigger lethal arrhythmias [1]. Although there is evidence that ventricular arrhythmias confer independent adverse prognostic effects [13], this may not hold true after adjusting for other variables, especially cardiac ejection fraction [14]. Importantly, the routine treatment of patients with antiarrhythmic drugs has not been shown to exert a protective effect and reduce mortality [15]. However, evidence recently reviewed elsewhere [11], especially the prematurely terminated COMPANION trial [16], suggests that when cardiac resynchronization therapy (with biventricular pacing) is combined with an implanted cardioverter–defibrillator, a significant survival benefit is conferred in patients with ischemic or nonischemic cardiomyopathy.

References

1. Givertz MM, Colucci WS, Braunwald E (2005) Clinical aspects of heart failure; pulmonary edema, high-output failure. In: Zipes DP, Libby P, Bonow RO, Braunwald E (eds) Braunwald's heart disease, 7th edn. Elsevier Saunders, Philadelphia, pp 539–568
2. Hunt SA, Baker DW, Chin MH et al (2001) ACC/AHA Guidelines for the evaluation and management of chronic heart failure in the adult: executive summary. A report of the American College of Cardiology/American Heart Association Task Force on Practice Guidelines (Committee to Revise the 1995 Guidelines for the Evaluation and Management of Heart Failure). Circulation 104:2996–3007
3. Chin MH, Goldman L (1997) Factors contributing to the hospitalization of patients with congestive heart failure. Am J Public Health 87:643–648
4. Mirvus DM, Goldberger AL (2005) Electrocardiography. In: Zipes DP, Libby P, Bonow RO, Braunwald E (eds) Braunwald's heart disease, 7th edn. Elsevier Saunders, Philadelphia, pp 107–185
5. Wagner GS (2001) Marriott's practical electrocardiography, 10th edn. Lippincott, Williams & Wilkins, Philadelphia, pp 72–94
6. Atlee JL (1996) Arrhythmias and pacemakers. Saunders, Philadelphia, pp 105–153
7. Olgin JE, Zipes DP (2005) Specific arrhythmias: diagnosis and treatment. In: Zipes DP, Libby P, Bonow RO, Braunwald E (eds) Braunwald's heart disease, 7th edn.

Elsevier Saunders, Philadelphia, pp 803–863
8. Menotti A, Seccareccia F (1997) Electrocardiographic Minnesota code findings predicting short-term mortality in asymptomatic subjects. The Italian RIFLE Pooling Project (Risk Factors and Life Expectancy). G Ital Cardiol 27:40–49
9. Sundstrom J, Lind L, Arnlov J, et al (2001) Echocardiographic and electrocardiographic diagnoses of left ventricular hypertrophy predict mortality independently of each other in a population of elderly men. Circulation 103:2346–2351
10. Jain A, Chandna H, Silber EN, et al (1999) Electrocardiographic patterns of patients with echocardiographically determined biventricular hypertrophy. J Electrocardiol 32:269–273
11. Atlee JL (2006) Pacemaker resynchronisation in the treatment of severe heart failure. In: Gullo A (ed) Anaesthesia, pain, intensive care and emergency medicine (A.P.I.C.E.) 20. Springer, Milan, pp 99–112
12. Opie LH (2005) Mechanisms of cardiac contraction and relaxation. In: Zipes DP, Libby P, Bonow RO, Braunwald E (eds) Braunwald's heart disease, 7th edn. Elsevier Saunders, Philadelphia, pp 457–489
13. La Rovere MT, Pinna GD, Maestri R, et al (2003) Short-term heart rate variability strongly predicts sudden cardiac death in chronic heart failure patients. Circulation 107:565–570
14. Singh SN, Fisher SG, Carson PE, Fletcher RD (1998) Prevalence and significance of nonsustained ventricular tachycardia in patients with premature ventricular contractions and heart failure treated with vasodilator therapy. Department of Veterans Affairs CHF STAT Investigators. J Am Coll Cardiol 32:942–947
15. Moss AJ, Zareba W, Hall WJ, et al (2002) Prophylactic implantation of a defibrillator in patients with myocardial infarction and reduced ejection fraction. N Engl J Med 346: 877–883
16. Salukhe TV, Francis DP, Sutton R (2003) Comparison of Medical Therapy, Pacing and Defibrillation in Heart Failure (COMPANION) trial terminated early; combined biventricular pacemaker-defibrillators reduce all-cause mortality and hospitalization. Int J Cardiol 87:119–120

10 Management of Patients with Acute Heart Failure

W.G. Toller, G. Gemes and H. Metzler

Introduction

With an aging population and improved therapeutic strategies in patients with coronary artery disease, hypertension, and diabetes mellitus, the prevalence of patients with chronically impaired myocardial performance is constantly increasing [1]. As a consequence, physicians are also frequently faced with the diagnosis and treatment of a rapid onset of symptoms and signs secondary to abnormal cardiac function. This clinical syndrome of acute heart failure (AHF) in general requires rapid diagnosis and is associated with challenging treatment and a high mortality. Unfortunately, steady improvements in the care of these patients have not been able to change the fact that heart failure is still a major cause of death in the intensive medicine setting. Because of the urgency and challenge of treatment, the number of randomized controlled clinical trials that include these patients is currently low, and therefore empirical rather than evidence-based therapeutic approaches dominate. In 2005, the European Society of Cardiology and the European Society of Intensive Care Medicine published guidelines on the diagnosis and treatment of AHF [2], in which clinical trials are reviewed and treatment algorithms are proposed. In this chapter the recommendations for diagnosis and treatment are summarized and new publications incorporated.

Department of Anesthesiology and Intensive Care Medicine, Medical University of Graz, Graz, Austria

Definition and Etiology of AHF

The clinical syndrome of AHF is the final pathway for various diseases of the heart and can present itself de novo, e.g., after myocardial infarction without previous myocardial dysfunction, as acute decompensation of chronic heart failure, or as end-stage chronic heart failure refractory to treatment. Although the underlying mechanisms of AHF may be diverse, including hypertensive AHF, cardiogenic shock, high output heart failure, pulmonary edema and right heart failure (Fig. 1), the final common denominator is a critical inability of the myocardium to maintain a cardiac output sufficient to meet the demands of the peripheral circulation. The resultant undersupply of peripheral organs with oxygen is responsible for the initiation and perpetuation of a vicious circle of AHF.

Particularly in the perioperative period, patients may be faced with numerous triggers of AHF, including withdrawal of heart failure drugs, hypertension, inadequate volume management, anemia, tachyarrhythmias, hypercoagulability, and myocardial ischemia. While some of these triggers may be avoided or treated relatively easily, myocardial ischemia certainly represents the most severe origin of AHF. The spectrum of complications associated with myocardial ischemia in this setting may range from asymp-

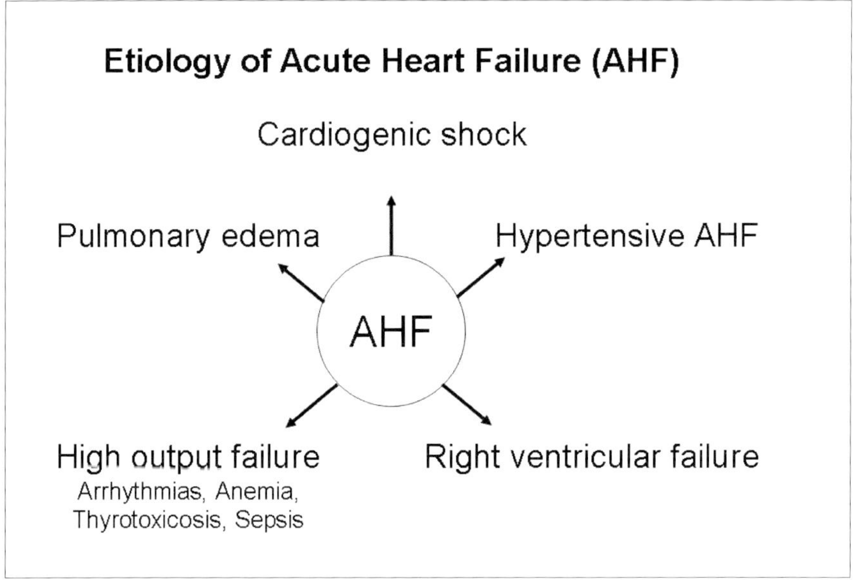

Fig. 1. Etiologies of acute heart failure (AHF)

tomatic elevation of cardiac enzymes to the development of cardiogenic shock. A constant rate of approximately 7% of acute myocardial infarctions (AMI) are complicated by cardiogenic shock, with a subsequent mortality rate of 70–80% [3]. Other less frequent but equally severe causes of perioperative cardiogenic shock include cardiac arrhythmias, acute or chronic heart valve insufficiencies, massive pulmonary embolism, and pericardial tamponade. Given this diversity, it is clear that no single pathophysiological model can cover these various clinical expressions, and that patient-adapted rather than standard diagnostic and therapeutic approaches are necessary.

Pathogenesis of AHF

In the early phase of AHF, compensatory mechanisms including sympathetic nervous and renin–angiotensin–aldosterone system activation aim to restore cardiac output by increasing heart rate, myocardial contractility, vasoconstriction, and shifting fluid into the vascular compartment. If the profound depression of myocardial contractility is not resolved, a vicious cycle of reduced cardiac output, low blood pressure, coronary insufficiency, and a further reduction in contractility and cardiac output is initiated. Eventually, decreased perfusion pressure results in further depression of myocardial contractility, and compensatory mechanisms are overwhelmed by the progressive deterioration of cardiac function.

Patients with AHF may have either systolic or diastolic dysfunction, or both. Systolic dysfunction relates to decreased myocardial contractility, with a decrease in ejection fraction and an impaired ability to increase stroke volume in response to increasing preload. The relationship between end-diastolic pressure and stroke volume is typically flattened. On the other hand, the ventricle is particularly sensitive to changes in afterload, i.e., small increases in afterload may severely decrease cardiac output. Diastolic dysfunction may occur either in combination with systolic contractile impairment or in the presence of a relatively normal ejection fraction and ventricular size. It is related to a variable combination of abnormal myocardial relaxation and reduced ventricular compliance.

At the level of the cardiac myocytes, downregulation of β-adrenergic receptors, abnormalities in the handling of calcium homeostasis and myofilament sensitivity to calcium, and disturbance of phosphodiesterase production and activity occur, which ultimately result in malfunction of myofilament contraction.

Diagnosis and Monitoring

The diagnosis of AHF is based on the symptoms and clinical findings and is supported by appropriate investigations. Typically, the systematic physical examination reveals hypotension, dyspnea, elevated jugular venous pressure, tachycardia, oliguria, cyanosis, cool extremities, and altered mentation. Clinical assessment with the help of four different patient profiles (warm-wet, warm-dry, cold-wet, cold-dry) has been demonstrated to predict outcome and guide therapy [4].

Basic Monitoring

Twelve-lead electrocardiography as well as continuous ECG monitoring may help identify the etiology of AHF, in particular in the assessment of acute coronary syndromes, ventricular hypertrophy, and arrhythmias. Chest X-radiography should be performed repeatedly to assess cardiac size, shape, pulmonary congestion, and the progress of therapy. Blood pressure measurements should be carried out routinely and regularly, as maintenance of a normal blood pressure is critical during initiation of therapy until the dosage of vasoactive drugs has been stabilized. While in the absence of high heart rates and intense vasoconstriction, noninvasive blood pressure measurement is reliable, hemodynamic instability or a requirement for multiple arterial blood gas analyses suggests the need for invasive arterial blood pressure monitoring. Pulse oximetry should be used continuously on any unstable patient who is being treated with supplemental oxygen.

Biochemical Markers

Determination of biochemical markers is useful in the diagnosis and guidance of treatment of patients with AHF. Assays for B-type natriuretic peptide (BNP) and its precursor molecule N-terminal pro-BNP (NT-proBNP), which are released from cardiac ventricles in response to increased wall stretch and volume overload, have recently been developed and may assist in the diagnosis and treatment of AHF in several clinical situations [5]. Decision cut-off points of 100 pg/ml for BNP and 300 pg/ml for NT-ProBNP have been proposed and good negative predictive values for the exclusion of AHF demonstrated. BNP and NT-proBNP are equally powerful diagnostic and prognostic markers in patients with heart failure and coronary artery disease [6, 7]. The value of these peptides in the diagnosis of AHF has to be interpreted in conjunction with other findings, including history, physical examination, and laboratory findings.

Echocardiography

Clinical practice heart failure guidelines to assist physicians in the diagnosis and management of patients with heart failure have been developed [8]. These and other guidelines [9] have emphasized the importance of echocardiography in the diagnosis and management of AHF. The clinical utility of echocardiography in patients with known or suspected heart failure, together with its widespread availability and safety, have made it one of the most useful cardiovascular diagnostic tools. The technique is an important adjunct for the diagnosis and management of patients with heart failure and has been shown to provide significant information that can be used for tailoring treatment and altering the prognosis in such patients. Echocardiography with Doppler imaging should be used to evaluate and monitor regional and global left and right ventricular function, valvular structure and function, possible pericardial pathology, and mechanical complications of acute myocardial infarction. Performance of Doppler echocardiography can allow estimation of pulmonary artery pressures and left ventricular preload.

Central Venous and Pulmonary Artery Catheterization

Central venous lines are useful to monitor central venous pressure and central venous oxygen saturation and may be used to administer fluids or drugs. In severely ill patients, right-sided filling pressures frequently do not correlate with left-sided pressures and may therefore be over-interpreted, especially in the presence of tricuspid regurgitation and positive end-expiratory pressure ventilation. Although controversies exist regarding the use of a pulmonary artery catheter [10], this device may assist in the diagnosis and treatment of the patient with AHF, including measurement of pulmonary artery wedge pressure, the possibility of obtaining mixed venous oxygen saturations (MVO_2), and (continuous) measurement of cardiac index. The diagnosis of AHF is suggested by the simultaneous presence of low cardiac index (< 2.2 l/m^2 per minute), low systolic blood pressure (< 90 mmHg), low mixed venous oxygen saturations (< 60%), elevated pulmonary capillary wedge pressure (> 15 mmHg), and elevated lactate concentrations (> 2 mg/dl). Under specific circumstances, determination of pulmonary capillary wedge pressure may not be an accurate reflection of left-ventricular filling pressures, e.g., in the presence of mitral stenosis, aortic regurgitation, high airway pressure, and hypertrophy of the left ventricle. The use of a pulmonary artery catheter is recommended in hemodynamically unstable patients who are not responding in a predictable fashion to traditional treatments, and in patients with a combination of congestion and hypoperfusion. Because the complications increase with the duration of its use, it is important to insert the pulmonary artery catheter only when specific data are needed and to remove it as soon as it is of no further help.

Angiography

As angiography-based revascularization therapy has been shown to improve prognosis, performance of this technique is important in AHF patients with unstable angina or myocardial infarction.

Therapeutic Approaches

General Principles

The immediate goals in the treatment of AHF are to improve symptoms and to stabilize the hemodynamic condition. These short-term benefits should be accompanied by favorable effects on long-term outcome, e.g., decreasing hospital readmission rates and time to readmission, improved quality of life and survival, and reducing the duration of intravenous vasoactive therapy. A distinction between the different etiologies of AHF should be made when resuscitative measures are initiated, because the subsequent therapeutic approach largely depends on the etiology of AHF and may prompt the use of specific therapies. For example, myocardial infarction requires rapid re-establishment of infarct-related, reduced arterial blood flow because early thrombolysis, percutaneous transluminal coronary angioplasty, coronary stent implantation, or coronary artery bypass graft are all superior to initial aggressive medical therapy [11]. Acute mitral regurgitation due to myocardial infarction may necessitate valve reconstruction or replacement, and rupture of the ventricular septum acute surgical correction. Acute right ventricular failure may require treatment of pulmonary hypertension by the removal of emboli or by the reduction of right ventricular afterload with inhaled or intravenous vasodilators [12]. Similarly, as patients with AHF are prone to infectious complications, meticulous infection control is mandatory by the obtaining of routine cultures and administration of antibiotics. Mild sedation should be performed by administering morphine or its analogues, especially if the patient suffers dyspnea and restlessness. In cases of acute coronary syndrome or atrial fibrillation, anticoagulation should be initiated using unfractionated or low-molecular-weight heparin. Normoglycemia should be achieved using insulin and albumin concentrations measured to maintain calorie balance. The importance of early metabolic support for the improvement of myocardial recovery in patients with AHF was highlighted by Berger and Mustafa [13].

Ventilatory Assistance

The improvement of oxygen delivery to the tissues is important in AHF patients in order to prevent end-organ dysfunction and multiple organ failure. The capillary oxygen saturation should be maintained in a normal range of 95–98%. This is best achieved by measures that aim to maintain patent airways, by the administration of supplemental oxygen, and by proper patient positioning. Patent airways may be achieved by the application of continuous positive end-expiratory pressures, either through continuous positive airway pressure (CPAP) devices or by noninvasive or invasive ventilation. These techniques frequently cause pulmonary recruitment, increase the functional residual capacity, and decrease the overall work of breathing and left ventricular afterload. In AHF patients, the use of CPAP reduced the need for endotracheal intubation and demonstrated a trend to decreased in-hospital mortality compared to standard therapy [14]. CPAP or noninvasive ventilation should be used before endotracheal intubation and mechanical ventilation are performed. Invasive mechanical ventilation should be applied only if acute respiratory failure does not respond to vasodilators, oxygen therapy, and CPAP or noninvasive ventilation.

Volume Management

Once therapy of hypoxia takes effect, intravascular volume management and correction of electrolyte and acid–base abnormalities are initiated, and sinus rhythm should be restored if possible by cardioversion and/or administration of antiarrhythmic drugs. For proper volume management, it is important to recognize that both cardiogenic pulmonary edema and peripheral edema may coexist with intravascular volume deficits. When this occurs, patients may benefit from careful fluid challenges under the guidance of appropriate hemodynamic monitoring.

Drugs for the Treatment of AHF

The recommended drugs for the treatment of AHF are presented in an algorithm by the European Society of Cardiology [2] (Fig. 2).

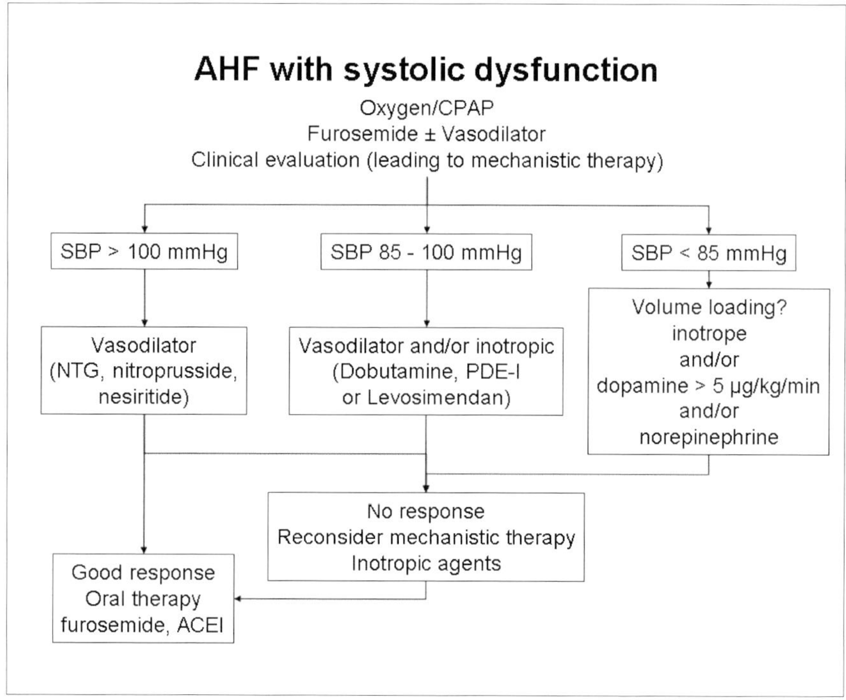

Fig. 2. Rationale for inotropic drugs in AHF. Reproduced from [2]

Diuretics

Administration of diuretics is indicated in patients with AHF in the presence of symptoms secondary to fluid retention, e.g., pulmonary edema. Loop diuretics are a universally accepted treatment in these patients and produce both an increase in urine volume and vasodilation. These effects reduce ventricular filling pressures as well as pulmonary resistances and frequently afford rapid relief of symptoms. In the treatment of AHF diuretics should be titrated according to the diuretic response and relief of congestive symptoms. Administration of a bolus followed by a continuous infusion is superior to repeated administration of boluses.

Vasodilators

Nitrates

Alternatively or in combination with diuretics, administration of nitrates has been shown to relieve pulmonary congestion, particularly in patients with AHF due to acute coronary syndrome. Using appropriate doses, nitrates produce vasodilation in veins and arteries, including coronary arteries. Combining the highest hemodynamically tolerable dose of nitrates with low-dose furosemide is superior to high-dose diuretic treatment alone [15]. A prospective outcome trial comparing diuretics and nitrates as first-line therapy in acute cardiogenic pulmonary edema demonstrated a decreased need for mechanical ventilation and a reduced incidence of myocardial infarction within 24 h of hospital admission and in-hospital death in patients treated with nitrates [15].

Nesiritide

Nesiritide is a recombinant human BNP with vasodilating properties in veins and arteries, including coronary arteries. This substance reduces pre- and afterload and may therefore improve cardiac output in the absence of direct inotropic effects. Although the improvement in hemodynamics was more effective when nesiritide was compared with nitroglycerin, this effect did not translate into a better clinical outcome of AHF patients [16]. Recently, nesiritide has been demonstrated to worsen renal function [17] and increase mortality [18], and the use of this substance has been criticized [19].

Sodium Nitroprusside

Sodium nitroprusside is recommended in patients with AHF if afterload is increased, e.g., hypertensive heart failure. In AHF caused by acute coronary syndrome, sodium nitroprusside may cause coronary steal. Controlled clinical trials of the use of sodium nitroprusside in AHF patients, however, are lacking.

Inotropic Agents

The decision to initiate administration of positive inotropic drugs depends on the blood pressure. While at systolic blood pressures above 100 mmHg augmentation of vasodilatory therapy is recommended, patients with systolic blood pressures between 85 mmHg and 100 mmHg should receive positive inotropic drugs in addition to vasodilators. Inotropic agents are particularly indicated in the presence of peripheral hypoperfusion with or without congestion or pulmonary edema refractory to diuretics and vasodilators at optimal doses. These substances include dobutamine, phosphodiesterase (PDE) inhibitors, or levosimendan. Although their use is potentially harmful due to an increase in myocardial oxygen demand and an arrhythmogenic effect, the improvements in hemodynamics may be useful and indeed lifesaving in the setting of AHF. Whether the risk–benefit ratio is the same for all positive inotropic substances is unclear. Patients with systolic blood pressures below 85 mmHg should additionally receive vasopressors, e.g., dopamine or norepinephrine, after adequate volume status has been confirmed.

Dobutamine

Dobutamine produces dose-dependent inotropic and chronotropic effects by stimulation of β_1-adrenergic receptors with a subsequent increase in intracellular cyclic adenosine monophosphate (cAMP). While the short-term use of this substance is effective in improving hemodynamic parameters, the longer-term use has been associated with tolerance, partial loss of hemodynamic effects, myocardial ischemia, and increased mortality [20]. Dobutamine is indicated when there is evidence of peripheral hypoperfusion with or without congestion or pulmonary edema refractory to diuretics and vasodilators at optimal doses. In patients receiving β-adrenoceptor antagonist therapy, dobutamine doses frequently have to be increased to restore its inotropic effect. Combinations of dobutamine with PDE inhibitors or levosimendan have been shown to have additive effects.

Phosphodiesterase Inhibitors

PDE inhibitors, which include milrinone and enoximone, increase intracellular cAMP by preventing cAMP degradation. This effect is independent of β_1-adrenergic stimulation and is therefore still effective when downregulation of these receptors has occurred. PDE inhibitors, however, increase cytosolic calcium levels and therefore ultimately also increase myocardial oxygen demand and the incidence of arrhythmias [21], particularly in the presence of concomitant ischemia [22]. These detrimental side effects of treatment with catecholamines and PDE inhibitors are well known and have been associated with a possible negative influence on mortality. Particularly in the setting of AHF caused by myocardial ischemia, the therapeutic concept of increasing myocardial contractility by increasing cytosolic calcium by stimulating the same intracellular cascade may therefore be challenged.

Levosimendan

Sensitization of cardiac myofilaments to calcium without further increasing intracellular calcium concentrations and myocardial oxygen demand [23], has recently evolved as an attractive therapeutic alternative in patients with AHF. This is accomplished either by replacing catecholamine with PDE inhibitor therapy, or by combining the two therapies. The latter approach should have neutral effects on myocardial oxygen demand by enabling a reduction in the dose of catecholamines or PDE inhibitors. Levosimendan, a myofilament calcium sensitizer, increases cardiac output without increasing myocardial oxygen demand and provoking significant arrhythmias [24], and has clinically been demonstrated to be superior to dobutamine for treatment of acute decompensation of chronic heart failure [25]. In addition, levosimendan also produces vasodilation in vascular smooth muscle cells. While this effect is important in the treatment of AHF, it also has the potential to decrease the blood pressure with all the associated side effects of decreased coronary perfusion pressure, e.g., arrhythmia or ischemia. In this situation, volume replacement and temporary addition of a vasopressor, e.g., norepinephrine, is recommended. Interestingly, parallel administration of β-adrenergic blockers does not attenuate the actions of levosimendan, whereas it naturally exerts this effect in patients receiving catecholamines. Levosimendan is indicated in patients with symptomatic low-output heart failure secondary to cardiac systolic dysfunction without severe hypotension.

Mechanical Assist Devices

The increasing incidence of chronic heart failure combined with the limited supply of hearts available for transplantation has prompted the development and pursuit of mechanical assist devices in order to maximize patient survival and minimize morbidity [26]. Experience with these techniques has also resulted in advances in mechanical assist devices in the perioperative period in addition to traditional devices, e.g., intra-aortic balloon counterpulsation. Many of these assist devices have been demonstrated to relieve the symptoms of AHF, to enable disconnection from extracorporeal circulation during cardiac surgery, or to bridge the time to transplantation following intraoperative myocardial infarction with subsequent AHF. For all of these mechanical assist devices, however, no definitive randomized prospective trials have been performed to confirm benefit. Most of these techniques are restricted to use in specialized cardiothoracic centers and require surgical insertion.

Temporary mechanical circulatory assistance may be indicated in patients with AHF who are not responding to conventional therapy and where there is a potential for myocardial recovery, or as a bridge to heart transplantation.

Intra-aortic Balloon Counterpulsation

This technique has become a standard component of treatment in AHF patients unresponsive to volume administration, vasodilation, and inotropic support. Intra-aortic balloon counterpulsation is performed by diastolic inflation and systolic deflation of a helium-filled balloon positioned in the descending aorta. As a result of this technique, hemodynamics are improved, coronary perfusion pressure and myocardial oxygen supply increased, and afterload decreased. In patients with severe peripheral vascular disease, uncorrectable causes of heart failure or multiorgan failure, this device should not be used.

Ventricular Assist Devices

These mechanical pumps partially replace the mechanical work of the ventricle. By this mechanism, they decrease myocardial work and may be used as a bridge to recovery or to transplantation. In clinical practice, expected support time is used to differentiate devices. Ventricular assist devices are categorized as paracorporeal (pumping device outside the patient) or implantable (e.g., preperitoneal or intraperitoneal) devices (Table 1), and additionally as short-, medium- or long-term devices. With the advent of axial flow pumps in clinical use, the distinction between pulsatile and non-pulsatile systems has become important.

Short-term support is instituted in acutely ill patients in profound cardiogenic shock. In this setting, paracorporeal devices are usually used as they can be implanted with a smaller surgical procedure. All of these devices have the option of biventricular support. The most common clinical settings in which recovery can be expected with a reasonable likelihood are acute myocardial infarction despite successful revascularization, patients with postcardiotomy low-output syndrome due to a long cross-clamp time, and patients with postpartum or viral myocarditis.

Table 1. Overview of the currently used cardiac assist devices. From [25]

Cardiac replacement devices	Models available
Paracorporeal devices	
Centrifugal Pumps	Sarns® centrifugal pump
	Bio-Medicus® Bio pump
	St. Jude Medical® Lifestream pump
	Nikkiso® centrifugal pump
	Jostra® centrifugal pump
Diagonal pumps	Medos® Deltastream pump
Pneumatic paracorporeal devices	Abiomed® BVS 5000
	Berlin Heart Excor®
	Thoratec®
	Medos®
Implantable pulsatile devices	HeartMate VE®
	Novacor®
	Thoratec®
Cardiac assist devices	
Implantable axial flow pumps	MicroMed DeBakey Heart®
	Jarvik 2000®
	Berlin Heart Incor®
Microaxial flow pumps	Impella® Recover

Devices for medium- and long-term support are usually implantable and are used to provide sufficient support to transplantation. The most important of these pulsatile devices are HeartMate I® and the Novacor® LVAD. Axial pumps for this use have recently been investigated.

In the case of intraoperative AHF during cardiac surgery with the need for mechanical support of the heart, use of intra-aortic balloon counterpulsation is a typical first-line approach. If AHF persists and disconnection from extracorporeal circulation is impossible despite an intra-aortic balloon pump, a centrifugal pump (e.g., Bio-Medicus® Bio pump) can be installed for short-term support. Special cannulas may be used for short-term support with the centrifugal pump, which allows a relatively uncomplicated switch to medium-term and long-term support with pneumatic paracorporeal devices (e.g., Berlin Heart Excor®), if necessary. An excellent overview of the currently available devices for mechanical circulatory assistance including key issues and problems associated with this technology has recently been published [26].

References

1. Levy D, Kenchaiah S, Larson, MG et al (2002) Long-term trends in the incidence of and survival with heart failure. N Engl J Med 347:1397–1402
2. Nieminen MS, Bohm M, CowieMR et al (2005) Executive summary of the guidelines on the diagnosis and treatment of acute heart failure: the Task Force on Acute Heart Failure of the European Society of Cardiology. Eur Heart J 26:384–416
3. Goldberg RJ, Samad NA, Yarzebski J et al (1999) Temporal trends in cardiogenic shock complicating acute myocardial infarction. N Engl J Med 340:1162–1168
4. Nohria A, Tsang SW, Fang JC et al (2003) Clinical assessment identifies hemodynamic profiles that predict outcomes in patients admitted with heart failure. J Am Coll Cardiol 41:1797–1804
5. Maisel AS, McCord J, Nowak RM et al (2003) Bedside B-Type natriuretic peptide in the emergency diagnosis of heart failure with reduced or preserved ejection fraction. Results from the Breathing Not Properly Multinational Study. J Am Coll Cardiol 41:2010–2017
6. Lainchbury JG, Campbell E, Frampton CM et al (2003) Brain natriuretic peptide and N-terminal brain natriuretic peptide in the diagnosis of heart failure in patients with acute shortness of breath. J Am Coll Cardiol 42:728–735
7. Morrow DA, de Lemos JA, Blazing MA et al (2005) Prognostic value of serial B-type natriuretic peptide testing during follow-up of patients with unstable coronary artery disease. JAMA 294:2866–2871
8. Hunt SA (2005) ACC/AHA 2005 guideline update for the diagnosis and management of chronic heart failure in the adult: a report of the American College of Cardiology/American Heart Association Task Force on Practice Guidelines (Writing Committee to Update the 2001 Guidelines for the Evaluation and Management of Heart Failure). J Am Coll Cardiol 46:81–82
9. Cheitlin MD, Armstrong WF, Aurigemma GP et al (2003) ACC/AHA/ASE 2003

Guideline Update for the Clinical Application of Echocardiography: summary article. A report of the American College of Cardiology/American Heart Association Task Force on Practice Guidelines (ACC/AHA/ASE Committee to Update the 1997 Guidelines for the Clinical Application of Echocardiography). J Am Soc Echocardiogr 16:1091–1110

10. Chittock DR, Dhingra VK, Ronco JJ et al (2004) Severity of illness and risk of death associated with pulmonary artery catheter use. Crit Care Med 32:911–915
11. Hochman JS, Sleeper LA, White HD et al (2001) One-year survival following early revascularization for cardiogenic shock. JAMA 285:190–192
12. Mebazaa A, Karpati P, Renaud E et al (2004) Acute right ventricular failure–from pathophysiology to new treatments. Intensive Care Med 30:185–196
13. Berger MM, Mustafa I (2003) Metabolic and nutritional support in acute cardiac failure. Curr Opin Clin Nutr Metab Care 6:195–201
14. Kelly CA, Newby DE, McDonagh TA et al (2002) Randomised controlled trial of continuous positive airway pressure and standard oxygen therapy in acute pulmonary oedema: effects on plasma brain natriuretic peptide concentrations. Eur Heart J 23:1379–1386
15. Cotter G, Metzkor E, Kaluski E et al (1998) Randomised trial of high-dose isosorbide dinitrate plus low-dose furosemide versus high-dose furosemide plus low-dose isosorbide dinitrate in severe pulmonary oedema. Lancet 351:389–393
16. Young JB, Abraham WT, Stevenson LW et al (2002) Intravenous nesiritide vs nitroglycerin for treatment of decompensated congestive heart failure: a randomized controlled trial. JAMA 287:1531–1540
17. Sackner-Bernstein JD, Skopicki HA, Aaronson, K.D. (2005) Risk of worsening renal function with nesiritide in patients with acutely decompensated heart failure. Circulation 111:1487–1491
18. Sackner-Bernstein JD, Kowalski M, Fox M et al (2005) Short-term risk of death after treatment with nesiritide for decompensated heart failure: a pooled analysis of randomized controlled trials. JAMA 293:1900–1905
19. Topol EJ (2005) Nesiritide–not verified. N Engl J Med 353:113–116
20. Thackray S, Easthaugh J, Freemantle N et al (2002) The effectiveness and relative effectiveness of intravenous inotropic drugs acting through the adrenergic pathway in patients with heart failure–a meta-regression analysis. Eur J Heart Fail 4:515–529
21. Cuffe MS, Califf RM, Adams KF Jr et al (2002) Short-term intravenous milrinone for acute exacerbation of chronic heart failure: a randomized controlled trial. JAMA 287:1541–1547
22. Felker GM, Benza RL, Chandler AB et al (2003) Heart failure etiology and response to milrinone in decompensated heart failure: results from the OPTIME-CHF study. J Am Coll Cardiol 41:997–1003
23. Kaheinen P, Pollesello P, Levijoki J et al (2004) Effects of levosimendan and milrinone on oxygen consumption in isolated guinea-pig heart. J Cardiovasc Pharmacol 43:555–561
24. Lilleberg J, Ylonen V, Lehtonen L et al (2004) The calcium sensitizer levosimendan and cardiac arrhythmias: an analysis of the safety database of heart failure treatment studies. Scand Cardiovasc J 38:80–84
25. Follath F, Cleland JG, Just H et al (2002) Efficacy and safety of intravenous levosimendan compared with dobutamine in severe low-output heart failure (the LIDO study): a randomised double-blind trial. Lancet 360:196–202

26. Siegenthaler MP, Martin J, Beyersdorf F (2003) Mechanical circulatory assistance for acute and chronic heart failure: a review of current technology and clinical practice. J Interv Cardiol 16:563–572

11 Pacemaker and Internal Cardioverter-Defibrillator Therapies

J. L. ATLEE

Cardiac rhythm management devices (CRMD) have evolved significantly since the late 1950s, when the first pacemakers (PM) were implanted [1]. However, transcutaneous electrical cardiac stimulation was used to treat symptomatic advanced second-degree or third-degree atrioventricular (AV) heart block (Stokes–Adams attacks) in the 1920s [1, 2]. The first implantable devices were asynchronous ventricular PM (VOO[1]) for patients with Stokes–Adams attacks, and then evolved into dual-chamber PMs (DDD) to preserve AV synchrony [1–4].[2] Next, intracardiac sensing was added to avoid competition between paced and intrinsic rhythms in patients with intermittent symptomatic bradycardia due to AV heart block or sinus node dysfunction. The response to sensed events (first ventricular–VVI; then, atrial or dual-chamber sensing–VAT, VDD, DVI, DDD) could be inhibition or the triggering of ventricular pacing stimuli. The next important evolution was adaptive rate pacing (ARP) in the 1980s, whereby a physiologic sensor detected the need for increased paced heart rates with exercise. Physiologic responses that have been investigated and are or might be used clinically in ARP are listed in Table 1.

[1] Generic PM code: V, ventricular; A, atrial; D, dual (A and V); and, O, none. First letter: chamber paced; second letter: chamber sensed; third letter: response to sensed events (T = triggered or I = inhibited pacing stimulation).
[2] As discussed in Chapter 9, loss of atrial transport function is most disadvantageous in patients with reduced ventricular compliance due to aging, cardiomyopathies, or restrictive disease (e.g., pericarditis, pericardial effusions, hemorrhagic tamponade).

Department of Anesthesiology, Medical College of Wisconsin, Milwaukee, WI 53226, USA

Table 1. Physiologic responses that have been investigated or might/could be[a] used clinically in adaptive rate pacing (ARP)

Response to exercise	Measures/derivatives	Sensors that are (or might be) used in ARP[a]
↑ Respiratory rate	↑ Minute ventilation	Respiratory rate (intercostal muscle contractions); altered chest wall bioimpedance or biomechanics
↑ Temperature	↑ Core body (blood) temperature	Thermistors (body heat production)
↑ Body motion	↑ Muscle contractions; changes in chest wall impedance	Skeletal (especially, intercostal) muscle contractions (chest wall motion artifacts); altered chest wall bioimpedance
↑ Venous return, preload and contractility	↑ Myocardial performance measures (any or derivatives thereof)	Peak endocardial activation; preejection interval; stroke volume; systolic ventricular wall motion and/or dP/dt
↓ Vagal discharge ↑ Sympathetic discharge	↑ Sinus node automaticity, sinoatrial conduction time, and/or ↓ AV node conduction time/refractoriness[b]	Heart rate (systolic time as R-R/S-S intervals); or direct sensing of vagal/cervicothoracic sympathetic efferent discharge ("traffic")
↑ Sympathetic discharge	Shortened repolarization (QTI); faster depolarization (PDI); ↑ myocardial contractility	Direct measurement of QTI from intrinsic cardiac electrograms; LV/RV contractile force (dP/dt) or wall motion; peak endocardial activation time; preejection interval; stroke volume; altered cardiac impedance
↑ Metabolism	↑ CO_2 production ↑ O_2 utilization	Direct pH; end-tidal or blood CO_2 analysis; MVO_2

Adapted and modified from Fig. 31-9 in [1], p 776

ARP, adaptive rate pacing/pacemaker; QTI, QT interval; PDI, paced depolarization integral; LV/RV, left/right ventricular; MVO_2, mixed venous O_2 saturation

[a] Some may be hypothetical or untested, based on the author's speculation and his knowledge of physiologic responses to exercise

[b] Might be detected by intrinsic atrial electrograms and used as an ARP measure (sensor) of the need to increase ventricular rate in patients with sinus node dysfunction (i.e., preset lower rate criteria for atrial electrograms), or with bradycardia due to high-degree sinoatrial heart block

Indications for pacemakers have greatly expanded, and the technology still is evolving. This includes the incorporation of sensors for hemodynamic monitoring in patients with heart failure (HF). These technologic advances have to some degree served as a catalyst for an even faster evolution with implantable cardioverter-defibrillators (ICDs) and cardiac resynchronization therapy (CRT) [1]. Contemporary ICDs do conventional pacing (or ARP), cardioversion (CV), or defibrillation (DF). Yet, all CRMDs are costly therapy. Thus, supportive evidence from large prospective clinical trials is now the driving force behind innovation in this field [1].

In this chapter, we focus on CRMD therapies used in patients with symptomatic HF; i.e., New York Heart Association (NYHA) class III or IV HF,[3] often accompanied by destabilizing atrial and/or ventricular tachyarrhythmias. Device nomenclature, indications for pacing, selection of appropriate pacing modes, PM timing cycles, CRMD function and malfunction, troubleshooting, and perioperative management are discussed elsewhere [1, 3–6]. Topics addressed here are:

- Pacing for hemodynamic improvement
- Cardiac resynchronization therapy
- Pacing to prevent atrial fibrillation
- Pacing in long QT interval syndromes
- Implantable cardioverter-defibrillator therapy (pacing–all types, CRT, CV, or DF)

Pacing for Hemodynamic Improvement

Pacing for Bradycardia

Pacing to increase heart rate in bradycardia improves hemodynamics, but restoration of AV synchrony in patients with high-degree heart block and/or lower escape rhythms (e.g., cardiac surgery or acute coronary syndromes) will further improve hemodynamic profiles by restoring atrial booster pump function ("the atrial kick").

Hypertrophic Obstructive Cardiomyopathy

Dual-chamber pacing is used to treat severely symptomatic patients with medically refractory hypertrophic obstructive cardiomyopathy (HCM) [1]. It

[3] NYHA class III HF =: symptoms with exercise; NYHA class IV =: symptoms at bed rest)

is based on the concept that altered septal activation caused by right ventricular (RV) apical pacing reduces narrowing of the left ventricular (LV) outflow tract (LVOT), and a subsequent reduction in the Venturi effect created by this narrowing, which is responsible for systolic anterior motion of the mitral valve [7]. Pacing in HCM has been the subject of several randomized single-center and multicenter trials, discussed elsewhere [1]. In one single-center randomized crossover trial, there was symptomatic improvement in 63% of patients with pacing (DDD mode), but 42% of these also had improvement with AAI pacing (i.e., effectively, no pacing), suggesting a placebo effect. Also, in one multicenter, randomized, crossover trial, dual-chamber pacing produced a 50% reduction of the LVOT gradient, a 21% increase in exercise duration, and improvement in NYHA functional class vs. baseline status. However, when clinical parameters (i.e., chest pain, dyspnea, and subjective health status) were compared between DDD and AAI pacing, there were no significant differences, again suggesting a placebo effect. In yet another multicenter study, no significant differences were evident with randomization between pacing and no pacing, either *subjectively* (quality-of-life score) or *objectively* (exercise capacity, treadmill exercise time, or peak O_2 consumption). Thus, pacing should not be viewed as a primary therapy in HCM, and a subjective benefit without objective evidence of improvement should be cautiously interpreted. Pacing for medically refractory HCM is a class IIb indication in the 2002 ACC/AHA/NASPE[4] guidelines [8].

Finally, when pacing is used to treat symptomatic HCM, programming of an optimally short AV interval is critical to achieving optimal hemodynamic improvement [1, 3]. Further, ventricular depolarization must be the result of pacing. Thus, the AV interval must be short enough to cause ventricular depolarization by pacing. Yet, the shortest AV interval is not necessarily the best. In fact, some experts have advocated AV node ablation to ensure paced ventricular activation if fast intrinsic AV conduction prevents total ventricular depolarization by pacing stimulation.

Cardiac Resynchronization Therapy

CRT is used to reestablish synchronous contraction between the LV free wall and the ventricular septum to improve LV efficiency and the functional status of patients with HF [1, 9, 10]. That CRT is effective therapy in patients with HF is not surprising, given that many present with left bundle branch

[4] ACC, American College of Cardiology; AHA, American Heart Association; NASPE, North American Society for Pacing and Electrophysiology (now the Heart Rhythm Society).

block (LBBB) or intraventricular conduction delays that affect LV function, along with intrinsic myocardial dysfunction due to ventricular remodeling. Wiggers was the first to recognize the importance of synchronized ventricular contractions [11], and described LV contraction as a "series of sequential fractionate contractions of muscle bundles." He proposed that interspersed areas of ischemia or fibrosis might cause the disturbed temporal sequence of LV contraction. Much later, Harrison noted "disorganized contractions" (termed "asynergy") on kinetocardiograms of patients with coronary disease [12]. Next, Herman and colleagues correlated the presence of LV asynergy with clinical HF [13]. Then, the impact of rate-dependent LBBB on LV function was tested with exercise radionuclide angiography [14]. With rate-dependent LBBB, but without demonstrable coronary artery disease, there was an abrupt reduction in LV function with exercise. In contrast, without rate-dependent LBBB (controls), LV function increased by 26%. Thus, historical evidence suggests that asynchronous ventricular activation leads to asynchronous and suboptimal LV contraction patterns.

Generally, the term "CRT" has been used to describe biventricular pacing (RV and LV) or multisite (right atrial + RV and LV, or separate LV sites) pacing, but CRT can be achieved by LV pacing alone in some patients [1, 9]. Prospective, randomized clinical trials have proven the safety and efficacy of CRT (Table 2). In the 2002 NASP/ACC/AHA guidelines [8], biventricular pacing (BVP) in patients with medically refractory, symptomatic NYHA class III or IV HF and idiopathic dilated or ischemic cardiomyopathy, QRS prolongation ≥ 130 msec, LV end-diastolic diameter ≥ 55 mm, and LV ejection fraction of 0,35 ore less, is a class IIa indication for CRT. Similarly, the current US Food and Drug Administration labeling criteria for CRT include the above, but also caution that the patient must be (1) receiving optimal medical therapy and (2) in normal sinus rhythm.

Over 20 randomized controlled trials of CRT (with or without other therapies, e.g., ICD:CRT–ICD) are in now in progress (still recruiting patients) or planned (approved, but not yet recruiting patients) based on web access: www.clinicaltrials.gov (April 2006). Others are observational trials of patients with implanted CRT or CRT–ICD devices, or test the expected benefit from CRT based on QRS duration (e.g., 120–150 msec vs. ≥ 150 msec). Other RCT are testing new methods and indications for CRT or CRT–ICD, methods to predict patients who will most benefit from CRT,[5] optimal LV lead positions, or other issues pertaining to CRT. Issues being adressed in these trials include the following:

1. What is the impact of pacing to prevent atrial fibrillation (AFB) or the

[5] As many as 30% of patients selected for CRT do not benefit from this costly form of therapy.

Table 2. Prospective clinical trials showing safety and efficacy of cardiac resynchronization therapy in patients with heart failurea

Trial	Patient inclusion criteria	Trial end points	Treatment arms	Key findings
InSync	NYHA class III or IV HF on stable drug regimen LVEDD > 60 mm, LVEF ≤ 0.35, QRS width ≥ 150 ms	QOL NYHA class Six-min hall walk	Nonrandomized	Sustained improvement in all three end points
MIRACLE	NYHA class III or IV HF on stable drug regimen LVEDD > 60 mm, LVEF ≤ 0.35; QRS width ≥ 130 ms	QOL; NYHA class; six-min hall walk	Randomized to pacing or no pacing for 6 months and then to pacing	Sustained improvement in all three end points
PATH-CHF	DCM of any cause NYHA class III or IV HF on stable drug regimen QRS ≥ 120 ms PR ≥ 150 ms	Acute maximum LV pressure derivative Aortic pulse pressure Chronic O_2 uptake Anaerobic threshold Six-min hall walk	Acute/chronic assessment of hemodynamics with RV pacing vs. LV pacing vs. BiV pacing	*Acute BiV and LV pacing:* ↑ LV pressure derivative and aortic pulse pressure more than with RV pacing Sustained chronic improvement in all end points
MUSTIC-NSR	NYHA class III HF Refractory symptoms on stable drug therapy LVEF < 0.35; LVEDD > 60 mm Six-min hall walk < 450 m NSR with QRS > 150 ms	Functional capacity; QOL Metabolic exercise performance Mortality or need for heart transplant or LVAD Hospital admission for CHF	BiV pacing vs. no pacing with crossover	Sustained improvement in all end points Fewer hospital admissions with CRT

MUSTIC-AF	NYHA class III HF Refractory symptoms on stable drug therapy LVEF < 0.35; LVEDD > 60 mm 6-min walk < 450 m AF with paced QRS > 200 ms	Functional capacity; QOL Metabolic exercise performance Mortality or need for heart transplant or LVAD Hospital admission for CHF	BiV pacing vs. no pacing with crossover	Sustained improvement in all end points Fewer hospital admissions with CRT
InSync-III	NYHA class III or IV HF on stable drug regimen LVEDD > 60 mm, LVEF ≤ 0.35 QRS width ≥ 130 ms	QOL NYHA class Six-min hall walk	BiV pacing with optimized AV and VV intervals vs. no pacing with crossover	Sustained improvement in all three end points
CARE-HF	NYHA class III or IV HF on stable drug regimen LVEDD > 60 mm, LVEF ≤ 0.35 QRS width ≥ 150 ms or > 120 ms with echo study	Mortality and QOL Economic outcomes Echo parameters Neurohormonal measurements	BiV pacing vs. no pacing with crossover	Fewer urgent hospitalizations for worsening HF Reduced all-cause mortality or any-cause hospitalizations
PACMAN	Functional NYHA class III CHF LVEF <0.35 DCM of any etiology QRS >150 ms Optimal medical management Hospitalization at least once in past 12 months	Functional capacity by 6-min walk Secondary end points of: QOL, adverse events, ventricular arrhythmias, hospitalizations	Observation over 1 year with 1:1 randomization of patients to CRT vs. no CRT	Trial completed in Dec 2005. No results disseminated at major meetings (ACC/AHA/HRS) or available on website (April 2006)

VecToR	NYHA class III or IV LVEF ≤ 0.35 QRS > 140 ms LVEDD > 54 mm	QOL Mortality Echo parameters	BiV pacing *vs.* no pacing with crossover	In progress[b]
ReLeVent	NYHA class III or IV LVEF ≤ 0.35 QRS > 140 ms LVEDD > 55 mm	6-min walk LVEDD LVESD Mortality QOL	BiV pacing vs. no pacing with crossover	In progress[b]
PAVE	NYHA class II or III Status post AV nodal ablation Able to complete 6-min hall walk On stable medical therapy (≥ 3 months)	Exercise tolerance QOL	BiV pacing vs. RV pacing	In progress[b]

[a] Table and format the same as used by Hayes and Zipes [1], and updated by the present author (18 April 2006) with PubMed, Yahoo, and Google searches

[b] Present author was unable to verify the current status of these trials by personal communication with David Hayes or at www.clinicaltrials.gov using the terms cardiac resynchronization therapy, clinical trials, and heart failure (18 April 2006).

ACC, American College of Cardiology; AF, atrial fibrillation; AHA, American Heart Association; BiV, biventricular; CARE-CHF, Cardiac Resynchronization in Congestive Heart Failure; CHF, congestive heart failure; CRT, cardiac resynchronization therapy; DCM, dilated cardiomyopathy; echo, echocardiography; EHA, European Heart Association; HF, heart failure; HRS, Heart Rhythm Society–formerly North American Society for Pacing and Electrophysiology (NASPE); LV, left ventricular; LVAD, left ventricular assist device; LVEDD, left ventricular end-diastolic dimension; LVEF, left ventricular ejection fraction; LVESD, left ventricular end-systolic dimension; MIRACLE, Multicenter InSync Randomized Clinical Evaluation; MUSTIC, Multisite Stimulation In Cardiomyopathy; NSR, normal sinus rhythm; NYHA, New York Heart Association; PACMAN, Pacing for Cardiomyopathy: a European Study; PATH-CHF, Pacing Therapy in Congestive Heart Failure; PAVE, Left Ventricular Post-AV Nodal Ablation Evaluation (in patients with atrial fibrillation); QOL, quality of life; ReLeVent, Remodeling of Cardiac Cavities by Long-Term Ventricular-Based Stimulation; RV, right ventricular; VecToR, Ventricular Resynchronization Therapy Randomized

addition of atrial cardioversion/defibrillation to CRT–ICD on the course of HF?

2. Several trials (MADIT-CRT; REVERSE) are testing whether combined ICD and CRT is a *preventive therapy* that will reduce risk of mortality and HF events by ≥ 25% in patients who do not meet current criteria for CRT or CRT–ICD (i.e., ejection fraction ≤ 0.40; NYHA functional class I or II HF; QRS duration ≥ 120 ms).
3. PEGASUS-CRT is examining the effectiveness of *atrial rate support* (by addition of ARP) on exercise capacity in patients with NYHA class III or IV HF.
4. Several ongoing studies ask whether *tissue Doppler echocardiography or imaging* can identify those subsets of patients who will not improve with CRT.
5. In patients who are candidates for CRT and an ICD, does the response to CRT differ with LV pacing only (also known as *univentricular*) compared to RV or BVP?
6. Another trial evaluates the benefit of *interventricular (V–V) delay optimization* in reducing nonresponder rates with CRT–ICD devices.
7. BLOCK HF examines the *possible benefit* of CRT–ICD in patients with AV heart block (including those with NYHA class I or II HF). Primary outcomes include improvement in cardiac function, reduced urgent HF care admissions, and patient longevity.
8. *CRT in children* (newborns to ≤ 18 years) is unexplored territory. One trial employs tissue Doppler imaging, tissue synchronization imaging, and three-dimensional echocardiography to determine whether CRT (BVP) benefits children with HF secondary to dilated cardiomyopathy (DCM). Ventricular dyssynchrony occurs in more than 50% of these patients.
9. An important cause of CRT failure is rapid ventricular rates with atrial tachyarrhythmias (especially AFB). Ventricular rate control in AFB can be difficult with drugs. The "An Art Study" will investigate whether patients with CRT or CRT–ICD devices benefit from radiofrequency (RF) AV node ablation vs. control (device with no AV node ablation).
10. Leads used for LV stimulation in BVP or "univentricular" CRT are fluoroscopically positioned in veins circumventing the LV. This can be time-consuming and difficult, and there are lead-related failures. Several studies are evaluating new CRT lead systems.
11. Another study looks at the correlation between ventricular rate regulation and percentage time of BVP, along with quality of life (QOL) and physical abilities in patients with CRT in AFB.
12. MASCOT (Europe) tests whether adding a proprietary atrial antitachyarrhythmia pacing algorithm to CRT improves HF prognosis with atrial tachyarrhythmias (mostly AFB).

13. Another algorithm being tested in Europe (The Conducted Atrial Fibrillation Response Algorithm (CAFR™) maximizes the amount of CRT (BVP) when AFB occurs.
14. Yet another study will evaluate CRT with β-blocker therapy in symptomatic HF patients who could tolerate β-blocker therapy (or optimal dosages thereof) before CRT.
15. LOCATE-Pilot will determine whether an echocardiogram before device implantation will improve responses to CRT. The hypothesis is that response to CRT can be optimized by guiding LV lead placement to the maximally delayed viable basal LV segment.
16. The ACC trial is evaluating the optimal atrial contribution to ventricular resynchronization in the event of right atrial (RA) pacing in patients with conventional CRT implant criteria.
17. Another study in Europe compares the efficacy of RV or biventricular antitachycardia pacing in candidates for CRT with a class I or IIA indication for ICD implantation.
18. A Canadian study asks whether ICD–CRT reduces mortality or hospitalizations for CHF.

Pacing to Prevent Atrial Fibrillation

Multisite and alternative site pacing–vs. right atrial appendage (RAA)–is used to prevent or reduce recurrent atrial tachyarrhythmias. They may reduce the dispersion of atrial refractoriness, conducive to reentry tachyarrhythmias [15]. Several strategies are used [1]. Biatrial synchronous pacing (leads in the RAA and coronary sinus) allows sensing from the RAA lead to be followed by immediate pacing from the coronary sinus. "*Dual-site atrial pacing*" is used to describe this lead configuration [1, 16]. With both RA leads connected to the same port, there is simultaneous pacing at both sites. This method has been shown in one randomized controlled trial and a follow-up report to reduce the number of AFB or atrial flutter (AFT) episodes, and to increase the time to recurrent arrhythmias [17, 18]. Single-site interatrial septal (at triangle of Koch) [19] or Bachmann's bundle pacing [20] have also been tested, and appear more effective than RAA pacing in preventing AFB in patients with standard bradycardia pacing indications.

In addition to biatrial pacing strategies, multiple pacing algorithms have been incorporated in CRMD to reduce the number of premature atrial beats and maintain constant atrial pacing. Some available or in-progress randomized controlled trials (2005) are summarized by Hayes and Zipes, and they illustrate an algorithm that alters the atrial pacing rate after a sensed premature atrial beat [1]. While some trials summarized were completed, others were still recruiting patients. Even so, these authorities considered it likely that programmable pacing strategies to reduce the number of triggering atrial events for AFT or AFB will be programmable features in most future dual-chamber pacing systems [1].

Pacing in Long QT Interval Syndromes

The long QT interval syndrome (LQTS), whether congenital (C-LQTS) or acquired (A-LQTS), is abnormally prolonged ventricular repolarization (represented by the QT interval and increased risk for life-threatening ventricular arrhythmias, especially *torsades de pointes* (TDP). TDP is any polymorphic ventricular tachycardia (PMVT) with QT-interval (QTI) prolongation [21, 22]. Without QTI prolongation, PMVT (often in acute coronary syndromes) is simply PMVT. A mainstay of therapy for TDP (A-LQTS) is withdrawal of drugs or substances (e.g., nutraceuticals or herbals) that prolong the QTI and cause TDP (http://www.torsades.org). Specific therapy includes intravenous magnesium and atrial or ventricular overdrive pacing [22]. Also, class IB antiarrhythmic drugs (e.g., lidocaine, procainamide) or isoproterenol (cautiously!) to increase heart rate can be tried.

For patients with the idiopathic LQTS (C-LQTS), but *without* syncope, complex ventricular arrhythmias (tachycardia/fibrillation–VT/VF), or a family history of sudden death, no treatment with β-blockers is often advised [22]. For *asymptomatic patients* with C-LQTS and VT/VF, or a family history of early sudden death, β-blockers at maximally tolerated doses are advised. Also, permanent pacing may be indicated to prevent bradycardia or pauses that may predispose to TDP. However, *with syncope due to ventricular arrhythmias or aborted sudden death,* an ICD is advised. In addition, such patients should be treated with β?-blockers and, perhaps, atrial overdrive pacing (via the ICD) to reduce the frequency of ICD shocks. Aside from shocks, contemporary ICDs are beneficial due to their ability to continually pace to prevent bradycardia-induced TDP, along with pacing algorithms that prevent post-premature ventricular beat pauses.

ICDs in C-LQTS patients without syncope but with a strong family history of sudden death remain controversial [22]. For those with syncope despite maximum drug therapy, left cervicothoracic sympathetic ganglionectomy (stellate ganglion + first 3–4 thoracic sympathetic ganglia) may be helpful. Finally, potassium-channel-activating drugs (cromakalim, pinacidil) may be useful in C-LQTS and A-LQTS with symptomatic VT or a history of resuscitated sudden death.

ICD Therapy

ICD Design and Function

ICD components include a power source, circuitry, memory, and a microprocessor to coordinate component functions [1, 3, 4, 23]. Capacitors transform battery voltages into discharges from ≤ 1 V to 750 V for VT or VF (CV or DF). ICDs incorporate a different sensing circuitry (to detect and discriminate tachyarrhythmias) from that of most CRMDs. However, all contemporary ICDs *are* PMs, and provide at least antibradycardia pacing during bradycardia or asystole that may follow CV or DF. Either of these postshock cardiac rhythm disturbances may facilitate or precipitate further tachyarrhythmias.

Almost all ICD systems implanted today have transvenous lead systems. In addition to shocks, they feature preprogrammed (during cardiac electrophysiologic studies) antitachycardia pacing to reduce the need for shocks in VT. Further, most are DDD devices and include adaptive-rate pacing. Increasingly, atrial CV/DF and CRT are also ICD features. ICD longevity depends on the frequency of shock delivery and need for PM therapies, but most last 5–9 years. All ICDs now use biphasic shocks. These are more efficient (use less energy) than monophasic shocks, but the specifics for biphasic shock waveforms varies among ICD device manufacturers [1].

An ICD continuously monitors the patient's heart rate and rhythm. It delivers therapy if the rate exceeds a programmed upper rate cutoff (e.g., VT ≥ 175 beats/min). If so, a "tiered therapy" may begin with antitachycardia pacing (ATP) or shocks, depending on the programming. ICDs incorporating "tiered therapy" have significant programming flexibility to adjust for the many aspects of tachycardia detection and discrimination (e.g., AFB or AFT vs. VT). In addition, different zones (or "tiers") of therapy can be programmed to allow confirmation of slower arrhythmias (often better tolerated[6]), so that ATP is attempted before shocks are delivered. Still, with tiered therapy, faster tachyarrhythmias are treated more aggressively (shocks first). Such therapy could include three zones of therapy for VT from 126 beats/min to up to ≥ 200 beats/min:

1. Zone 1 (126–160 beats/min): two different sequences of ATP (ATP-1; ATP-2), then shocks of 1 J, 5 J and 34 J
2. Zone 2 (161–200 beats/min): ATP, then 10 J and 34 J shocks
3. Zone 3 (> beats/min): 34 J shocks [1]

Shocks are synchronized (CV) if tachycardia has distinct R and S waves. Otherwise, they are nonsynchronized (DF), high-energy shocks for PMVT (or TDP) and VF. Finally, zones and detection rates for tachyarrhythmias, specifics of the different therapies, and antibradycardia pacing are program-

[6] In some devices, this is confirmed by hemodynamic measures of cardiac performance

mable. However, programming flexibility varies significantly between ICD devices, regardless of manufacturer.

Indications for ICD Therapy

The ACC/AHA/NASPE guidelines for PMs and ICDs were last updated in 2002 [8], and ICD indications are summarized in Table 3. Given the expanded indications for pacing in HF, technological advances and findings of recent prospective clinical trials in CRT, combined CRT–ICD and now "atrioverter" therapies, these guidelines will soon be or are being updated–see www.americanheart.org, www.acc.org, www.hrsonline.org. Important changes from the 1998 guidelines are discussed below under the headings "Randomized Clinical Trials of ICD therapy" and "Who is Expected to Benefit from ICD Therapy?" Also discussed is combined ICD–CRT therapy. However, device selection, issues unique to ICD implantation, complications, etc., are detailed in standard works on CRMD or cardiac arrhythmias and their management. Common to all CRMDs are: (1) malfunction secondary to electromagnetic interference, (2) interference due to drugs or metabolic causes, and (3) device follow-up. These topics have recently been discussed elsewhere [1, 3, 4, 6].

Randomized Clinical Trials of ICD Therapy

ICD therapy has been determined efficacious for: (1) *secondary prevention* of sudden death (SD) in patients who have experienced SD due to VT or VF, or (2) *primary prevention* for SD in patients who have not yet experienced SD due to VT or VF, but are at high risk of same. Criteria that have been used to determine patient suitability for inclusion in primary prevention ICD trials include [1]:

1. Q-wave myocardial infarction (MI) ≥ 3 weeks previously
2. Asymptomatic nonsustained VT (NSVT)
3. LV ejection fraction ≤ 0.40 or ≤ 0.36
4. Induced VT–VF at electrophysiologic study (EPS) not suppressed by procainamide
5. NYHA HF classes I–III
6. Abnormal signal-averaged ECG (SAECG)
7. Patient scheduled for elective coronary artery bypass surgery
8. Nonischemic, dilated cardiomyopathy
9. Acute MI + EF ≤ 0.40 + SDRR[7] < 70 ms or ≥ 109 premature ventricular

[7] Standard deviation of the R-R interval

Table 3. Summary of indications for implantation of an internal cardioverter–defibrillator from the 2002 ACC/AHA/NASPE guidelines.

Class I	Class II	Class III
Cardiac arrest (VT or VF) not due to a transient or reversible cause	Patients with a LVEF ≤ 30% and at least 1 month post-MI, 3 months past coronary artery revascularization surgery or successful PCCI	Syncope of undetermined origin in a patient without inducible ventricular tachyarrhythmias and without SHD
Spontaneous sustained VT in patients with SHD	Cardiac arrest presumed due to VF when EP testing is precluded by coexisting disease	Incessant VT or VF
Syncope of undetermined origin with clinically relevant VT or VF induced at EPS when drug therapy is ineffective, or not tolerated or preferred	Severe symptoms (e.g., syncope) that can be attributed to sustained ventricular VT or VF while awaiting cardiac transplantation	VF or VT consequent to arrhythmias that are amenable to surgical or catheter ablation (e.g., atrial tachyarrhythmias associated with WPW, RVOT VT, idiopathic LV tachycardia, or fascicular VT
NSVT in patients with coronary disease, prior MI, LV dysfunction, and inducible VF or sustained VT at EPS that is not suppressed by a class I antiarrhythmic drug (i.e., quinidine-like)	Familial or inherited conditions with a high risk of life-threatening tachyarrhythmias (e.g., A-LQTS or hypertrophic cardiomyopathy)	Ventricular tachyarrhythmias due to a transient or reversible disorder (e.g., AMI, electrolyte imbalance, drugs, or trauma) if correction of the disorder is believed feasible and likely to substantially reduce the risk of recurrent tachyarrhythmias
Spontaneous, sustained VT in patients with SHD not amenable to other therapies	NSVT with CAD, prior MI, LV dysfunction, and inducible VT or VF at EPS	Significant psychiatric illnesses that may be aggravated by device implantation or may preclude systematic follow-up
	Recurrent syncope of undetermined cause in the presence of ventricular dysfunction and inducible ventricular tachyarrhythmias at EPS when other causes of syncope have been excluded	Terminal illnesses with a projected life-expectancy of < 6 months
	Syncope of unexplained origin or family history of unexplained sudden cardiac death associated with typical or atypical RBBB and ST segment elevation (i.e., the Brugada syndrome)	Patients with CAD with LV dysfunction and prolonged QRS duration in the absence of spontaneous or inducible sustained VT or NSVT who are undergoing coronary bypass surgery or PCCI
	Syncope in patients with advanced SHD in whom thorough invasive and noninvasive investigations have failed to define a cause	NYHA class IV, drug-refractory heart failure in patients who are not candidates for cardiac transplantation[a]

From [8] and [1], p 787

VT, ventricular tachycardia; VF, ventricular fibrillation; LVEF, left ventricular ejection fraction; MI, myocardial infarction; SHD, structural heart disease; PCCI, percutaneous coronary intervention; EP, electrophysiologic; EPS, electrophysiologic study; WPW, Wolff–Parkinson–White syndrome; RVOT, right ventricular outflow tract; LV, left ventricle/ventricular; NSVT, nonsustained VT; A-LQTS, acquired long QT interval syndrome; AMI, acute myocardial infarction; CAD, coronary artery disease; NYHA, New York Heart Association

a Given now-available evidence for combined cardiac resynchronization and ICD therapy (one implantable device), when the 2002 guidelines are updated, this supposition will/should include (in addition to cardiac transplantation) "or an ICD–CRT device" (present author)

beats (PVBs) per hour or abnormal SAECG; or, these with a heart rate ≥ 80 beats/min
10. Ischemic or nonischemic cardiomyopathy + EF ≤ 0.35 + NYHA class II or III HF + appropriate angiotensin-converting enzyme inhibitor + no history of sustained VT/VF
11. Survivor of sudden cardiac arrest from resuscitated VT/VF or probable sudden cardiac arrest with right bundle branch block and ST-segment elevation
12. VT, VF, or nonischemic cardiomyopathy + EF < 0.35 + NSVT or positive SAECG

Who Is Expected to Benefit from ICD Therapy?

In the AVID trial, a prospective, multicenter RCT, patients with CAD and a reduced LVEF (≤ 0.40) experienced a survival benefit with ICDs vs. class III antiarrhythmic drugs (ADs–mainly, amiodarone) ± β-blockers [24]. Unadjusted survival estimates were 89.3% for ICD vs. 82.3% with AD at 1 year, 81.6% vs. 74.7% at 2 years, and 75.4% vs. 64.1% at 3 years ($P < 0.02$). Mortality reductions (± 95% confidence limits) with ICD vs. drugs at 1, 2, and 3 years, respectively, were 39 ± 20%, 27 ± 21%, and 31 ± 21%. Similarly, the MADIT trial results confirm a survival benefit in patients at high risk of VT/VF [25]. MADIT's premise was that documented NSVT was known to confer a 2-year mortality rate of around 30% in patients with prior MI and LV dysfunction (EF ≤ 0.35). MADIT asked whether prophylactic ICD therapy vs. conventional medical therapy (amiodarone, β-blockers, or other AD) would improve survival in this high-risk patient subset. Over a 5-year period, 196 patients with NYHA class I, II, or III HF, prior MI, and LVEF ≤ 0.35, as well as inducible, nonsuppressible VT or VF at electrophysiologic study (EPS), were randomly assigned to receive an ICD (n = 95) or conventional medical therapy (n During average follow-up of 27 months, there was a significant average 46% reduction in the hazard ratio for all-cause death with ICD vs. medical therapy. In addition, there was no evidence that medical therapy alone had a significant influence on the observed hazard ratio. Thus, prophylactic ICD appears to improve survival vs. medical therapy in patients with prior MI, NSVT, and LVEF ≤ 0.35.

MADIT-II was a multicenter sequel trial in 1232 patients with previous MI and a reduced LVEF (≤ 0.30) at risk of life-threatening ventricular arrhythmias [26]. ICD use as primary prevention was evaluated in these patients. Patients were randomized to receive ICD (n = 742) or conventional medical therapy (n = 490). Invasive EPS for risk stratification was not required. The primary end point was any-cause death. Clinical characteristics and prevalence of medications used at last follow-up were similar in both groups. During an average 20-month follow-up, mortality rates were 19.8% with medical therapy vs. 14.2% with ICD. There was a significant reduction in the hazard ratio for risk of any-cause death with ICD (31%) vs. conventional therapy. The ICD survival benefit was similar in stratified subgroup analyses (i.e., age, sex, LVEF, NYHA class, and QRS interval). Based largely on these findings, the 2002 ACC/AHA/NASPE guidelines include patients meeting MADIT-II inclusion criteria as having a class IIa indication for ICD implantation, provided their QRS is greater than 120 ms.

MADIT-II tested patients with reduced LVEF due to an ischemic event, but not those with HF and symptoms or with idiopathic dilated cardiomyopathy (IDCM). However, patients with IDCM, poor LV function, and NSVT too are at increased risk of sudden cardiac death [24]. Completed or ongoing trials of combined ICD–CRT therapy as primary prevention in dilated cardiomyopathy, whether due to ischemic heart disease or idiopathic causes, are reviewed elsewhere [1]. Two are discussed below.

Combined ICD-CRT Therapy

Several trials have included patients with either IDCM or ischemic cardiomyopathy with criteria for CRT and ICD implantation for secondary prevention [1]. Among these, COMPANION [27] and MIRACLE-ICD [38] were the largest and most conclusive. COMPANION was terminated early following recruitment of 1634 patients out of an expected 2200 [27, 28]. Patients (1520) with ischemic cardiomyopathy or IDCM in NYHA class III or IV HF, and with a QRS interval of ≥ 0.12 s, were randomly assigned (1:2:2 ratio) to receive optimal drug therapy for HF alone or with CRT (PM–CRT or ICD–CRT). The primary end point was time to death or any-cause hospitalization. Compared to drug therapy alone, PM–CRT reduced this risk (hazard ratio, 0.81; $P = 0.014$), as did ICD–CRT (hazard ratio, 0.80; $P = 0.01$). Also, compared to optimal drug therapy for HF, the risk of hospitalization for or death from HF was significantly reduced with PM–CRT (34%) or ICD–CRT (40%), as was the risk of death from any cause (by 24% or 36%, respectively). In MIRACLE-ICD, 369 patients at high risk of life-threatening VT or VF with QRS ≥ 130 ms, EF ≤ 0.35, and NYHA class III–IV HF (despite optimal medical therapy) were randomized to control (ICD activated, CRT off; $n = 182$) or to CRT (ICD activated, CRT on; n YHA functional class, and 6-min hall walk distance. Survival, incidence of ventricular arrhythmias, and rates of hospitalization were also compared. At 6 months, patients with CRT had greater improvement in QOL and NYHA functional class, but 6-min hall walk distance was not different between groups. Treadmill exercise duration increased by 56 s in the CRT group vs. an 11-s decrease in controls. There were no significant differences between groups in LV size or function, overall HF status, survival, and rates of hospitalization.

Summary and Conclusions

PM–CRT and ICD–CRT are novel *adjunct* device therapies for management of NYHA class III or IV HF. They *do not replace the need for optimal drug therapy.* Not only does CRT improve hemodynamics, exercise tolerance, and QOL for patients with severe HF over the short term, it also confers a survival benefit. And, based on the COMPANION trial results, this may be even greater for patients with ICD–CRT vs. PM–CRT, probably because the former patient subset is at higher risk of sudden death from VT/VF. However, today, CRT therapy is costly, and combined CRT–ICD therapy is even more so. Thus, these life-saving therapies won't be affordable for most of the world for some time. Yet, if these therapies could be shown to significantly reduce overall healthcare costs in patients meeting well-defined criteria for CRT and/or ICD therapies, this might reduce the need for even costlier therapies (e.g., ventricular assist devices; total artificial heart; heart transplantation). If this happens, there will be greater use of PM–CRT or ICD–CRT devices globally.

References

1. Hayes DL, Zipes DP (2005) Cardiac pacemakers and cardioverter-defibrillators. In: Zipes DP, Libby P, Bonow RO, Braunwald E (eds) Braunwald's heart disease, 7th edn. Elsevier Saunders, Philadelphia, pp 767–96
2. Atlee JL (1996) Arrhythmias and pacemakers. Saunders, Philadelphia, pp 205–46
3. Atlee JL, Bernstein AD (2001) Cardiac rhythm management devices. Part 1. Indications, device selection and function. Anesthesiology 95:1265–80
4. Atlee JL, Bernstein AD (2001) Cardiac rhythm management devices. Part 2. Perioperative management. Anesthesiology 95:1492–1506
5. Lee TH (2005) Guidelines: cardiac pacemakers and cardioverter-defibrillators. In: Zipes DP, Libby P, Bonow RO, Braunwald E (eds) Braunwald's heart disease, 7th edn. Elsevier Saunders, Philadelphia, pp 796–802
6. American Society of Anesthesiologists Task Force on Perioperative Management of Patients with Cardiac Rhythm Management Devices (2005) Practice advisory for the perioperative management of patients with cardiac rhythm management devices: pacemakers and implantable cardioverter-defibrillators: a report by the American Society of Anesthesiologists Task Force on Perioperative Management of Patients with Cardiac Rhythm Management Devices. Anesthesiology 103:186–98
7. Sorajja P, Elliott PM, McKenna WJ (2000) Pacing in hypertrophic cardiomyopathy. Cardiol Clin 18:67–79

8. Gregoratos G, Abrams J, Epstein AE, et al (2002) American College of Cardiology/American Heart Association Task Force on Practice Guidelines/North American Society for Pacing and Electrophysiology Committee to Update the 1998 Pacemaker Guidelines. Circulation 106:2145–61
9. Atlee JL (2005) Pacemaker resynchronisation in the treatment of severe heart failure. In: Gullo A (ed) Anaesthesia, Pain, Intensive Care and Emergency Medicine (A.P.I.C.E.) 20. Springer, Milan, pp 99–112
10. Fantoni C, Auricchio A (2006) Cardiac resynchronisation therapy: do we know everything? In: Gullo A (ed) Anaesthesia, Pain, Intensive Care and Emergency Medicine (A.P.I.C.E.) 20. Springer, Milan, pp 257–66
11. Wiggers C (1926) Are ventricular conduction changes important in the dynamics of left ventricular contraction? Am J Physiol 74:12–30
12. Harrison T (1965) Some unanswered questions concerning enlargement and failure of the heart. Am Heart J 69:100–115
13. Herman MV, Heinle RA, Klein MD, et al. (1967) Localized disorders in myocardial contraction. Asynergy and its role in congestive heart failure. N Engl J Med 277:222–32
14. Bramlet DA, Morris KG, Coleman RE, et al (1983) Effect of rate-dependent left bundle branch block on global and regional left ventricular function. Circulation. 67:1059–65
15. Gillis AM (2000) Pacing to prevent atrial fibrillation. Cardiol Clin 18:25–36
16. Misier AR, Beukema WP, Willems R (2003) Multisite atrial pacing for atrial fibrillation prevention: where to go from here? Card Electrophysiol Rev 7:329–32
17. Saksena S, Prakash A, Ziegler P, et al (2002) Improved suppression of recurrent atrial fibrillation with dual-site right atrial pacing and antiarrhythmic drug therapy. J Am Coll Cardiol 40:1140–50
18. Prakash A, Saksena S, Ziegler P, et al (2005) Dual site right atrial pacing can improve the hemodynamic impact of standard dual-chamber on atrial and ventricular mechanical function in patients with symptomatic atrial fibrillation: further observations from the dual site atrial pacing for prevention of atrial fibrillation trial. J Intervent Card Electrophysiol 12:177–87
19. Padeletti L, Pieragnoli P, Ciapetti C, et al (2001) Randomized crossover comparison of right atrial appendage pacing versus interatrial septum pacing for prevention of paroxysmal atrial fibrillation in patients with sinus bradycardia. Am Heart 142:1047–55
20. Bailin SJ, Adler S, Giudici M (2001) Prevention of chronic atrial fibrillation by pacing in the region of Bachmann's bundle: results of a multicenter randomized trial. J Cardiovasc Electrophysiol 12:912–7
21. Atlee JL (2004) Decision-making in critical care: cardiac arrhythmias and related topics. In: Gullo A (ed) Anaesthesia, Pain, Intensive Care and Emergency Medicine (A.P.I.C.E.) 19. Springer, Milan, Springer-Verlag Italia Compiler/Production: page numbers<<QA16>>?
22. Olgin JE, Zipes DP (2005) Specific arrhythmias: diagnosis and treatment. In: Zipes DP, Libby P, Bonow RO, Braunwald E (eds) Braunwald's heart disease, 7th edn. Elsevier Saunders, Philadelphia, pp 803–863
23. Pinski SL, Fahey GJ (1999) Implantable cardioverters-defibrillators. Am J Med 106:446–58
24. The Antiarrhythmics Versus Implantable Defibrillators (AVID) Investigators (1997) A comparison of antiarrhythmic drug therapy with implantable defibrillators in patients resuscitated from near-fatal ventricular arrhythmias. N Engl J Med 337:1576–83

25. Moss AJ, Hall WJ, Cannom DS, et al (1996) Multicenter Automatic Defibrillator Implantation Trial Investigators: improved survival with an implanted defibrillator in patients with coronary disease at high risk for ventricular arrhythmia. N Engl J Med 335:1933–40
26. Moss AJ, Zareba W, Hall WJ, et al, for the Multicenter Automatic Defibrillator Implantation Trial II Investigators (2002) Prophylactic implantation of a defibrillator in patients with myocardial infarction and reduced ejection fraction. N Engl J Med 346:877–83
27. Bristow MR, Saxon LA, Boehmer J, et al (2004) Comparison of Medical Therapy, Pacing, and Defibrillation in Heart Failure (COMPANION) Investigators. Cardiac-resynchronization therapy with or without an implantable defibrillator in advanced chronic heart failure. N Engl J Med 350:2140–50
28. Young JB, Abraham WT, Smith AL, et al (2003) Combined cardiac resynchronization and implantable cardioversion defibrillation in advanced chronic heart failure: the MIRACLE ICD Trial. JAMA 289:2685–94

12 Updates on Cardiac Arrest and Cardiopulmonary Resuscitation

G. Ristagno[1], A. Gullo[2], W. Tang[1,3] and M. H. Weil[1,3,4]

Introduction

Cardiac arrest is a dramatic clinical event that can occur suddenly, often without premonitory signs. The condition is characterized by sudden loss of consciousness due to the lack of cerebral blood flow, which occurs when the heart ceases to pump. This phenomenon is potentially reversible if cardiopulmonary resuscitation (CPR) procedures are started early, but it becomes irreversible without interventions or when initiation of CPR is delayed [1].

The majority of cardiac arrests are "sudden death" due to coronary or other vascular events. Accordingly, sudden death is defined as a natural event since traumatic causes are excluded. Sudden death often occurs in individuals who had no prior awareness of life-threatening disease. Before starting CPR, the rescuer must identify the absence of a heart beat. Prompt intervention is then necessary to secure temporary circulation and ventilation and allow for the potential of reestablishing spontaneous circulation. Indeed, CPR is likely to be successful only if it is instituted within 5 min after the heart stops beating [2, 3].

As many as 400 000 Americans and 700 000 Europeans sustain cardiac arrests each year [4]. Despite major efforts to improve outcomes from sudden cardiac death, including worldwide publication of new cardiopulmonary resuscitation guidelines every 5–8 years for the past three decades, only 4–9% of victims survive [5–8] (Table 1). In both heavily populated larger cities and sparsely populated rural communities, delayed response by rescue

[1]Weil Institute of Critical Care Medicine, Rancho Mirage, CA, USA; [2]UCO Anestesia e Rianimazione, Azienda Ospedaliero-Universitaria, Policlinico di Catania; [3]Keck School of Medicine of the University of Southern California, Los Angeles, CA, USA; [4]Northwestern University Medical School, Chicago, IL, USA

Table 1. History of guidelines for cardiac resuscitation

1974	Cardiopulmonary resuscitation training extended to general public
1980	ACLS guidelines
1986	Pediatric BLS and ALS, neonatal ALS
1992	ILCOR founded
2000	First international guidelines
2005	International Consensus on Science followed by American Heart Association guidelines

BLS, basic life support; ALS, advanced life support; Advanced Cardiovascular Life Support, International Liaison Committee on Resuscitation

services compromises outcomes such that survival is even more disappointing, namely between 1% and 5% [9, 10]. Bystander-initiated CPR by minimally trained nonprofessional rescuers or by well-organized professional emergency medical response providers has increased survival from out-of-hospital cardiac arrest by as much as ten-fold [11–13].

In 1991, Cummins et al. introduced the concept of the "chain of survival" for the victims of out-of-hospital cardiac arrest [14]. This chain has four links, namely: (1) early access to qualified rescuers; (2) basic life support (BLS); (3) early defibrillation; and (4) advanced life support (ALS). The first three links are especially focused on out-of-hospital cardiac resuscitation. The critical time interval, in part based on the Utstein templates [15], begins with the call for emergency assistance and documents arrival time of the response team at the site of the victim. If BLS has not been initiated, it is started immediately after cardiac arrest has been confirmed. However, emergency medical service (EMS) systems usually require more than 5 min to respond. Greater survival will therefore depend on bystander-initiated CPR. Current evidence supports the importance of well-organized public access defibrillation programs in which CPR by lay rescuers is combined with automated defibrillation [16].

Major Changes in the 2005 Cardiopulmonary Resuscitation Guidelines

International experts followed a consistent and thorough process for evolging updated resuscitation guideline. They searched the literature, evaluated studies, quantitated levels of evidence and developed consensus on classes of recommendations. The new 2005 American Heart Association (AHA) guidelines for CPR represent an international scientific document, which is individualized at the discretion of regions or country. Three major changes may be summarized including the priority of CPR, and especially of precordial compression; the new algorithm for defibrillation; and the lesser use of drugs and especially including vasopressor agents.

Precordial Compression

The highest priority after "sudden death" is to start external cardiac compression to maintain at least minimal coronary and cerebral perfusion. The exception may be the majority of neonatal, pediatric, and young adult victims in whom failure of ventilation is the primary cause of cardiac arrest. It is likely that opening of the airway and externally assisted ventilation take the highest priority in these cases which present in settings other than those characteristic of "sudden death." Airway obstruction and other causes of asphyxia, including traumatic injuries, drowning, or drug overdose, are the predominant causes. For initial management of "sudden death," however, the new 2005 guidelines focus on the importance of chest compression as the highest-priority treatment to sustain both coronary and cerebral blood flows. Sustaining cerebral blood flow by effective chest compression minimizes ischemic brain damage [17]. There is no challenge to the documentation that outcomes from sudden death primary depend on the effectiveness of chest compression. Wik et al. [18] found that "good bystander CPR," defined as generating a palpable carotid or femoral pulse and intermittent lung inflation such as to expand the chest, improved outcomes in victims of sudden death. Whereas 23% of victims were resuscitated with "good CPR", only 1% were resuscitated with "not good CPR." Accordingly, in both in-hospital and out-of-hospital settings, the quality of CPR is a major determinant of outcomes. Based on a study on 176 victims of out-of-hospital cardiac arrest, only 28% of rescuers performed competent chest compressions in which the anterior–posterior diameter was decreased by between 38 and 51 mm as recommended in the guidelines [19, 20]. Based on 67 instances of in-hospital cardiac arrest, Abella et al. [21] confirmed failure to provide adequate depth of compression in conformance with existing guidelines. Suboptimal rates of compression have also been associated with less favorable outcomes [22].

Nevertheless, the guidelines may not be applicable in some settings. For instance the frequency and the depth of artificial ventilation is one example. Aufderheide et al. [23] observed that professional rescues frequently ventilate patients with excessive tidal volume and frequency during out-of-hospital CPR. The average ventilation rate was 30 per min. In animal studies, such excesses of ventilation yield unfavorable outcomes, presumably due to increases in intrathoracic pressure, which account for decreases in cardiac filling and therefore decreases in forward blood flow during lung inflation. Failure to achieve threshold levels of forward blood flow, aortic pressure, and consequently coronary perfusion pressure are consistently identified as predictive of unfavourable outcomes based on both experimental and clinical studies [24, 25–28].

To obtain shorter interruptions of chest compression during CPR, the 2005 guidelines mandate compression/ventilation ratios of 30:2 in lieu of 15:2. Although secure clinical proof of ultimate benefit of these revised compression/ventilation ratios has not yet been published, experimental studies have provided evidence that more frequent ventilations did not improve outcomes [29, 30]. However, increasing the compression/ventilation ratios increased pulmonary blood flow and end-tidal CO_2 without compromise of arterial oxygen content or acid–base balance [30]. Only more recently have we fully appreciated that the cardiac output and therefore pulmonary blood flow produced by chest compression during CPR is actually less than one-third of normal physiological levels. Accordingly, fewer ventilations are required to maintain optimal ventilation/perfusion ratios. Even more important, gas exchange may be sufficient in the absence of external ventilation. Precordial compression itself provides sufficient gas exchange for the small pulmonary blood flow, especially if high flow oxygen is passively delivered into the airway [31, 32]. Spontaneous gasping provides another and probably important source of pulmonary gas exchange during CPR [33, 34]. We now also recognize that earlier guidelines overestimated the tidal and minute volumes required during conventional CPR and failed to appreciate the adverse effects of interruptions of chest compression and descreased venous return [35]. Ventilation has indeed become of much lesser importance except in asphyxial cardiac arrest [36]. In a swine model, adverse outcomes followed prolonged interruptions in chest compressions during simulated mouth-to-mouth ventilation [37]. During lung inflation, venous return is transiently decreased such that preload and ultimately the aortic diastolic pressure are decreased. Systemic blood flow and organ perfusion are correspondingly reduced. It has also been apparent that after interrupting chest compression, full restoration of forward blood flow is not promptly achieved. As many as seven chest compressions are required prior to achieving maximal effect. Accordingly, uninterrupted chest compression would be expected to, and in fact did, produce better 24-h survival and neurological recovery [38].

Timing of Defibrillation and Defibrillation Algorithm

The international guidelines 2000 advised electrical defibrillation as soon as VF was detected regardless of the estimated duration of untreated cardiac arrest [39]. The 2005 guidelines mandated chest compressions as the initial intervention prior to attempted defibrillation. In istances other than witnessed onset of cardiac arrest or when the duration of untreated cardiac arrest exceeded 5 minutes. Evidence supported the likelihood of successful defibrillation if compression preceded defibrillation attempts in such setting and especially when the duration of untreated VF was prolonged beyond 5 min. Improvements in survival of human victims after prolonged cardiac arrest from 24% to 30%, were reported by Cobb et al. [43] and more favorable neurological recovery, from 17% to 23%, when 90 s of CPR preced the defibrillation attempts. In a separate clinical trial, Wik et al. [19] randomized patients after out-of-hospital cardiac arrest to immediate defibrillation or to a 3-min interval of chest compression and ventilation prior to defibrillation. The authors confirmed that when the response time was less than 5 min, no benefit of chest compression was observed. However, when intervention was delayed for more than 5 min, significantly better 1-year survivals was documented in victims in which CPR preceded defibrillation. The new international guidelines 2005, therefore, mandate a 1.5 min to 3 min interval of CPR prior to attempted defibrillation in adults after either unwitnessed out-of-hospital sudden death or when CPR is estimated to have been delayed for 5 min or more [47].

The rationale for instituting chest compression prior to attempted defibrillation is best explained by the high energy cost of VF. During cardiac arrest, coronary blood flow ceases, accounting for a progressive and severe energy imbalance. Intramyocardial hypercarbic acidosis is associated with depletion of high-energy phosphates and correspondingly severe global myocardial ischemia, resulting in myocardial contractile dysfunction [48, 49]. After prolonged, untreated VF, the right ventricle becomes distended and fails to expel its stroke volumes. Consequently, the ischemic left ventricle becomes contracted [50]. Progressive reductions in left ventricular diastolic and stroke volumes have been well documented, together with increases in left ventricular free-wall thickness, ushering in the "stone heart" [51]. "Stone heart", therefore represents ischemic contracture of the myocardium of the left ventricle and terminates in the noncontractile and noncompressible left ventricle earlier, as described by our group [52]. After the onset of contracture, the probability of successful defibrillation is remote. Early CPR, such as to restore coronary perfusion pressure and myocardial blood flow, delays onset of ischemic myocardial injury and contracture and facilitates defibrillation [53].

Weisfeld and Becker [54] described three time-sensitive phases: (1) the electrical phase of 0–4 min, (2) the circulatory phase of 4–10 min, and (3) the metabolic phase of > 10 min. During the electrical phase, immediate defibrillation is likely to be successful. As ischemia progresses, the likely success of attempted defibrillation diminishes without CPR. This phase is characterized by transition to slow VF wavelets during accumulation of ischemic metabolites in the myocardium. Slow VF often fails defibrillation attempts because there is no longer an excitable gap to interrupt the reentry that sustains VF, which implies electrically silent (unexcitable) myocardium. In the metabolic phase, there is therefore no likelihood of successful restoration of a perfusing rhythm.

Among the greatest perceived advances of the past decade has been the introduction of automated external defibrillators (AEDs). These devices "jump start" the heart by allowing rapid conversion of VF or ventricular tachycardia when applied by minimally trained layperson [10]. However, we have also recognized that the severity of postresuscitation myocardial dysfunction is also related to the magnitude of the electrical energy delivered during attempted defibrillation [55]. These include interruptions for electrocardiographic analyses of rhythm, "hands-off intervals" during capacitor charge of the defibrillator prior to delivery of an electrical shock and the AED-related "hands-off" intervals for protection of the rescuer. These intervals require discontinuance of chest compression for as long as 28 s [56] and translate into major compromises in outcomes. Moreover, with the defibrillation algorithm of the earlier guidelines, which allowed for a sequence of up to three electrical shocks, these interruptions could reach more than 80 s (Fig. 1).

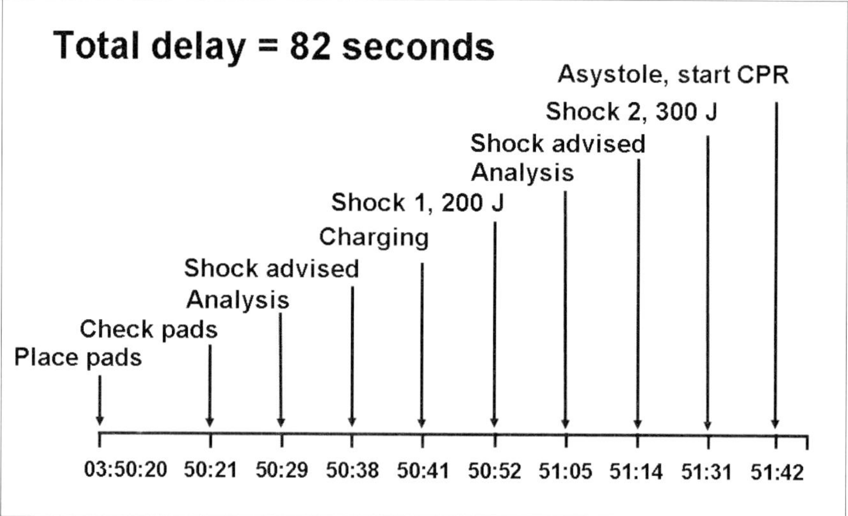

Fig. 1. AEDs-imposed interruption in CPR with the algorithm of up to three consecutive electrical shocks

Current data provide evidence that interruptions of chest compression that exceed as little as 15 s significantly reduce the success of initial resuscitation (Table 2), increase the severity of postresuscitation myocardial dysfunction, and accordingly reduced survival [57, 58]. In response thereto, the new guidelines mandate that for routine resuscitation, only a single rather than a sequence of up to three shocks be delivered, thereby minimized interruptions of chest compression. In addition, the new guidelines advise resumption of chest compression immediately after delivery of a shock, foregoing delays for visual confirmation of rhythm. Even if there is delayed recognition that a perfusing rhythm has been restored, continuing chest compressions is not in fact by itself likely to be damaging [59]. This change is further supported by the availability of more effective biphasic waveform shocks, which have yielded a first-shock 89% success rate in comparison with lesser success with monophasic shocks [60–63]. Moreover, when compared to conventional higher-energy monophasic shocks, biphasic shocks are advantageous in that they better preserve postresuscitation myocardial function [64, 65].

Table 2. Adverse effects of interruption of CPR prior to defibrillation attempt. Adapted from [57]

Delay (s)	Resuscitated (*n*/total)	CPR (min)	Post-CPR EF
3	5/5	3.3	0.57
10	4/5	8.2[a]	0.44[b]
15	2/5[a]	10.8[a]	0.42[b]
20	0/5	–	–

EF, ejection fraction
[a] $P < 0.05$ vs. 3-s interruption
[b] $P < 0.05$ vs. 3-s interruption

Limitations of Epinephrine

One of the most contentious topics debated during the development of the new 2005 guidelines for CPR related to the use of vasopressor agents during advanced life support. In settings of cardiac arrest, reestablishing vital organ perfusion plays an important role for initial CPR. As a pharmacologic intervention, the rationale for the administration of vasopressor agents during CPR is to restore threshold levels of myocardial and cerebral blood flow and consequently increase the success of initial resuscitation [66]. Epinephrine has been the preferred adrenergic amine for the treatment of human cardiac arrest for almost 40 years [67, 68]. However despite the widespread use of epinephrine and several studies supporting the use of vasopressin, no placebo-controlled study has that routine administration of any vasopressor at any stage during human cardiac arrest increases survival to hospital discharge. Several animal studies instead pinpointed the possible detrimental effects in outcome due to administration of epinephrine during CPR. Epinephrine increases myocardial lactate concentration and decreases myocardial ATP content even though coronary blood perfusion may be doubled [69]. We also previously demonstrated that administration of epinephrine during cardiopulmonary resuscitation increases the severity of postresuscitation myocardial dysfunction [70]. This is primarily related to the β-adrenergic action of epinephrine. Epinephrine, in fact, has not only α-adrenergic agonist action, which increases peripheral vascular resistance (this could paradoxically reduce myocardial and cerebral blood flow and perfusion), but also has β-adrenergic agonist actions (inotropic and chronotropic) to increase myocardial oxygen consumption during ventricular fibrillation during VF. These β-adrenergic actions also prompt increases in ectopic ventricular arrhythmias, and cause transient hypoxemia due to pulmonary arteriovenous shunting. Experimentally, when β-adrenergic effects of epinephrine were blocked by a rapid β-adrenergic blocker, esmolol, administered during CPR, initial cardiac resuscitation was significantly improved, postresuscitation myocardial dysfunction was minimized, and lengthened duration of postresuscitation survival was observed [71, 72]. In addition, β_1-adrenergic receptors which, like β-receptors, mediate increase in both inotropic and chronotropic responses, augment myocardial oxygen requirements, and thereby increase the severity of global ischemic injury [73]. β_1-Adrenergic agonists may also constrict coronary arteries such that there is superimposed reduction in myocardial perfusion. When β_1-adrenergic receptors were blocked by a selective β_1-adrenergic blocker, myocardial function was significantly improved after acute myocardial infarction [74]. We have also previously shown that the equivalent of selective α_2- vasopressor agonists, administered during CPR, resulted in better postresuscitation cardiac and neurological recovery and longer survival, compared to epinephrine [66, 75, 76] (Fig. 2). These selective α_2-agonists are as effective as epinephrine for initial cardiac resuscitation but do not increase myocardial oxygen consumption and therefore result in strikingly better postresuscitation myocardial function and survival. In addition, α_2-adrenergic agonists increase endothelial nitric oxide production and therefore counterbalance the α_2-adrenergic vasoconstrictor effects in coronary arteries [77]. These reports suggest the rationale for the use of selective α_2-adrenergic agonists as a better vasopressor agent in settings of cardiac arrest, but at this stage no published human studies have been identified.

Recently, we investigated the effects of epinephrine on microcirculatory blood flow on sublingual tissue flow in a porcine model of cardiac arrest and

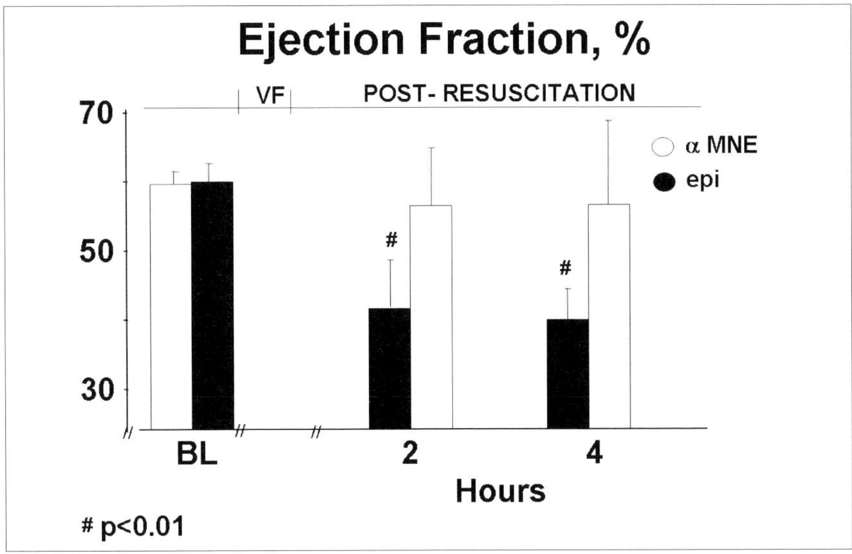

Fig. 2. Ejection fraction at baseline (BL) and postresuscitation in animals treated with α-methylnorepinephrine (α-MNE) and epinephrine (epi). # $P < 0.01$ (adapted from Klouche K, Weil NH, Tang W et al (2002) A selective alpha 2 adrenergic agonist for cardiac resuscitation. J Lab Clin Med 140:27-34)

resuscitation [78]. In pigs treated with epinephrine, microcirculatory flow was significantly reduced compared to that in untreated animals. These effects were present for at least 5 min and persisted even when return of spontaneous circulation was achieved. This impairment of microcirculatory blood flow was also confirmed in cortical cerebral microcirculation [79]. Dissociation between the increases in large pressure vessel flow and microcirculatory flow, which is the last determinant of outcome under conditions of circulatory failure, was reported.

Additional Measurements to Improve Outcome of CPR

To further limit the "hands-off" interval and minimize the damaging effects of repetitive electrical shocks during CPR—thereby reducing postresuscitation myocardial dysfunction—we now recognize the importance of electrocardiographic signal analyses for predicting whether an electrical shock would successfully reverse VF. Previous reported, the electrical property of VF wavelets, and in particular the amplitude of VF wavelets, reflect the capability to predict the success of a defibrillation attempt. The approach used by our group is the so called "amplitude spectrum area" (AMSA). AMSA represents a numerical value based on the sum of the magnitude of the weighted frequency spectrum between 3 and 48 Hz. Under experimental conditions, in a porcine model of cardiac arrest and resuscitation [80], AMSA predicted with a high negative predictive value (0.96) when an electrical shock would fail to restore spontaneous circulation. This approach also showed a positive predictive value of 0.78. Recently, we confirmed the efficacy of the AMSA method in a retrospective analysis of human electrocardiograms presenting VF using the same method. At an AMSA value of > 13.0 mV-Hz, successful defibrillation yielded a sensitivity of 91% and a specificity of 94% [81]. AMSA therefore, represents a clinically applicable method for a real-time prediction of the success of defibrillation during uninterrupted compression and ventilation. AMSA analysis has the advantage that it requires no more than conventional surface electrocardiogram, which is part of the routine current practice of advanced cardiac life support.

End-tidal carbon dioxide ($EtCO_2$) has emerged as a very good measure for quantifying the cardiac output produced by chest compression [82, 83]. This would explain its potential usefulness as a quantitative indicator of the effectiveness of perfusion during CPR. It also provides almost immediate detection of return to spontaneous circulation, reducing the need to stop chest compression to interpret ECG or check for the presence of a pulsatile rhythm. $EtCO_2$ also serves as a monitor to detect operator fatigue during manual chest compression [84]. Moreover, $EtCO_2$ is also predictive of survival from cardiac arrest [85]. When $EtCO_2$ declines below 10 mmHg after 20 min of CPR, it uniformly predicts death and therefore is used to facilitate decisions about discontinuing resuscitative efforts. However, there are exceptions; e.g., bolus infusion of sodium bicarbonate increases $EtCO_2$, and epinephrine produces a transient ventilation/perfusion mismatch accounting for reductions in $EtCO_2$ [86].

Another useful tool for determining the efficacy of chest compression and for predicting outcomes is represented by orthogonal polarization spectral (OPS) imaging, which allows for noninvasive and real-time measurement of the microcirculatory blood flow in the buccal and/or sublingual mucosa of patients. Experimentally we investigated changes in sublingual microcirculation during cardiac arrest and cardiopulmonary resuscitation [87]. With OPS imaging we observed that microvascular blood flow was highly correlated with coronary perfusion pressure (CPP) during CPR (r = 0.82; P < 0.01); and, like CPP, the magnitude of microcirculatory blood flow was indicative of the effectiveness of the resuscitation intervention and of outcome. In animals that were resuscitated, microvascular flow was significantly greater after 1 and 5 min for the efficacy of chest compressions than in animals in which resuscitation attempts failed.

Conclusions

The evidence supports quality-controlled chest compression as the initial intervention after "sudden death" prior to attempted defibrillation, if the duration of cardiac arrest is more than 5 min. Chest compressions of themselves provide forward blood flow and thereby restoration of myocardial and cerebral blood flows. The resulting restorations of coronary (and therefore myocardial) blood flow increase the success of initial resuscitation, and secure better postresuscitation myocardial function, neurological outcomes, and survival. The new guidelines therefore mandate fewer interruptions including ventilation and defibrillatory shocks, and single rather than multiple defibrillatory shocks prior to resuming chest compressions.

CPR quality is best measured. CPP remains the gold standard predictor of successful CPR, but is usually inapplicable in preclinical settings. Surrogates including end-tidal CO_2, which has already been shown by our group to be highly correlated with the cardiac output generated by chest compression are readily available. Unsuccessful and potentially injurious electrical shocks may be avoided by the use of electrocardiographic predictors like AMSA [88]. The direct and noninvasive visualization of the sublingual or buccal microcirculatory blood flow may prove useful to confirm the efficacy of chest compression and to predict outcomes.

References

1. Gullo A (2002) Cardiac arrest, chain of survival and Utstein style. Eur J Anaesthesiol 19:624–633
2. Weil MH, Sun S (2005) Clinical review: Devices and drugs for cardiopulmonary resuscitation—opportunities and restraints. Crit Care 9:287–290
3. Cummins RO, Eisenberg MS (1985) Prehospital cardiopulmonary resuscitation; is it effectiveβ JAMA 253:2408–2412
4. International Liaison Committee on Resuscitation (2005) Part 2: Adult basic life support. Resuscitation 67:187–201
5. Sanders AB, Ewy GA (2005) Cardiopulmonary resuscitation in the real world: when will the guidelines get the message? JAMA 293:363–365
6. Nichol G, Stiell IG, Laupacis A et al (1999) A cumulative meta-analysis of the effectiveness of defibrillator-capable emergency medical services for victims of out-of-hospital cardiac arrest. Ann Emerg Med 34:517–525
7. Engdahl J, Bang A, Lindqvist J et al (2003) Time trends in long-term mortality after out-of-hospital cardiac arrest, 1980 to 1998, and predictors for death. Am Heart J 145:749–750
8. Eisenberg MS, Horwood BT, Cummins RO et al (1990) Cardiac arrest and resuscitation: a tale of 29 cities. Ann Emerg Med 19:179–186
9. Becker LB, Ostrander MP, Barrett J et al (1991) Outcome of cardiopulmonary resuscitation in a large metropolitan area: where are the survivors? Ann Emerg Med 20:355–361

10. Caffrey SL, Willoughby PJ, Pepe PE et al (2002) Public use of automated external defibrillators. N Engl J Med 347:1242–1247
11. Larsen MP, Eisenberg MS, Cummins RO, et al. (1993) Predicting survival from out-of-hospital cardiac arrest: a graphic model. Ann Emerg Med 22:1652–1658
12. Rea TD, Eisenberg MS, Culley LL et al (2001) Dispatcher-assisted cardiopulmonary resuscitation and survival in cardiac arrest. Circulation 104:2513–2516
13. White RD (1997) Optimal access to—response by—public and voluntary services, including the role of bystanders and family members, in cardiopulmonary resuscitation. New Horiz 5:153–157
14. Cummins RO, Ornato JP, Thies WH et al (1991) Improving survival from sudden cardiac arrest: the "chain of survival" concept. A statement for health professionals from the 20 Advanced Cardiac Life Support Subcommittee and the Emergency Cardiac Care Committee, American Heart Association. Circulation 83:1832–1847
15. Jacobs I, Nadkarni V, Barh J et al (2004) Cardiac arrest and cardiopulmonary resuscitation outcome reports: update and simplification of the Utstein templates for resuscitation registries: a statement for healthcare professionals from a task force of the International Liaison Committee on Resuscitation. Circulation 110:3385–3397
16. American Heart Association (2005) 2005 American Heart Association Guidelines for Cardiopulmonary Resuscitation and Emergency Cardiovascular Care. Part 3: Overview of CPR. Circulation 112(24Suppl):IV-12–18
17. Herlitz J, Ekstrom L, Wennerblom B et al (1994) Effects of bystander initiated cardiopulmonary resuscitation on ventricular fibrillation and survival after witnessed cardiac arrest outside hospital. Br Heart J 72:408–412
18. Wik L, Steen PA, Bircher NG (1994) Quality of bystander cardiopulmonary resuscitation influences outcome after prehospital cardiac arrest. Resuscitation 28:195–203
19. Wik L, Kramer-Johansen J, Myklebust H et al. (2005) Quality of cardiopulmonary resuscitation during out-of-hospital cardiac arrest. JAMA 293:299–304
20. No authors listed (2000) Guidelines 2000 for cardiopulmonary resuscitation and emergency cardiovascular care: international consensus on science. Circulation 102(8Suppl):I1-I403
21. Abella BS, Sandbo N, Alvarado JP et al (2005) Quality of cardiopulmonary resuscitation during in-hospital cardiac arrest. JAMA 293:305–310
22. Abella BS, Sandbo N, Vassilatos P et al (2005) Chest compression rates during cardiopulmonary resuscitation are suboptimal. Circulation 111:428–434
23. Aufderheide TP, Sigurdsson G, Pirrallo RG et al (2004) Hyperventilation-induced hypotension during cardiopulmonary resuscitation. Circulation 109:1960–1965
24. Deshmukh HG, Weil MH, Gudipati CV et al (1989) Mechanism of blood flow generated by precordial compression during CPR. I: Studies on closed chest precordial compression. Chest 95:1092–1099
25. Sanders AB, Kern KB, Atlas M et al (1985) Importance of the duration of inadequate coronary perfusion pressure on resuscitation from cardiac arrest. J Am Coll Cardiol 6:113–118
26. Sanders AB, Ogle M, Ewy GA (1985) Coronary perfusion pressure during cardiopulmonary resuscitation. Am J Emerg Med 2:11–14
27. Yu T, Weil MH, Tang W et al (2002) Adverse outcome of interrupted precordial compression during automated defibrillation. Circulation 106:368–372
28. Paradis NA, Martin GB, Rivers EP et al (1990) Coronary perfusion pressure and the return of spontaneous circulation in human cardiopulmonary resuscitation. JAMA

263:1106–1113
29. Sanders AB, Kern KB, Berg RA et al (2002) Survival and neurologic outcome after cardiopulmonary resuscitation with four different chest compression-ventilation ratios. Ann Emerg Med 40:553–562
30. Yannopoulos D, McKnite SH, Tang W et al (2005) Reducing ventilation frequency during cardiopulmonary resuscitation in a porcine model of cardiac arrest. Respir Care 50:628–635
31. Tang W, Weil MH, Sun S et al (1994) Cardiopulmonary resuscitation by precordial compression but without mechanical ventilation. Am J Respir Crit Care Med 150(6Pt1):1709–1713
32. Noc M, Weil MH, Tang W et al (1995) Mechanical ventilation may not be essential for initial cardiopulmonary resuscitation. Chest 108:821–827
33. Noc M, Weil MH, Tang W et al (1994) Spontaneous gasping during cardiopulmonary resuscitation without mechanical ventilation. Am J Respir Crit Care Med 150:861–864
34. Fukui M, Weil MH, Tang W et al (1995) Airway protection during experimental CPR. Chest 108:1663–1667
35. Babbs CF, Kern KB (2002) Optimum compression to ventilation ratios in CPR under realistic, practical conditions: a physiological and mathematical analysis. Resuscitation 54:147–157
36. Weil MH, Tang W (1997) Cardiopulmonary resuscitation: a promise as yet largely unfulfilled. Dis Mon 43:429–501
37. Kern KB, Hilwig RW, Berg RA et al (2002) Importance of continuous chest compressions during cardiopulmonary resuscitation. Improved outcome during a simulated single lay-rescuer scenario. Circulation 105:645–649
38. Berg RA, Sanders AB, Kern KB et al (2001) Adverse hemodynamic effects of interrupting chest compressions for rescue breathing during cardiopulmonary resuscitation for ventricular fibrillation cardiac arrest. Circulation 104:2465–2470
39. No authors listed (2000) Guidelines 2000 for Cardiopulmonary Resuscitation and Emergency Cardiovascular Care. Part 3: Adult basic life support. The American Heart Association in collaboration with the International Liaison Committee on Resuscitation. Circulation 102(8Suppl):I22-I59
40. Eisemberg MS, Copass MK, Hallstrom AP et al (1980) Treatment of out-of-hospital cardiac arrests with rapid defibrillation by emergency medical technicians. N Engl J Med 302:1379–1383
41. Valenzuela TD, Roe DJ, Nichol G et al (2000) Outcomes of rapid defibrillation by security officers after cardiac arrest in casinos. N Engl J Med 343:1206–1209
42. White R, Asplin B, Bugliosi T et al (1996) High discharge survival rate after out-of-hospital ventricular fibrillation with rapid defibrillation by police and paramedics. Ann Emerg Med 28:480–485
43. Cobb LA, Fahrenbruch CE, Walsh TR et al (1999) Influence of cardiopulmonary resuscitation prior to defibrillation in patients with out-of-hospital ventricular fibrillation. JAMA 281:1182–1188
44. Wik L, Hansen TB, Fylling F et al (2003) Delaying defibrillation to give basic cardiopulmonary resuscitation to patients with out-of-hospital ventricular fibrillation. JAMA 289:1389–1395
45. Niemann JT, Cairns CB, Sharma J et al (1992) Treatment of prolonged ventricular fibrillation: immediate countershock versus high-dose epinephrine and CPR preceding countershock. Circulation 85:281–287
46. Berg RA, Hilwig RW, Ewy GA et al (2004) Precountershock cardiopulmonary resu-

scitation improves initial response to defibrillation from prolonged ventricular fibrillation: a randomized, controlled swine study. Crit Care Med 32:1352–1357
47. International Liaison Committee on Resuscitation (2005) Part 3: Defibrillation. Resuscitation 67:203–211
48. Johnson BA, Weil MH, Tang W et al (1995) Mechanisms of myocardial hypercarbic acidosis during cardiac arrest. J Appl Physiol 78:1579–1584
49. Kern KB, Garewal HS, Sanders AB et al (1990) Depletion of myocardial adenosine triphosphate during prolonged untreated ventricular fibrillation: effect on defibrillation success. Resuscitation 20:221–229
50. Steen S, Liao Q, Pierre L et al (2003) The critical importance of minimal delay between chest compressions and subsequent defibrillation: a haemodynamic explanation. Resuscitation 58:249–258
51. Klouche K, Weil MH, Sun S et al (2000) Echo-Doppler observations during cardiac arrest and cardiopulmonary resuscitation. Crit Care Med 28(11 Suppl):N212-N213
52. Klouche K, Weil MH, Sun S et al (2002) Evolution of the stone heart after prolonged cardiac arrest. Chest 122:1006–1011
53. Deshmukh HG, Weil MH, Gudipati CV et al (1989) Mechanism of blood flow generated by precordial compression during CPR. I: Studies on closed chest precordial compression. Chest 95:1092–1099
54. Weisfeldt ML, Becker LB (2002) Resuscitation after cardiac arrest: a 3-phase time-sensitive model. JAMA 288:3035–3038
55. Xie J, Weil MH, Sun S et al (1997) High-energy defibrillation increases the severity of postresuscitation myocardial dysfunction. Circulation 96:683–688
56. Snyder D, Morgan C (2004) Wide variation in cardiopulmonary resuscitation interruption intervals among commercially available automated external defibrillators may affect survival despite high defibrillation efficacy. Crit Care Med 32(9 Suppl):S421-S424
57. Yu T, Weil MH, Tang W et al (2002) Adverse outcome of interrupted precordial compression during automated defibrillation. Cirulation 106:368–372
58. Sato Y, Weil MH, Sun S et al (1997) Adverse effects of interrupting precordial compression during cardiopulmonary resuscitation. Crit Care Med 25:733–736
59. Hess EP, White RD (2005) Ventricular fibrillation is not provoked by chest compression during post-shock organized rhythms in out-of-hospital cardiac arrest. Resuscitation 66:7–11
60. Bain AC, Swerdlow CD, Love JC et al (2001) Multicenter study of principles-based waveforms for external defibrillation. Ann Emerg Med 37:5–12
61. Poole JE, White RD, Kanz KG et al (1997) Low-energy impedance-compensating biphasic waveforms terminate ventricular fibrillation at high rates in victims of out-of-hospital cardiac arrest. LIFE investigators. J Cardiovasc Electrophysiol 8:1373–1385
62. Greene HL, Di Marco JP, Kudenchuk PJ et al (1995) Comparison of monophasic and biphasic defibrillating pulse waveforms for transthoracic cardioversion. Am J Cardiol 75:1135–1139
63. Schneider T, Martens PR, Paschen H et al (2000) Multicenter, randomized, controlled trial of 150-J biphasic shocks compared with 200- to 360-J monophasic shocks in the resuscitation of out-of-hospital cardiac arrest victims. Circulation 102:1780–1787
64. Tang W, Weil MH, Sun S et al (2001) A comparison of biphasic and monophasic waveform defibrillation after prolonged ventricular fibrillation. Chest 103:948–954
65. Tang W, Weil MH, Sun S et al (1999) The effects of biphasic and conventional monophasic defibrillation on postresuscitation myocardial function. J Am Coll

Cardiol 34:815–822
66. Pellis T, Weil MH, Tang W et al (2003) Evidence favoring the use of an β2-selective vasopressor agent for cardiopulmonary resuscitation. Circulation 108:2716
67. Lewis CM, Weil MH (1969) Hemodynamic spectrum of vasopressor and vasodilator drugs. JAMA 208:1391–1398
68. No authors listed (2005) 2005 International Consensus on Cardiopulmonary Resuscitation and Emergency Cardiovascular Care Science with Treatment Recommendations. Circulation 112:25–54
69. Ditchey RV, Lindenfeld J (1988) Failure of epinephrine to improve the balance between myocardial oxygen supply and demand during closed-chest resuscitation in dogs. Circulation 78:382–389
70. Tang W, Weil MH, Sun S et al (1995) Epinephrine increases the severity of postresuscitation myocardial dysfunction. Circulation 92:3089–3093
71. Cammarata G, Weil MH, Sun S et al (2004) Betal-adrenergic blockade during cardiopulmonary resuscitation improves survival. Crit Care Med 32(9 Suppl):S440-S443
72. Huang L, Weil MH, Cammarata G et al (2004) Nonselective beta-blocking agent improves the outcome of cardiopulmonary resuscitation in a rat model. Crit Care Med 32(9 Suppl):S378-S380
73. Grupp IL, Lorenz JN, Walsh RA et al (1998) Overexpression of alpha 1B-adrenergic receptor induces left ventricular dysfunction in the absence of hypertrophy. Am J Physiol 275:H1338-H1350
74. Gregorini L, Marco J, Kozakova M et al (1999) Alpha-adrenergic blockade improves recovery of myocardial perfusion and function after coronary stenting in patients with acute myocardial infarction. Circulation 99:482–490
75. Sun S, Weil MH, Tang W et al (2001) Alpha-methylnorepinephrine, a selective alpha-2 adrenergic agonist for cardiac resuscitation. J Am Coll Cardiol 37:951–956
76. Klouche K, Weil MH, Sun S et al (2003) A comparison of alpha-methylnorepinephrine, vasopressin and epinephrine for cardiac resuscitation. Resuscitation 57:93–100
77. Ishibashi Y, Duncker DJ, Bache RJ (1997) Endogenous nitric oxide masks alpha2-adrenergic coronary vasoconstriction during exercise in the ischemic heart. Circ Res 80:196–207
78. Fries M, Tang W, Castillo C et al (2004) Detrimental effects of epinephrine on microcirculatory blood flow in a porcine model of cardiac arrest. Crit Care Med 32(Suppl):A56
79. Ristagno G, Sun S, Chang YT et al (2005) Epinephrine reduces cerebral microcirculatory blood flow during CPR. Crit Care Med 33(Suppl):A95
80. Povoas HP, Weil MH, Tang W et al (2002) Predicting the success of defibrillation by electrocardiographic analysis. Resuscitation 53:77–82
81. Young C, Bisera J, Gehman S et al (2004) Amplitude spectrum area: measuring the probability of successful defibrillation as applied to human data. Crit Care Med 32 (9 Suppl):S356-S358
82. Weil MH, Bisera J, Trevino RP et al (1985) Cardiac output and end-tidal carbon dioxide. Crit Care Med 13:907–909
83. Pernat A, Weil MH, Sun S et al (2003) Stroke volumes and end-tidal carbon dioxide generated by precordial compression during ventricular fibrillation. Crit Care Med 31:1819–1823
84. Kalenda Z (1978) The capnogram as a guide to the efficacy of cardiac massage. Resuscitation 6:259–263

85. Falk JL, Rackow EC, Weil MH (1988) End-tidal carbon dioxide concentration during cardiopulmonary resuscitation. N Engl J Med 318:607–611
86. Tang W, Weil MH, Gazmuri RJ et al (1991) Pulmonary ventilation/perfusion defects induced by epinephrine during cardiopulmonary resuscitation. Circulation 84:2101–2107
87. Fries M, Weil MH, Chang YT et al (2006) Capillary blood flow during cardiopulmonary resuscitation is predictive of outcome. Resuscitation (in press<<QA5>>)
88. Pernat A, Weil MH, Tang W et al. (2001) Optimizing timing of ventricular defibrillation. Crit Care Med 29:2360–2365

13 Circulatory Shock: Hypovolemic, Distributive, Cardiogenic, Obstructive

J.-L. Vincent and A. Rapotec

Introduction

Circulatory shock is the clinical picture associated with generalized, acute circulatory insufficiency, which is a frequent complication of many pathological states as diverse as severe sepsis, extensive myocardial infarction, polytrauma, or massive pulmonary embolism. Whatever the cause of the shock, cells no longer possess enough oxygen to function optimally, and this condition is associated with high mortality rates. Even in patients who survive the acute episode of shock, protracted cellular damage frequently results in organ dysfunction. Prompt recognition of shock is essential to enable appropriate therapy to be instituted rapidly and tissue damage limited.

According to the landmark proposal by Weil and Shubin many years ago [1], there are four major categories of shock, based on the underlying pathophysiological defects. Although we will discuss these individually, several forms of shock may coexist in one patient.

Pathophysiological Classification of Shock

Essentially, shock can be classified according to four pathophysiological phenomena [1]:

Hypovolemic shock. Hypovolemic shock occurs as a consequence of inadequate circulating volume, whether as a result of internal or of external fluid loss, and causes include hemorrhage, associated, for example, with trauma,

Department of Intensive Care, Erasme University Hospital, Free University of Brussels, Belgium

surgery, severe upper gastrointestinal bleeding, ruptured aortic aneurysm, etc., and severe dehydration, as can occur, for example, with severe vomiting or diarrhea, or prolonged coma. Hypovolemic shock is the most common form of circulatory shock seen in surgical and trauma patients; indeed most forms of shock include some hypovolemic component. The hemodynamic pattern is characteristically one of a low cardiac output (due to reduced venous return), associated with low cardiac filling pressures and increased systemic vascular resistance (SVR).

Cardiogenic shock. This is caused by primary pump failure. Cardiogenic shock is most commonly the result of acute myocardial infarction, occurring when the infarction involves at least 40% of the total myocardium, and affecting some 6–7% of patients hospitalized with acute myocardial infarction [2, 3]. Other causes of cardiogenic shock include severe cardiac valvular disease, end-stage cardiomyopathy, severe myocarditis, or severe cardiac arrhythmia (e.g., ventricular tachycardia, rapid supraventricular tachycardia). Of the four types of shock, cardiogenic shock carries the worse prognosis, with mortality rates in the region of 75%. It is the leading cause of death in patients hospitalized with myocardial infarction. Cardiogenic shock is characterized by a low cardiac output (due to pump failure), elevated cardiac filling pressures, and raised SVR.

Obstructive shock. This form of shock occurs as the result of an obstruction to the normal flow of blood; the most common causes are massive pulmonary embolism and cardiac tamponade. Other causes include severe aortic stenosis, tension pneumothorax, and aortic dissection. Obstructive shock is typically characterized by a low cardiac output and increased SVR. Right cardiac filling pressures are raised in pulmonary embolism and right and left pressures are raised in tamponade. Pulmonary arterial hypertension is also present in cardiogenic shock associated with pulmonary embolism.

Distributive shock. Of the four forms of shock, the distributive type has the most complex pathophysiology and is most commonly due to sepsis, and secondary to the release of inflammatory mediators. Other causes include anaphylactic shock, neurogenic shock, and acute adrenal insufficiency. Characteristically, vascular tone is reduced. Unlike the other three shock types, cardiac output is characteristically normal or raised (Table 1). SVR and cardiac filling pressures are reduced.

In all types of acute circulatory failure, there is an imbalance between the oxygen requirements and tissue oxygen availability. In hypovolemic, cardiogenic, and obstructive types of shock, the primary abnormality is the reduced cardiac output and hence inadequate oxygen transport. However, in septic shock, the main anomaly lies on the other side of the equation, with oxygen needs being increased, due to the inflammatory response, in addition to altered oxygen extraction capabilities and myocardial contractility. Hence,

Table 1. Typical clinical and biological characteristics of septic shock and other forms of shock

	Septic (distributive) shock	Hypovolemic, cardiogenic, and obstructive shock
Arterial hypotension	Present	Present
Tachycardia	Present	Present
Cardiac output	Normal or elevated	Reduced
Cutaneous vasoconstriction	Often absent	Present
Oliguria	Usually present	Present
Altered mental status	Present	Present
Intestinal peristalsis	Often absent	Often absent
Altered coagulation status	Sometimes present	Often present
Hyperlactatemia	Present	Present

although the cardiac output may be normal or even elevated in such patients, it may still be insufficient to provide adequate oxygen for the cells' increased requirements.

Importantly, in some pathologies, more than one type of shock may be present. For example, anaphylactic shock or severe pancreatitis are often associated with both distributive and hypovolemic types of shock, and patients with septic shock often have a combination of distributive, hypovolemic, and even cardiogenic, shock types.

Diagnosis and Monitoring

The diagnosis of acute circulatory failure is based on the presence of arterial hypotension with signs of altered tissue perfusion. Clinical examination is essential and will reveal features of inadequate tissue perfusion including altered mental status, decreased capillary refill and oliguria. This must then be combined with hemodynamic parameters and monitors of tissue hypoxia to enable a complete assessment of each patient.

Clinical Signs of Shock

Alterations in organ perfusion are most easily identified for three organs: the kidney, the brain and the skin.

- Oliguria (urine output < 20 ml h^{-1}): reduced renal perfusion limits the glomerular filtration rate and hence urine output. Obviously this symptom will only be noted in patients in whom urinary output is monitored.
- Altered mental status: this often shows as moderate confusion with drowsiness or agitation.
- Reduced skin perfusion: typically characterized by a cold, mottled, clammy skin. These cutaneous alterations are not always present in distributive shock.

Hemodynamic and Laboratory Parameters of Shock

Heart Rate

Cardiac output is dependent on both stroke volume and heart rate, and tachycardia is thus a hallmark of shock, regardless of the etiology. In hyperkinetic states (distributive types), heart rate must increase to allow the cardiac output to increase above normal. In hypokinetic states, when stroke volume decreases due to decreased intravascular volume, the body typically increases the heart rate to maintain cardiac output. In all cases, tachycardia is due to increased sympathetic tone, and can be further enhanced by the administration of β-adrenergic agents.

Arterial Hypotension

A fall in arterial pressure may be due to a reduction in cardiac output, a reduction in blood volume (and hence also in cardiac output), or a reduction in vascular tone. The development of arterial hypotension is not an early sign and thus represents a serious marker of patient condition. Importantly, the arterial pressure is not always as low as one may expect to be associated with shock, particularly in patients with chronic hypertension. A systolic pressure of less than 90 mmHg (or a mean arterial pressure less than 70 mmHg) or a fall in mean arterial pressure of greater than 30 mmHg are indications of circulatory failure.

Cardiac Output

Low cardiac output is associated with hypovolemic, cardiogenic, and obstructive types of circulatory shock. The low cardiac output causes marked vasoconstriction mediated by stimulation of α-adrenergic receptors, with the aim of restoring and maintaining an adequate tissue perfusion pressure. The heart and the brain have fewer α-adrenergic receptors and, therefore, there is less marked vasoconstriction of the coronary and cerebral circulations. In contrast, the renal and splanchnic circulations are affected to a much greater extent. The reasons for these differences are obvious: correct cardiac and intellectual functions are more important for the immediate survival of an individual in shock than the adequate function of the intestine, and decreased diuresis may even be beneficial at preserving volemia. Nevertheless, although these observations could lead us to think that intestinal perfusion is of little importance in circulatory shock, intestinal hypoperfusion may result in translocation of bacteria and their products (notably endotoxin) across the ischemic intestinal wall or in local activation of the immune system.

The measurement of cardiac output provides an assessment of total body blood flow but provides no information on regional flow. It adapts according to the oxygen demands of the body and must, therefore, not be considered in isolation. An apparently normal or even high cardiac output may be insufficient if accompanied by increased tissue oxygen demand, e.g., a "normal" cardiac output may be sufficient for an anesthetized, hypothermic, mechanically ventilated patient, while in an agitated patient with severe sepsis oxygen requirements will be much greater and a "normal" cardiac output may well be inadequate.

Mixed Venous Oxygen Saturation

In the absence of anemia and hypoxemia, mixed venous oxygen saturation (SvO_2) reflects the relationship between oxygen uptake (VO_2) and cardiac output, since $SvO_2 = SaO_2 - VO_2/(\text{cardiac output} \times Hb)$ where SaO_2 is the arterial oxygen saturation and Hb the hemoglobin concentration. Thus, SvO_2 is typically reduced in low-flow states and normal or even high in hyperkinetic states. However, although a reduction in SvO_2 represents an imbalance between VO_2 and oxygen delivery (DO_2), it provides no indication as to which factor has altered. In addition, while a low SvO_2 may be a global indicator of inadequate oxygenation and has prognostic value, it cannot be considered in isolation as a healthy individual can have a low SvO_2 during exercise, and a low SvO_2 may be a usual feature in a cardiac-compromised patient. The interpretation of SvO_2 must, therefore, be made in the context of other variables including cardiac output and blood lactate levels.

Blood Lactate Levels

Tissue hypoxia results in anaerobic metabolism and an increase in blood lactate levels, which are, therefore, a marker of inadequate oxygenation. The blood lactate level is a reflection of the balance between lactate production and elimination, and as elimination occurs primarily in the liver, lactate levels in patients with liver failure may remain raised for longer. The physician should also be aware of other possible causes of hyperlactatemia, including prolonged seizures or shivering and extensive neoplastic disease, but these are uncommon and usually obvious (Table 2). In addition, while anaerobic metabolism is the prime cause of raised blood lactate levels in low-output shock, the situation is more complex in sepsis, with metabolic alterations including a decrease in pyruvate dehydrogenase activity and increased glycolysis probably playing a contributory role [4]. In the absence of other factors, a blood lactate level above 2 mEq l^{-1} should raise the suspicion of tissue hypoxia. Although blood lactate levels only provide a global index of oxygenation, they correlate well with survival in various groups of patients [5, 6] and have a greater prognostic significance than oxygen-derived variables [7]. Serial measurements provide more valuable information than a single level.

Table 2. Factors influencing the interpretation of blood lactate levels in shock

Condition	Comment
Hepatic failure	Acute or chronic hepatic failure can slow the elimination of lactate. Although blood lactate levels are usually normal even in severe hepatic failure, additional circulatory failure will result in persistently raised blood lactate levels.
Severe sepsis	Hyperlactatemia in severe sepsis can be due to factors other than (or in addition to) anaerobic metabolism, including: – Increased aerobic glycolysis – Altered pyruvate metabolism as a result of decreased pyruvate dehydrogenase activity
Intense muscular activity	For example, prolonged epileptic fits, severe shivering, severe agitation
Hyperventilation	Hyperventilation can result in hyperlactatemia as a result of combined increased respiratory muscle contraction, reduced hepatic perfusion, and activation of phosphofructokinase by the accompanying alkalosis.
Alcohol intoxication	
Advanced, disseminated cancer	
Decompensated diabetes	

Regional Circulatory Changes

All the above parameters provide information on systemic oxygenation and circulation, but offer no information on regional perfusion, believed to be of critical importance in the development of organ dysfunction and multiple organ failure. Various techniques have been developed to monitor the regional circulation, but further study is required to refine and validate them. The gut is particularly sensitive to reductions in blood flow and has been a key target of monitoring systems, notably gastric tonometry. A number of studies have demonstrated that regional splanchnic ischemia may persist in circulatory failure when global hemodynamic and oxygen-derived variables have apparently returned to normal [8, 9]. The measurement of gastric intramucosal pH (pHi) was widely investigated as a means of obtaining a more local indicator of hypoxia [5, 10]. To avoid potential problems in the calculation of pHi associated with the assumption that the arterial bicarbonate is identical to the intramucosal bicarbonate, it was later suggested that the PCO_2 value itself should be used. The PCO_2 of the gastric lumen ($PgCO_2$) is, however, directly influenced by the $PaCO_2$ so that it may be altered by changes in ventilatory status in the absence of any changes in regional blood flow. The use of the PCO_2 gap–the difference between $PgCO_2$ and $PaCO_2$–avoids any potential confusion in the presence of respiratory acidosis, and facilitates the correct interpretation of $PgCO_2$ values [11]. However, gastric tonometry has serious limitations, including interruption of enteral feeding and concomitant use of H_2-blockers, which limit its practical application in the intensive care unit (ICU).

Microcirculatory Alterations

Recently, the more easily accessible sublingual circulation has become a target for regional monitoring. Using orthogonal polarization spectral imaging, the sublingual microcirculation can be visualized. In patients with septic or cardiogenic shock, alterations in the microcirculation are observed, including a decrease in vessel density and an increased proportion of nonperfused or intermittently perfused capillaries [12, 13]. These alterations were more severe and more persistent in nonsurvivors, and, importantly, could be fully reversed by the topical application of acetylcholine [12–14]. Sublingual capnometry has been shown to track the microcirculatory changes in patients with septic shock and correlated well with $PgCO_2$ [15]. Drotrecogin alfa (activated) was recently shown to benefit the sublingual microcirculation in patients with severe sepsis [16]. Although further study is needed, monitoring the sublingual microcirculation at the bedside does seem to be a promising approach to assess the severity of disease, to predict outcome, and to follow the effects of therapy in patients with shock.

Treatment

There are two essential aspects to the treatment of acute circulatory failure: first, aggressive cardiorespiratory resuscitation and support, and, second, correction of the underlying cause. Importantly, it may take some time to determine the underlying cause, and hence active resuscitation must be started immediately while other tests are being conducted and results awaited to identify the cause.

Cardiorespiratory Support

Intensive cardiorespiratory support is vital to restore the imbalance between oxygen supply and demand. This support should follow the basic VIP rule, initially proposed by Weil and colleagues: *v*entilation, *i*nfusion, *p*ump [17].

Ventilation

Even if the patient is not very hypoxemic, oxygen should be started immediately to increase DO_2 and reduce hypoxic pulmonary vasoconstriction, and should aim to maintain PaO_2 well above 8 kPa (60 mmHg), and SaO_2 above 90%. Prolonged administration of high inspired oxygen fractions (FiO_2) can be toxic, but this not a problem in the acute situation. Once blood gas results are available, oxygen therapy can be adjusted accordingly, remembering that hyperoxia can, paradoxically, reduce tissue oxygenation by causing peripheral vasoconstriction and reduced regional perfusion. DO_2 is primarily a product of the hemoglobin oxygen saturation, and once this is close to 100%, further increases in PaO_2 may, therefore, be useless if not detrimental. If mask ventilation is problematic or provides inadequate oxygenation, mechanical ventilation should be commenced without too much hesitation. Indeed, in addition to ensuring adequate oxygenation, mechanical ventilation also reduces left ventricular afterload by increasing intrathoracic pressures, and rests the respiratory muscles, thus reducing the patient's oxygen requirements.

Infusion

Fluid therapy is an essential part of the treatment of any form of shock, aimed at improving microvascular blood flow by increasing plasma volume, and increasing cardiac output by the Frank–Starling effect. Persistent hypovolemia will result in organ dysfunction and multiple organ failure, the end result of critically reduced organ perfusion. However, too much fluid also carries risks, primarily of pulmonary edema. The quantity of fluid necessary will vary and each patient must be assessed individually. Precise endpoints for fluid resuscitation are difficult to define as we do not yet have sensitive tools for monitoring the regional microcirculation and oxygenation, and changes may persist at a local level while systemic parameters appear to have stabilized. A fluid challenge technique is the best method of determining a patient's ongoing need for fluids [18]. The fluid challenge technique incorporates four phases:

1. *The type of fluid.* The type of fluid to be administered remains controversial. Colloid molecules (albumin, gelatin, hydroxyethylstarch) are often preferred in patients with shock as they are retained within the intravascular compartment for longer intervals than crystalloids, and less fluid is required to achieve the same hemodynamic goal. However, colloid solutions are more expensive, especially human albumin. In the recent SAFE study [19], the mortality rate was identical among ICU patients who received albumin and those who received crystalloid solution as the initial resuscitation fluid. However, hypoalbuminemia is associated with higher morbidity [20], and a meta-analysis indicated that albumin administration may reduce complications in critically ill patients [21]. Until further evidence becomes available, the choice is best made contingent on the underlying disease, the type of fluid that has been lost, the severity of the circulatory failure, the serum albumin concentration of the patient, and the risk of bleeding.
2. *The rate of fluid administration.* It is important to define the amount of fluid to be administered over a defined interval. The Surviving Sepsis Campaign Guidelines for the management of severe sepsis and septic shock recommend 500–1000 ml of crystalloids or 300–500 ml of colloids over 30 min [22].
3. *The goal to be achieved.* The primary defect or defects that prompt the fluid challenge should be identified and quantitated so that a goal can be determined; most commonly this will be restoration of an adequate mean arterial pressure.
4. *Safety limits.* Pulmonary edema due to congestive heart failure is the most serious complication of fluid infusion. A safety limit, generally the central venous pressure (CVP), must be set to avoid this complication.

Blood transfusions should be given as necessary, and are predominantly used in the bleeding patient with hypovolemic shock. Hemoglobin-based oxygen carriers may be of benefit in the early resuscitation of trauma patients, but further study is needed to clarify their role.

Pump

Vasopressors are commonly required in the early stages of shock to restore blood pressure. Some debate continues about the relative efficacy of the available agents, and decisions must be made according to the underlying disease process. Epinephrine is the drug of choice in anaphylactic shock and can be given at a dose of 0.5 mg intramuscularly. In cardiac arrest, epinephrine is also used and can be given at a dose of 0.1 mg intravenously. However, in others forms of shock, other vasopressors are generally preferred as there are concerns about epinephrine's effects on the regional circulation. Dopamine combines α-adrenergic, β-adrenergic, and dopaminergic effects, depending on the dose given. Dopaminergic effects are limited to low-dose dopamine infusions (less than 3 μg kg^{-1} min^{-1}). Low-dose dopamine theoretically should selectively increase renal and splanchnic blood flow, but clinical studies have not confirmed a beneficial effect on renal function [23] and its routine use for this purpose is not recommended. At larger doses (8–12 μg kg^{-1} min^{-1}), β-adrenergic effects predominate, and at higher doses, α effects come to the fore. The combination of α- and β-adrenergic effects leads to an increase in blood pressure while maintaining cardiac inotropy, and hence cardiac output. Generally dopamine is well tolerated, with arrhythmias seen less frequently than with other vasopressor drugs. The dose of dopamine should not exceed 20–25 μg kg^{-1} min^{-1}. Norepinephrine is a potent α-agonist with some β_1, but minimal β_2, activity, making it one of the most powerful of the vasopressors. It causes marked peripheral vasoconstriction with a rise in blood pressure, but often at the expense of cardiac output. The increased afterload causes an increased myocardial workload, and norepinephrine can precipitate acute cardiac failure, myocardial ischemia, and pulmonary edema. Norepinephrine is of use in severely hypotensive patients, especially when dopamine is not effective. The normal dose range is 0.05–2 μg kg^{-1} min^{-1}. Some studies have suggested that in septic shock, norepinephrine may be preferable to dopamine as a first-line vasopressor. A randomized controlled trial is being conducted across Europe to compare these two agents as first-line vasopressors in the management of shock.

Inotropic agents are indicated in the presence of reduced myocardial contractility, and dobutamine has become the agent of choice. Dobutamine is a mixture of two isomers, one acting on β-receptors and the other on α-receptors. It increases myocardial activity while having little effect on blood pressure. Dobutamine does increase heart rate, but the increase in coronary blood flow usually matches the raised heart rate, so myocardial ischemia is uncommon provided that doses of 20 μg kg^{-1} min^{-1} are not exceeded. Dobutamine is frequently used in addition to vasopressor agents and, in this situation, increases cardiac index, oxygen uptake and DO_2 [24]. It may raise blood pressure somewhat in patients with low output due to altered myocardial contractility, but a fall in blood pressure should raise the possibility of underlying hypovolemia. Usual doses are 5–15 (maximum 20) μg kg^{-1} min^{-1}. Dopexamine is available in some countries as an alternative to dobutamine with β-adrenergic and dopaminergic effects, but no effect on α-receptors. Its use is limited by the development of marked tachycardia, particularly at higher doses. The maximum dose is 4–5 μg kg^{-1} min^{-1}.

Correction of the Underlying Cause

- *Hypovolemic shock.* Hemorrhage, vomiting, or diarrhea must be controlled, and appropriate fluid replacement instituted. Although restoration of intravascular volume is a priority to limit the development of tissue hypoxia and multiple organ system failure, in hemorrhaging patients increased blood pressure can increase bleeding [25], and these patients must be closely monitored.
- *Cardiogenic shock.* Correction of the primary cause is often not possible in cardiogenic shock, which is commonly the result of myocardial infarction; but thrombolytic therapy, percutaneous coronary intervention, or emergency coronary artery bypass grafting may be beneficial [26]. Intra-aortic balloon pump and ventricular assist devices may also be used.
- *Obstructive shock.* Pericardial fluid should be drained in pericardial tamponade. Where possible, the pulmonary thrombus should be removed by thrombolysis or surgery with pulmonary embolization. Pneumothorax will require insertion of a chest drain.
- *Distributive shock.* The septic source should be identified and removed by surgery whenever possible. Appropriate bacteriological cultures should be taken, and then broad-spectrum antibiotics administered early to cover all possible organisms [22]. As microbiological results become available, antimicrobial regimens should be adjusted accordingly. Drotrecogin alfa (activated) should be considered in patients with no contraindications [27]. Intravenous corticosteroids (hydrocortisone 200–300 mg per day for 7 days, in three or four divided doses or by continuous infusion) are recommended in patients with septic shock who, despite adequate fluid replacement, require vasopressor therapy to maintain adequate blood pressure.

Complications of Circulatory Shock

Circulatory shock can have important effects on all organ systems, including:

- *Coagulation system.* Disseminated intravascular coagulation (DIC) is a common complication of shock. DIC resolves as the hemodynamic status resolves and rarely needs specific treatment.
- *Pulmonary system.* Acute respiratory distress syndrome occurs within 24–72 h after the onset of circulatory shock and can last several weeks.
- *Renal system.* Reduced renal perfusion leads to oliguria, one of the classical signs of shock. Alterations in renal function will result in an increase in the blood urea and creatinine concentrations.
- *Hepatic system.* Liver function tests are often altered, primarily showing

hyperbilirubinemia with no signs of cholestasis. Other liver enzymes are also often raised, but this may also be due to release from other organs.

- *Central nervous system.* Altered mental status is one of the clinical signs of shock, but cerebrospinal fluid analysis and computed tomography scans are typically normal (unless CNS pathology is the cause of the shock).

The complications of circulatory shock may develop into multiple organ failure, a syndrome with mortality rates in excess of 50%. Multiple organ failure may be the result of excessive initial release of proinflammatory mediators in response to the sepsis or trauma that caused the episode of shock. These mediators can increase oxygen requirements and alter cellular oxygen extraction capabilities, thus worsening the tissue hypoxia already present due to the circulatory shock. Hypoxia in turn can cause the release of further proinflammatory mediators. Thus, a vicious cycle is created, spiraling on to worsening multiple organ system failure and death.

Conclusion

Acute circulatory failure, whatever the cause, is associated with an imbalance in oxygen supply and demand. Early aggressive treatment with oxygen, fluid administration, and adrenergic agents when needed, combined with methods to correct the underlying cause, help to limit the damage. Repeated clinical examination, with appropriate hemodynamic and oxygenation parameters, is important to monitor the patient's progress and response to treatment. The development of improved monitoring techniques, including strategies to visualize and quantify microcirculatory changes, will enable us to better assess and target regional perfusion; and by so doing, improve patient outcomes.

References

1. Weil MH, Shubin H (1971) Proposed reclassification of shock states with special reference to distributive defects. Adv Exp Med Biol 23:13–23
2. Goldberg RJ, Gore JM, Thompson CA, Gurwitz JH (2001) Recent magnitude of and temporal trends (1994–1997) in the incidence and hospital death rates of cardiogenic shock complicating acute myocardial infarction: the second national registry of myocardial infarction. Am Heart J 141:65–72
3. Lindholm MG, Kober L, Boesgaard S et al (2003) Cardiogenic shock complicating acute myocardial infarction; prognostic impact of early and late shock development. Eur Heart J 24:258–265
4. De Backer D (2003) Lactic acidosis. Intensive Care Med 29:699–702

5. Friedman G, Berlot G, Kahn RJ, Vincent JL (1995) Combined measurements of blood lactate concentrations and gastric intramucosal pH in patients with severe sepsis. Crit Care Med 23:1184–1193
6. Manikis P, Jankowski S, Zhang H et al (1995) Correlation of serial blood lactate levels to organ failure and mortality after trauma. Am J Emerg Med 13:619–622
7. Bakker J, Coffernils M, Leon M et al (1991) Blood lactate levels are superior to oxygen derived variables in predicting outcome in human septic shock. Chest 99:956–962
8. Gutierrez G, Clark C, Brown SD, Price K, Ortiz L, Nelson C (1994) Effect of dobutamine on oxygen consumption and gastric mucosal pH in septic patients. Am J Respir Crit Care Med 150:324–329
9. Maynard N, Bihari D, Beale R et al (1993) Assessment of splanchnic oxygenation by gastric tonometry in patients with acute circulatory failure. JAMA 270:1203–1210
10. Doglio GR, Pusajo JF, Egurrola MA et al (1991) Gastric mucosal pH as a prognostic index of mortality in critically ill patients. Crit Care Med 19:1037–1040
11. Vincent JL, Creteur J (1998) Gastric mucosal pH (pHi) is definitely obsolete–please tell us more about gastric mucosal PCO_2 ($PgCO_2$). Crit Care Med 26:1479–1481
12. De Backer D, Creteur J, Preiser JC et al (2002) Microvascular blood flow is altered in patients with sepsis. Am J Respir Crit Care Med 166:98–104
13. De Backer D, Creteur J, Dubois MJ et al (2004) Microvascular alterations in patients with acute severe heart failure and cardiogenic shock. Am Heart J 147:91–99
14. Sakr Y, Dubois MJ, De Backer D et al (2004) Persistent microcirculatory alterations are associated with organ failure and death in patients with septic shock. Crit Care Med 32:1825–1831
15. Creteur J, De Backer D, Sakr Y et al (2006) Sublingual capnometry tracks microcirculatory changes in septic patients. Intensive Care Med 32:516–523
16. De Backer D, Verdant C, Chierego M et al (2006) Effects of drotrecogin alfa activated on microcirculatory alterations in patients with severe sepsis. Crit Care Med 34:1918–1924
17. Weil MH, Shubin H (1969) The "VIP" approach to the bedside management of shock. JAMA 207:337–340
18. Vincent JL, Weil MH (2006) Fluid challenge revisited. Crit Care Med 34:1333–1337
19. Finfer S, Bellomo R, Boyce N, et al (2004) A comparison of albumin and saline for fluid resuscitation in the intensive care unit. N Engl J Med 350:2247–2256
20. Vincent JL, Dubois MJ, Navickis RJ, Wilkes MM (2003) Hypoalbuminemia in acute illness: is there a rationale for intervention? A meta-analysis of cohort studies and controlled trials. Ann Surg 237:319–334
21. Vincent JL, Navickis RJ, Wilkes MM (2004) Morbidity in hospitalized patients receiving human albumin: a meta-analysis of randomized, controlled trials. Crit Care Med 32:2029–2038
22. Dellinger RP, Carlet JM, Masur H et al (2004) Surviving Sepsis Campaign guidelines for management of severe sepsis and septic shock. Crit Care Med 32:858–873
23. Bellomo R, Chapman M, Finfer S et al (2000) Low-dose dopamine in patients with early renal dysfunction: a placebo-controlled randomised trial. Australian and New Zealand Intensive Care Society (ANZICS) Clinical Trials Group. Lancet 356:2139–2143
24. Vincent JL, Roman A, Kahn RJ (1990) Dobutamine administration in septic shock: addition to a standard protocol. Crit Care Med 18:689–693
25. Kwan I, Bunn F, Roberts I (2001) Timing and volume of fluid administration for patients with bleeding following trauma. Cochrane Database Syst Rev CD002245

26. Duvernoy CS, Bates ER (2005) Management of cardiogenic shock attributable to acute myocardial infarction in the reperfusion era. J Intensive Care Med 20:188–198
27. Bernard GR, Vincent JL, Laterre PF et al (2001) Efficacy and safety of recombinant human activated protein C for severe sepsis. N Engl J Med 344:699–709

14 Prevention and Management of Cardiac Dysfunction during and after Cardiac Surgery

W. MOOSBAUER, A.HOFER AND H. GOMBOTZ

Introduction

Surgery is analogous to an extreme stress test. It initiates inflammatory, hypercoagulable, stress, and hypoxic states, which may be associated with elevations in troponin levels leading to postoperative myocardial dysfunction and failure [1]. Cardiac surgery, especially, is associated with the inherent risk of myocardial ischemia and myocardial infarction; and consequently, with postoperative heart failure. The degree of permanent postoperative myocardial injury is determined by the severity and duration of ischemia. A progressive pattern of myocardial dysfunction–apart from ongoing ischemia–suggests that additional underlying mechanisms, which are at least partially different from those of myocardial stunning, may also exist [2].

The risk profile of patients undergoing cardiac surgery has steadily accelerated over the last decade due to increasing patient age combined with increasing comorbidities. Patients have higher mortality and morbidity risks in direct relation to their age, left ventricular function, extent of coronary disease, comorbid conditions, and whether the procedure is urgent, emergent, or a reoperation [3]. In general, cardiac-related variables are major predictors of short-term mortality, whereas non-cardiac-related variables are more or less major predictors of intermediate-term mortality. In consequence, previous heart surgery, angina class III or IV, previous myocardial infarction, and preoperative use of an intra-aortic balloon pump have greater effects in the short-term postoperative period; whereas impaired

Department of Anesthesiology and Intensive Care, General Hospital Linz, Austria functional status, chronic obstructive pulmonary disease, and renal dysfunction have greater effects in the intermediate-term postoperative period [4]. As morbidity and mortality are directly related to the proportion between preserved and damaged myocardium, myocardial protection is of central importance throughout the perioperative period. More complex procedures and critically ill patients require even more optimized myocardial protection.

Despite improvements in surgical and anesthetic technique, a large proportion of patients undergoing open heart surgery (up to 96%) still suffer from early, at least transient postoperative ventricular dysfunction and failure, regardless of the type of procedure. After surgical repair, left ventricular or biventricular function (when measured) improves initially, but then declines, reaching a nadir between 4 and 6 h after surgery, with gradual recovery occurring during the next 8–24 h postoperatively (Fig. 1) [5]. In low-risk patients, ventricular dysfunction occurs to comparable degrees after *off-pump* and *on-pump* surgery. However, in patients with ischemic left ventricular dysfunction or those with multivessel disease, *off-pump* surgery causes less myocardial damage and also a lower incidence of postoperative atrial fibrillation [6]. Patients with preexisting heart failure undergoing cardiac or noncardiac surgery still suffer substantial morbidity and mortality despite advances in perioperative care [7]. In patients with preexisting ventricular dysfunction–best identified by preoperative left ventricular ejection fraction (LVEF)–the myocardial depression is more severe and recovery is prolonged. For example, patients with LVEF < 45% or preexisting ventricular dyssynergy exhibited more prolonged dysfunction than did those with normal ventricles [8]. The importance of heart failure as an independent risk factor is also underlined by the fact that patients with coronary artery disease but without heart failure have a similar 30-day mortality rate to the general population.

After valve repair or replacement, preexisting hemodynamic alterations of co-existing disease may persist - at least in part - throughout the postoperative period. Although afterload has been markedly reduced, left ventricular hypertrophy and reduced left ventricular compliance still remain after aortic valve replacement for moderately severe aortic stenosis [9]. Similarly, left ventricular dilatation induced by long-standing aortic insufficiency persists immediately after successful aortic valve replacement. With mitral stenosis, preoperative atrial fibrillation and pulmonary hypertension may limit the potential for recovery of full function, whereas with mitral regurgitation, valve replacement may acutely increase afterload in a dilated heart [10].

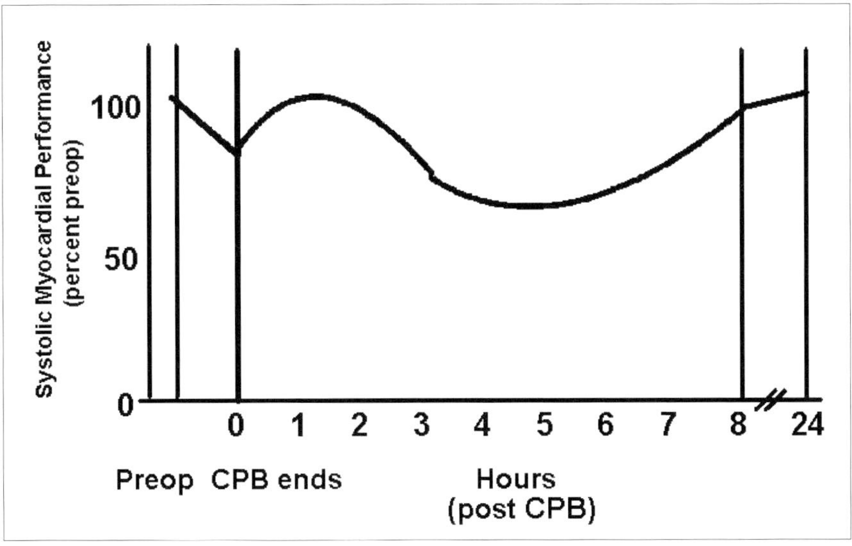

Fig. 1. Time course of ventricular function after cardiopulmonary bypass. Reproduced with permission from [5]

Causes of Postoperative Myocardial Dysfunction and Failure

Increasing severity of surgical trauma and anesthesia can initiate increasing inflammatory and hypercoagulable states [1]. The *inflammatory state* involves increases in tumor necrosis factor-α, interleukin-1 (IL-1), IL-6, and C-reactive protein. These factors may have a direct role in initiating plaque fissuring and acute coronary thrombosis. The hypercoagulable *state* involves increases in plasminogen activator inhibitor-1, factor VIII and platelet reactivity, as well as decreases in antithrombin III. All these factors can lead to acute coronary thrombosis. The *stress state* involves increased levels of catecholamines and cortisol. Increased stress hormone levels result in increases in blood pressure, heart rate, coronary artery sheer stress, relative insulin deficiency, and free fatty acid levels. Coronary artery shear stress may trigger plaque fissuring and acute coronary thrombosis. The other factors increase oxygen demand and can result in perioperative myocardial ischemia, which is strongly associated with perioperative myocardial infarction. Factors that can initiate a *hypoxic state* include anemia, hypothermia (through shivering), and suppression of breathing.

Cardiac surgery *per se* may cause additional myocardial damage by numerous mechanisms such as diffuse ischemia from inadequate myocardial protection and myocardial reperfusion injury, inadequate repair, myocardial infarction, inflammation, coronary spasm, local trauma by surgical manipulation, air embolism, or residual hypothermia. Myocardial injury during cardiac surgery can be divided into three phases: *prebypass ischemia*, including preoperative disease status (unprotected ischemia); *protected ischemia*, electively initiated by cardioplegia and hypothermic extracorporeal circulation (ECC); and *reperfusion injuries* after ECC. After brief periods of myocardial ischemia the myocardial depression is usually mild and transient, but it becomes worse as the ischemic episodes that precede it are more severe and longer-lasting. Patients with preexisting severe underlying disease, poor ischemic conditions, and reduced cardiac reserves have limited ability to cope with ischemia-related myocardial dysfunction. Ischemia is more prevalent postoperatively than preoperatively or before ECC.

Prebypass Ischemia

Patients with severe coronary artery disease continue to have frequent episodes of silent myocardial ischemia despite intensive medical therapy. Before induction of anesthesia almost half the–mostly silent–ischemic episodes occur randomly as well as in response to hemodynamic abnormalities. Myocardial ischemia before the start of cardiopulmonary bypass (CPB) has been observed in 38% of coronary artery bypass graft (CABG) patients, and myocardial infarction was three times more frequent than in patients without ischemia (6.9% vs. 2.5%) [11]. Although perioperative myocardial ischemia appears not always to be induced by hemodynamic stress, it has been shown that patients with perioperative myocardial ischemia had previous tachycardia more frequently [12]. A preoperative heart rate above 100 bpm was also associated with increased risk of perioperative myocardial infarction. Preoperative regional wall motion score index and new regional wall motion abnormalities immediately after CPB have been shown to be the most important independent predictor for the use of inotropes after cardiac surgery [13].

Elevated serum troponin I (cTnI) concentrations as sensitive markers of myocardial damage measured 24 h before surgery have been demonstrated to identify patients at high risk for developing perioperative myocardial infarction or low cardiac output syndrome, and at increased risk of in-hospital death. Perioperative myocardial infarction and low cardiac output syndrome occurred at rates of 5.9% and 1.6% respectively in patients with preoperative cTnI levels less than 0.1 ng/ml, compared to 17.2% and 10.9% in patients with preoperative cTnI levels greater than 1.5 ng/ml [14].

ECC and Cardiac Arrest

In most cardiac surgical patients, the use of ECC is a precondition for surgical cardiac repair. However, during ECC the heart is subjected to a number of events that eventually lead to myocardial ischemia: inadequate myocardial perfusion, ventricular distension or collapse, coronary embolism, and ventricular fibrillation, as well as aortic cross-clamping and reperfusion. In addition, ECC per se may cause myocardial dysfunction as a result of severe hemodilution and hyperkalemia or as a result of cardioplegia-induced systemic hypocalcemia. Thus, the operation originally designed to preserve or improve myocardial function may be associated with deleterious effects. Those adverse effects may be well tolerated in patients with normal ventricular function, but may become serious in patients with compromised ventricular function.

During ECC, perfusion of the coronary arteries may be compromised by perfusion via the aortic route or direct cannulation of the arteries or elevated vascular resistance. In addition, autoregulation may be lost due to hypothermia. Ventricular distension and the use of catecholamines may upset the oxygen supply/demand ratio. Ventricular fibrillation increases myocardial wall tension and oxygen consumption and impairs subendocardial blood flow. Aortic cross-clamping *per se* is potentially a major cause of myocardial injury. The extent of necrosis in unprotected myocardium is directly related to the duration of aortic cross-clamping and cardiac reperfusion **injury**[15]. Increased aortic cross-clamp time and longer duration of CPB are indeed associated with a significant reduction in ventricular function [16].

Inadequate Cardioplegic Arrest

Cardioplegic arrest provides protected ischemia by reducing the oxygen demand below 10% of the demand of the working heart and also avoids reperfusion injury by specifically targeting the pathophysiologic mechanism and mediators of postischemic injury. Effective myocardial protection through either cold or warm blood cardioplegia is essential, because late survival is significantly reduced in patients with even nonfatal perioperative cardiac outcomes [17]. Cardioplegic arrest neutralizes some negative aspects of hypothermia including a paradoxical increase in the inotropic state and oxygen demands per beat or the induction of ventricular fibrillation [18]. The greatest degree of myocardial protection is achieved by combining (tepid) hypothermia with chemical cardioplegia. Normothermic cardioplegia may be used to overcome some of the disadvantages of hypothermia.

Inability to establish or maintain electromechanical quiescence is a signal that cardioplegic solution does not reach some regions in adequate concentration. This can be the consequence of the underlying artery disease, inadequate pressure in the aortic root, or even steal phenomena. An insufficient cardioplegic procedure results in anaerobic metabolism during cardiac arrest with subsequent lactate accumulation, which is regarded as a predictor of low cardiac output syndrome. In addition, the type of cardioplegia and route of administration may play a role in protecting the myocardium. Blood cardioplegia provides a closer approximation to normal physiology and superior myocardial protection compared to crystalloid cardioplegia, including lower rates of hospital stay and myocardial-bound creatine kinase increase, whereas the incidence of myocardial infarction and death is similar [19].

During cardiac surgery the right ventricle is at special risk of inadequate protection by disparate distribution of cardioplegia and cooling. Especially in the presence of a significant stenosis or obstruction of the right coronary artery (RCA), uneven cooling of the right ventricle has been reported [20]. In a group of patients with RCA occlusion the right ventricular ejection fraction (RVEF), right ventricular stroke work index (RVSWI) and cardiac index (CI) were significantly reduced after CPB. In patients with severe right coronary stenosis, off-pump cardiac surgery seemed to provide better right ventricular protection because of the avoidance of cardioplegic arrest. Inadequate cardioplegic protection of the atria, myocardial ischemia, and also atrial cannulation may increase the frequency of postoperative atrial fibrillation. Compared to patients operated on off-pump, the incidence of postoperative atrial fibrillation was significantly higher in on-pump patients, and ECG during cardioplegic arrest has been found to be the main independent predictor of postoperative atrial fibrillation in CABG patients.

Hypothermia

Hypothermic ECC decreases metabolic rate and oxygen requirements and in consequence increases tolerance of ischemia. Hypothermia also helps to preserve high-energy phosphate stores and reduces excitatory neurotransmitter release, which is especially important for protection of the central nervous system. Strict maintenance of normothermia during ECC is in fact associated with increased neurologic risk. However, hypothermia is also associated with several disadvantages for the myocardium. Transient, readily reversible edema of the myocardium after reperfusion may occur. In addition, topical cooling injury of extracardiac structures is a matter of concern. Topical cooling yielded no additional benefit but increased the incidence of diaphragm paralysis and associated pulmonary edema [21]. Furthermore, citrate toxicity may be augmented, leading to additional myocardial depression and thrombocytopenia.

Reperfusion

Reperfusion injury is defined as additional myocardial injury occurring after restoration of blood flow to ischemic myocardium. It causes inflammatory cell activation from cytokine generation, up-regulation of neutrophil adhesion molecules with neutrophil activation, oxygen free radical formation, and lipoperoxidation, and enables important pathways for postoperative myocardial dysfunction. Reperfusion injury has an early phase (< 4 h) based on early neutrophil and adhesion molecule-dependent interaction and a later phase (4–6 h) with still unknown mediators. Reperfusion injuries include structural deterioration (edema, platelet deposition, etc.) and biochemical (decreased oxygen utilization, complement activation, acidosis, etc.) and electromechanical pathologies (dysrhythmias, impaired systolic/diastolic function). Experimental studies showed possible prevention of myocardial dysfunction by using free radical scavengers. However, whether this protection confers meaningful clinical benefits is uncertain [22]. There is also a time link between cytokine release and the timing of ventricular dysfunction. Cytokines can release nitric oxide from endothelium, resulting in myocardial dysfunction.

Reperfusion injury can cause atrial and ventricular dysrhythmias, reversible systolic and diastolic dysfunction (stunning), endothelial dysfunction, myocardial necrosis, and apoptosis [23]. After short periods of ischemia the negative effect on contractile function is benign but might be injurious to other targets like endothelium or neutrophil accumulation. Long periods of ischemia cause injury of the myocardium, leading to persistent contractile dysfunction. In the absence of morphologic injury, postischemic contractile dysfunction may be reversible within hours (stunned myocardium). *Stunning* is common after ECC and is defined as prolonged postischemic contractile dysfunction of the myocardium salvaged by reperfusion. In a number of studies increased chamber stiffness and dilatation were found after blood reperfusion following normothermic or hypothermic ischemia [24]. Acute increases in postischemic chamber stiffness are caused by myocardial edema and abnormal calcium handling in the myocardium. A decrease in diastolic relaxation impairs diastolic filling and reduces stroke volume independently of any postischemia or postcardioplegia abnormalities in inotropic state or contractility.

The question of whether reperfusion causes myocardial necrosis is still a matter of discussion. However, endothelial dysfunction in the pathogenesis of reperfusion injury is well documented. Endothelial damage occurs during reperfusion rather than after short periods of global and/or regional ischemia, but more prolonged periods of ischemia also cause endothelial damage. Apart from ischemia–reperfusion, inflammatory mediators and gaseous microemboli may also induce endothelial damage during ECC. For example, pulmonary endothelial dysfunction may be impaired until 3–4 days after exposure to ECC [25].

Reperfusion dysrhythmias manifest themselves as premature ventricular contractions and ventricular fibrillation. Poor myocardial protection (global or distal to severe coronary artery occlusions) causes failure to spontaneously resume sinus rhythm or persistence of arrhythmias requiring therapeutic interventions. The incidence and severity of reperfusion arrhythmias is strongly related to the severity of the preceding ischemia. The induction of calcium-dependent arrhythmias by accumulation of intracellular calcium during ischemia is another mechanism. Furthermore, oxygen-derived free radicals may cause reperfusion arrhythmias by altering membrane lipids and various transport proteins. The combination of oxygen-derived free radicals and calcium-related events especially might act as a trigger for reperfusion dysrhythmias.

Prevention of Postoperative Myocardial Dysfunction and Failure

The healthy heart has enormous functional reserve. However, when ventricular performance is marginally matched to the individual patient's physiologic needs, even small decrements in myocardial function may cause an increase in morbidity and mortality. Therefore, in addition to the surgical procedure, efficient myocardial protection should to be one of the main goals for all members of the surgical team throughout the perioperative period. Surgical myocardial protection includes optimal surgical technique, adequate performance of ECC and cardioplegic arrest, as well as liberal (prophylactic) use of assist devices in patients who are severely hemodynamically unstable. Perioperative stress protection by the anesthesiologist includes preoperative optimization, adequate treatment of pain and anxiety, and precise hemodynamic management including heart rate control and ("early goal") volume management. Also, additional cardioprotective drugs may be used. However, the best approach to medical protection of patients from cardiovascular complications during surgery is still a matter of discussion.

Role of the Anesthesiologist in Myocardial Protection

Although brief periods of ischemia can contribute to prolonged left ventricular dysfunction and even heart failure, they paradoxically play a cardioprotective role. Episodes of ischemia as short as 5 min, followed by reperfusion, protect the heart from a subsequent longer coronary artery occlusion by markedly reducing the amount of necrosis that results from the test episode of ischemia. This phenomenon, called *ischemic preconditioning*, has been observed in virtually every species in which it has been studied and has a powerful cardioprotective effect [23, 26]. Volatile anesthetics appear to be related to better and earlier recovery of myocardial function and lesser myocardial damage manifested as minor elevation in myocardial enzymes. CABG patients on a sevoflurane-based anesthetic regimen demonstrated more preserved cardiac performance, reduced requirement of inotropic support, and lower serum concentrations of cardiac enzymes compared to those on an intravenously based anesthetic regimen [27, 28]. In addition, a decreased inflammatory response to CPB–measured as reduced release of IL-6, CD11b/CD18, and TNF-α–as well as significant reduction in new regional wall motion abnormalities after sevoflurane anesthesia suggest effective protection against ischemia reperfusion injury [29]. The cardiac protective property of volatile anesthetics may depend on the duration and timing of administration [27].

Increasing evidence shows that perioperative β-blocker treatment significantly reduces the risk and the incidence of perioperative cardiac complications after cardiac and noncardiac surgery [30]. In *noncardiac* surgery β-blockers were shown to reduce the number of deaths from cardiac events, as well as nonfatal myocardial infarction but did not have a significant impact on the total number of deaths. β-blockers reduce sympathetic tone, heart rate, and contractility, decrease share stress, and reduce the prothrombotic effect of sympathetic activation. Despite extensive investigations, important questions such as the ideal target population, ideal dose, route of administration, duration of therapy, or even type of β-blocker remain unresolved [31]. In addition, the observation that there may be some disadvantages associated with β-blocker therapy in low-risk patients has not been fully explained. Furthermore, in patients receiving *chronic* β-blocker therapy the adequacy of cardiac protection has been questioned. The required dose of isoproterenol needed to increase heart rate by 25 bpm was similar in patients receiving chronic β-blocker treatment compared to those without. It has been suggested that patients undergoing chronic β-blocking therapy compensate to such a degree that cardiovascular β-receptor function actually becomes normal (receptor up-regulation). As a matter of fact, chronic β-blocker therapy has been shown to be associated with higher risk of myocardial infarction, cardiac death, and major cardiac complications in noncardiac surgery [32]. On the other hand, discontinuing β-blocker therapy immediately after surgery may increase the risk of postoperative cardiovascular morbidity and mortality and may be associated with a higher risk of ventricular heart failure. Additional perioperative β-blockade and the combination of β-blockers with statin therapy may be beneficial in patients receiving chronic β-blocker therapy and high-risk patients with coronary artery disease. The combined use of β-blocker and simvastatin may prevent the up-regulation of β-adrenoceptors induced by chronic β-blocker therapy and therefore enable better stress protection [33]. In noncardiac surgery beneficial effects have been shown to be greatest in patients with higher cardiac risk factors and in those with more wall motion abnormalities. Bisoprolol treatment before noncardiac surgery significantly decreased the rate of cardiac death (3.4% vs. 17%) and nonfatal myocardial infarction (0% vs. 17%). A recent meta-analysis relating to ?-blocker use in noncardiac surgery has demonstrated a 65% reduction in perioperative myocardial ischemia (11.0% vs. 25.6%), a 56% reduction in myocardial infarction (0.5% vs. 3.9%), and a 67% in the composite endpoint of cardiac death and nonfatal myocardial infarction reduction (1.1% vs. 6.1%) [34].

Faster heart rate may be a marker of the under-use of β-blocker therapy. A preinduction heart rate of 80 bpm or higher was indeed associated with increased in-hospital mortality after CABG surgery (Fig. 2) [12]. The deleterious consequences of tachycardia may be particularly aggravated by systemic hypotension and increased ventricular filling pressures. Yet, β-blocker therapy is still titrated to a heart rate of 80 bpm or higher in many patients [35].

In the setting of CABG surgery preoperative β-blocker therapy was associated with a small but consistent survival benefit for patients, except among those with an LVEF of less than 30% [36]. After coronary surgery chronic *preoperative* β-blocker therapy reduces 30-day mortality. Death was even more likely after nitrate therapy than after β-blocker therapy [37]. Prophylactic treatment with β-blockers also reduces the incidence of postoperative atrial fibrillation, particularly in elderly patients.

In patients with overt or underlying cardiac disease the actions of α_2-adrenoceptor agonists, which include maintenance of stable systemic blood pressure and low heart rate and a reduction in overall oxygen consumption, can be expected to reduce the risk of procedure-related cardiac events. This expectation has been corroborated in clinical trials with clonidine, dexmedetomidine, and mivazerol in *noncardiac* surgery. Large controlled tri-

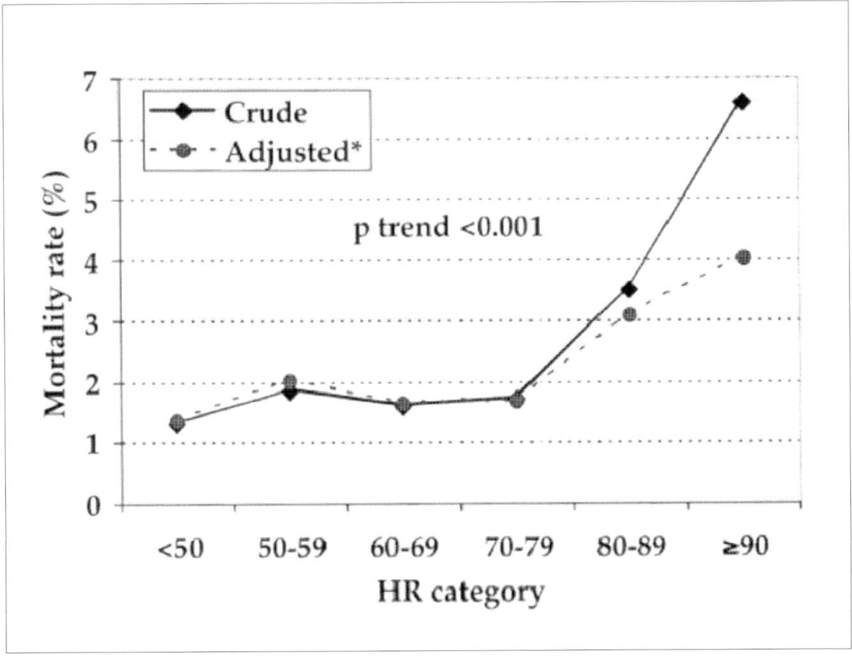

Fig. 2. Preinduction heart rate (HR) and in-hospital mortality. Reproduced with permission from [12]

als would be instructive in establishing a robust estimate of the benefit. These drugs could be used as an alternative or as second-line agents when β-blocker therapy is contraindicated.

Several clinical trials clearly demonstrated that, although inotropic agents like α_2-agonists and phosphodiesterase (PDE) inhibitors may improve hemodynamic parameters, their use may be associated with increased morbidity and mortality [38]. The new calcium-sensitizing agent levosimendan protects against myocardial ischemia and reperfusion injury and may serve as a promising alternative to conventional therapy in cardiac surgery. In comparison to dobutamine in patients with low-output heart failure the primary hemodynamic endpoint–defined as an increase of 30% or more in cardiac output and a decrease of 25% or more in pulmonary capillary wedge pressure–was achieved in 28% of patients in the levosimendan group and 15% of those in the dobutamine group [39]. Because levosimendan decreases pulmonary capillary wedge pressure more effectively than dobutamine, the substance may be of value in patients with reversibly increased pulmonary pressures or right ventricular dysfunction (Fig. 3) [39, 40]. When compared to milrinone as well as dobutamine in patients undergoing elective coronary artery surgery, treatment with levosimendan was associated with significantly higher cardiac index and mixed venous oxygen saturation, whereas pulmonary capillary wedge pressure, systemic vascular resistance, and oxygen extraction ratios were significantly higher in the milrinone treatment group [41]. Furthermore, despite improved myocardial performance in patients undergoing CABG, no increase in myocardial oxygen consumption has been observed. Significant cardioprotection by levosimendan may also be provided by the vasodilatory effects as a result of opening ATP-dependent potassium channels and reducing the calcium sensitivity of contractile proteins in vascular smooth muscles. Decreases in vascular resistance and augmented blood flow in coronary arteries and internal mammary artery have been demonstrated in cardiac surgery as having a potentially protective effect in patients with compromised coronary blood flow and vasospasm in the arterial grafts after coronary bypass grafting.

After levosimendan treatment, a reduction of the number of hypokinetic segments and an improvement in left ventricular function without impairment of diastolic function have been reported in patients with acute coronary syndrome immediately after reperfusion during angioplasty [42]. In the setting of off-pump coronary artery bypass surgery, increases in stroke vol-

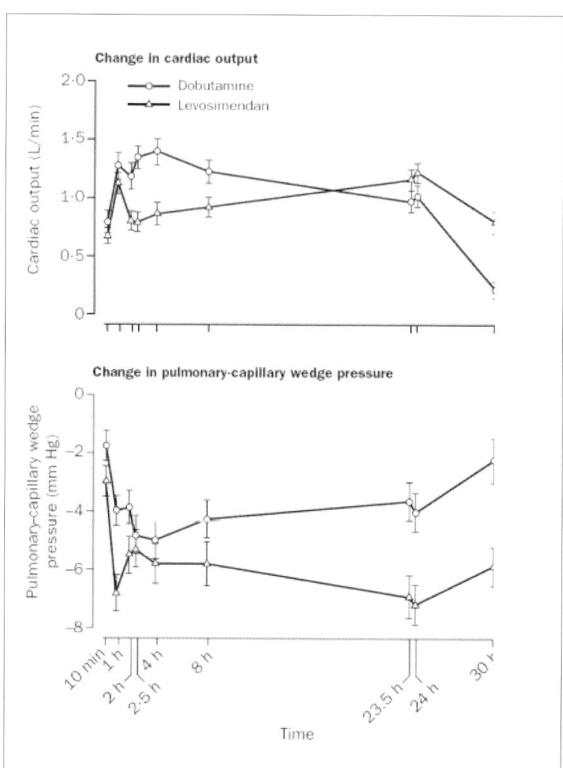

Fig. 3. Comparison of hemodynamic effects of levosimendan and dobutamine. Changes in cardiac output and pulmonary capillary wedge pressure were recorded from baseline to 30 h in patients with low-output heart failure. Reproduced with permission from [39]

ume and cardiac output and decreases in systemic vascular resistance were observed when levosimendan was administered [43]. Levosimendan administered 15 min before separation of CPB and continued for 6 h had beneficial effects on cardiac performance in low-risk patients but no detrimental effects on arterial oxygenation and perioperative arrhythmias [44]. Levosimendan also appears to be useful in failure-to-wean from CPB after cardiotomy when conventional inotropic therapy proves inadequate. There is also evidence that patients receiving a short infusion of levosimendan before their CABG surgery have less myocardial damage as expressed by lower troponin I levels [45]. Although the efficacy of levosimendan has repeatedly been demonstrated in the perioperative setting, the number of patients investigated is still rather small. Therefore, further trials will be necessary to investigate the effectiveness and indications for preemptive use of levosimendan alone or in combination with other inotropic drugs or assist devices in patients with severely compromised ventricular function.

Role of the Surgeon in Myocardial Protection

Myocardial protection is not necessarily the primary goal and purpose of cardiac surgery, but a prerequisite for successful postoperative outcome. In addition to careful avoidance of myocardial ischemia and optimal surgical repair, myocardial protection techniques (i.e., cardioplegia) are of central importance, especially for the critically ill patients. Cornerstones of cardioplegic myocardial protection are rapid cardiac arrest, maintenance of electromechanical quiescence, minimizing myocardial ischemia, and control of reperfusion. Each of these variables has to be considered together with the type and conduct of ECC. Because of the pathophysiologic complexity of cardioplegic arrest in combination with ECC, and because of the variety of surgical techniques, it is almost impossible to provide a general recipe for myocardial protection. In hypothermic conditions, longer intervals between readministering cardioplegic solutions allow the team to focus more on the surgical procedure. However, the benefit of hypothermia has to be weighed against hypothermia-associated disadvantages such as longer ECC times or greater postoperative diastolic function. More normothermic techniques, on the other hand, need readministration at more frequent intervals for cardioplegia, but have the advantage of more rapid restoration of myocardial function, decreased reperfusion time, and less use of inotropic drugs and assist devices. Because of the increased danger of ischemia, with use of normothermic cardioplegia techniques, more care must be exercised when "normothermic" cardioplegia is delivered. Further, the degree of care that must be exercised increases, depending on more close to "normothermic" the cardioplegia used is.

Rapid cardiac arrest is necessary to avoid depletion of high-energy phosphates. After cardiac arrest further ischemia and loss of energy are mainly determined by the extent to which electromechanical quiescence is maintained. Inability to obtain electromechanical quiescence may be a consequence of the coronary artery disease, inadequate pressure on the aortic root, or steal phenomena. Additional retrograde cardioplegia may help to facilitate the maintenance of electromechanical quiescence. To further minimize myocardial ischemia, cold cardioplegic solution can be administered intermittently, whereas warm solutions should be administered more frequently or continuously. If ischemia can be eliminated, reperfusion injury is minimized and myocardial protection enhanced.

Worsening ischemia and/or left ventricular systolic dysfunction, with resultant hemodynamic instability, inability to wean off CPB, and death, may complicate cardiac surgery. In patients at risk of these complications, intra-aortic balloon pump (IABP) support may have beneficial hemodynamic and anti-ischemic effects. The use of an IABP provides circulatory support by augmenting diastolic coronary perfusion pressure and by afterload reduction. This increases myocardial oxygen supply and decreases myocardial oxygen demands, leading to improved systolic and diastolic function, decreased pulmonary capillary wedge pressure, and reduced heart rate. A large body of evidence suggests that preoperative (prophylactic) IABP support should be part of a strategy to protect high-risk patients undergoing cardiac surgery. The implementation of IABP may reduce periods of long-duration subendocardial ischemia and help avoid postoperative myocardial injury and complications. As a matter of fact, in high risk-patients, placement of IABP before surgery is associated with better short- and long-term survival. Hospital mortality in patients with elevated cardiac risk (LVEF $\leq 40\%$, left main stem stenosis $\geq 70\%$, or undergoing CABG was significantly lower when the IABP was inserted before the start of surgery [46].

In conclusion, meticulous myocardial protection is a must in cardiac surgery in order to avoid postoperative myocardial dysfunction and failure, especially in patients with compromised myocardial function. More complex procedures and critically ill patients require even more and better optimized myocardial protection. This can only be achieved through close cooperation between surgeons, anesthesiologists, and technicians and using modern cardioplegic and pharmacologic strategies.

References

1. Devereaux PJ, Goldman L, Cook DJ et al (2005) Perioperative cardiac events in patients undergoing noncardiac surgery: a review of the magnitude of the pro-

blem, the pathophysiology of the events and methods to estimate and communicate risk. CMAJ 173:627–634

2. Liakopoulos OJ, Muhlfeld C, Koschinsky M et al (2005) Progressive loss of myocardial contractile function despite unimpaired coronary blood flow after cardiac surgery. Basic Res Cardiol 100:75–83
3. Surgenor SD, O'Connor GT, Lahey SJ et al (2001) Predicting the risk of death from heart failure after coronary artery bypass graft surgery. Anesth Analg 92:596–601
4. Gardner SC, Grunwald GK, Rumsfeld JS et al (2001) Risk factors for intermediate-term survival after coronary artery bypass grafting. Ann Thorac Surg 72:2033–2037
5. Royster RL (1993) Myocardial dysfunction following cardiopulmonary bypass: recovery patterns, predictors of inotropic need, theoretical concepts of inotropic administration. J Cardiothorac Vasc Anesth 7:19–25
6. Khan NE, De Souza A, Mister R et al (2004) A randomized comparison of off-pump and on-pump multivessel coronary-artery bypass surgery. N Engl J Med 350:21–28
7. Argenziano M, Spotnitz HM, Whang W et al (1999) risk stratification for coronary bypass surgery in patients with left ventricular dysfunction: analysis of the Coronary Artery Bypass Grafting Patch Trial database. Circulation 100:119II–124
8. Mangano DT (1985) Biventricular function after myocardial revascularization in humans: deterioration and recovery patterns during the first 24 hours. Anesthesiology 62:571–577
9. Vanky FB, Hakanson E, Tamas E et al (2006) Risk factors for postoperative heart failure in patients operated on for aortic stenosis. Ann Thorac Surg 81:1297–1304
10. Corin WJ, Sutsch G, Murakami T et al (1995) Left ventricular function in chronic mitral regurgitation: preoperative and postoperative comparison. J Am Coll Cardiol 25:113–121
11. Slogoff S, Keats AS (1985) Does perioperative myocardial ischemia lead to postoperative myocardial infarction? Anesthesiology 62:107–114
12. Fillinger MP, Surgenor SD, Hartman GS et al (2002) The association between heart rate and in-hospital mortality after coronary artery bypass graft surgery. Anesth Analg 95:1483–1488
13. Leung JM, O'Kelly B, Browner WS et al (1989) Prognostic importance of postbypass regional wall-motion abnormalities in patients undergoing coronary artery bypass graft surgery. SPI Research Group. Anesthesiology 71:16–25
14. Thielmann M, Massoudy P, Neuhauser M et al (2006) Prognostic value of preoperative cardiac troponin I in patients undergoing emergency coronary artery bypass surgery with non-ST-elevation or ST-elevation acute coronary syndromes. Circulation 114: I448–I453
15. Kirklin JW, Conti VR, Blackstone EH (1979) Prevention of myocardial damage during cardiac operations. N Engl J Med 301:135–141
16. Kay HR, Levine FH, Fallon JT et al (1978) Effect of cross-clamp time, temperature, and cardioplegic agents on myocardial function after induced arrest. J Thorac Cardiovasc Surg 76:590–603
17. Fremes SE, Tamariz MG, Abramov D et al (2000) Late results of the Warm Heart Trial: the influence of nonfatal cardiac events on late survival. Circulation 102:339III–345
18. Fukunami M, Hearse DJ (1989) The inotropic consequences of cooling: studies in the isolated rat heart. Heart Vessels 5:1–9
19. Guru V, Omura J, Alghamdi AA et al (2006) Is blood superior to crystalloid cardioplegia?: a meta-analysis of randomized clinical trials. Circulation 114: I-331

20. Banach M, Rysz J, Drozdz JA et al (2006) Risk factors of atrial fibrillation following coronary artery bypass grafting: a preliminary report. Circ J 70:438–441
21. Tripp HF, Bolton JW (1998) Phrenic nerve injury following cardiac surgery: a review. J Card Surg 13:218–223
22. Kevin LG, Novalija E, Stowe DF (2005) Reactive oxygen species as mediators of cardiac injury and protection: the relevance to anesthesia practice. Anesth Analg 101:1275–1287
23. Kloner RA, Jennings RB. (2001) Consequences of brief ischemia: stunning, preconditioning, and their clinical implications: Part 1. Circulation 104:2981–2989
24. Casthely PA, Shah C, Mekhjian H et al (1997) Left ventricular diastolic function after coronary artery bypass grafting: a correlative study with three different myocardial protection techniques. J Thorac Cardiovasc Surg 114:254–260
25. Glavind-Kristensen M, Brix-Christensen V, Toennesen E et al (2002) Pulmonary endothelial dysfunction after cardiopulmonary bypass in neonatal pigs. Acta Anaesthesiol Scand 46:853–859
26. Toller WG, Kersten JR, Pagel PS et al (1999) Sevoflurane reduces myocardial infarct size and decreases the time threshold for ischemic preconditioning in dogs. Anesthesiology 91:1437–1446
27. De Hert SG, Van der Linden PJ, Cromheecke S et al (2004) Cardioprotective properties of sevoflurane in patients undergoing coronary surgery with cardiopulmonary bypass are related to the modalities of its administration. Anesthesiology 101:299–310
28. Conzen PF, Fischer S, Detter C et al (2003) Sevoflurane provides greater protection of the myocardium than propofol in patients undergoing off-pump coronary artery bypass surgery. Anesthesiology 99:826–833
29. Nader ND, Li CM, Khadra WZ et al (2004) Anesthetic myocardial protection with sevoflurane. J Cardiothorac Vasc Anesth 18:269–274
30. Mangano DT, Layug EL, Wallace A et al (1996) Effect of atenolol on mortality and cardiovascular morbidity after noncardiac surgery. N Engl J Med 335:1713–1721
31. Fleisher LA, Beckman JA, Brown KA et al (2006) ACC/AHA 2006 Guideline update on perioperative cardiovascular evaluation for noncardiac surgery: focused update on perioperative beta-blocker therapy: a report of the American College of Cardiology/American Heart Association Task Force on Practice Guidelines (Writing Committee to Update the 2002 Guidelines on Perioperative Cardiovascular Evaluation for Noncardiac Surgery). Circulation 113:2662–2674
32. Giles JW, Sear JW and Foex P. (2004) Effect of chronic beta-blockade on peri-operative outcome in patients undergoing non-cardiac surgery: an analysis of observational and case control studies. Anaesthesia 59:574–583
33. Nette AF, Abraham G, Ungemach FR et al (2005) Interaction between simvastatin and metoprolol with respect to cardiac beta-adrenoceptor density, catecholamine levels and perioperative catecholamine requirements in cardiac surgery patients. Naunyn Schmiedebergs Arch Pharmacol 372:115–124
34. Poldermans D, Boersma E, Bax JJ et al (1999) The effect of bisoprolol on perioperative mortality and myocardial infarction in high-risk patients undergoing vascular surgery. N Engl J Med 341:1789–1794
35. Akhtar S, Amin M, Tantawy H et al (2005) Preoperative beta-blocker use: is titration to a heart rate of 60 beats per minute a consistently attainable goal? J Clin Anesth 17:191–197
36. Ferguson TB Jr, Coombs LP, Peterson ED (2002) Preoperative beta-blocker use and mortality and morbidity following CABG surgery in North America. JAMA

287:2221–2227

37. ten Broecke PWC, De Hert SG, Mertens E et al (2003) Effect of preoperative ?-blockade on perioperative mortality in coronary surgery. Br J Anaesth 90:27–31
38. Toller WG, Stranz C (2006) Levosimendan, a new inotropic and vasodilator agent. Anesthesiology 104:556–569
39. Follath F, Cleland JG, Just H et al (2002) Efficacy and safety of intravenous levosimendan compared with dobutamine in severe low-output heart failure (the LIDO study): a randomised double-blind trial. Lancet 360:196–202
40. Morelli A, Teboul JL, Maggiore SM et al (2006) Effects of levosimendan on right ventricular afterload in patients with acute respiratory distress syndrome: a pilot study. Crit Care Med 34:2287–2293
41. Al-Shawaf E, Ayed A, Vislocky I et al (2006) Levosimendan or milrinone in the type 2 diabetic patient with low ejection fraction undergoing elective coronary artery surgery. J Cardiothorac Vasc Anesth 20:353–357
42. Sonntag S, Sundberg S, Lehtonen LA et al (2004) The calcium sensitizer levosimendan improves the function of stunned myocardium after percutaneous transluminal coronary angioplasty in acute myocardial ischemia. J Am Coll Cardiol 43:2177–2182
43. Barisin S, Husedzinovic I, Sonicki Z et al (2004) Levosimendan in off-pump coronary artery bypass: a four-times masked controlled study. J Cardiovasc Pharmacol 44:703–708
44. Nijhawan N, Nicolosi AC, Montgomery MW et al (1999) Levosimendan enhances cardiac performance after cardiopulmonary bypass: a prospective, randomized placebo-controlled trial. J Cardiovasc Pharmacol 34:219–228
45. Tritapepe L, De S, V, Vitale D et al (2006) Preconditioning effects of levosimendan in coronary artery bypass grafting–a pilot study. Br J Anaesth 96:694–700
46. Christenson JT, Cohen M (2002) Preoperative IABP in high-risk patients reduces postoperative lactate release and subsequent mortality. Ann Thorac Surg 73:1026–1027

15 Management of Systemic and Pulmonary Hypertension

P. GIOMARELLI, S. SCOLLETTA AND B. BIAGIOLI

Systemic Hypertension

Introduction

Systemic hypertension is a very frequent condition in developed countries and therefore constitutes a common problem in the perioperative period. In the Unites States nearly 29% of adults in 1999 and 2000 were affected by hypertension (age-adjusted prevalence of hypertension): 30% of hypertensive individuals are not aware of their diagnosis, 59% are being treated for hypertension, and only 34% have a blood pressure below 140/90 mmHg [1, 2].

The definition of a hypertensive state is uncertain. Really, it is of crucial importance to consider definitions and charts from studies based on large patient populations, especially when both age and associated diseases are taken into account (Fig. 1). The first problem in the classification of hypertension is the definition of the upper limit of normality (systolic, diastolic, or systolic plus diastolic); most clinicians are aware of this, and several papers may help to clarify the pathophysiologic condition [2]. The second problem is that this classification is set by the peak and trough of a pressure wave in a peripheral (brachial) artery in which the arterial pulse is amplified to a variable degree [3, 4]. In subjects older than 70 years and in small children, systolic pressure (brachial or radial) is a good guide to systolic pressure in the ascending aorta and the left ventricle, whereas in adolescents and young adults, systolic pressure (brachial or radial) may overestimate the systolic central pressure by 30–35 mmHg or more (Fig. 1). Thus, systolic pressure is

Department of Anesthesia and Intensive Care Unit, University of Siena, Italy

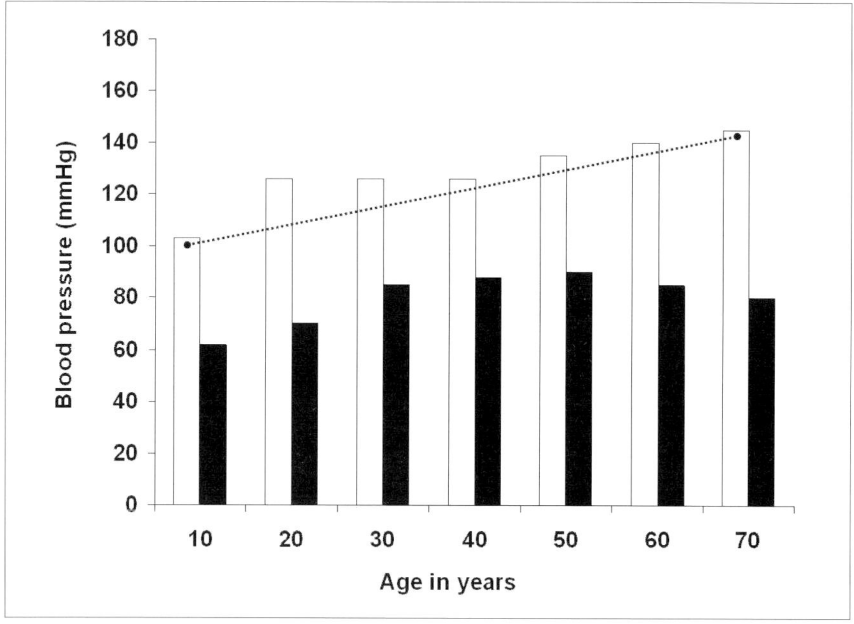

Fig. 1. *Changes in arterial blood pressure with age.* The figure shows the relationship between age and arterial blood pressure in USA population. The apparent plateau in systolic pressure between age 20 and 40 years appears to be artifactual and attributable to extreme amplification of the brachial systolic pressure peak in young adults. White and black bars represent systolic and diastolic blood pressure values, respectively. The dotted line is the regression line for directly measured aortic systolic pressure in a group of apparently normal persons undergoing cardiac catheterization (Adapted from McDonald's Blood Flow in Arteries: Theoretical, Experimental and Clinical Principles. Nichols WW and O'Rourke MF, 5th edn, 2005, Hodden Arnold, London [3])

an accurate index of cardiovascular risk in the elderly but a poor guide in the young [3, 4].

Hypertension and Pulse Wave Analysis

The basic problem in hypertension is the increase in peripheral resistance and the decrease in arterial distensibility. With aging, vascular resistance is also increased because of vascular rarefaction and stiffened arteries, with low to normal cardiac output and mean arterial pressure usually only moderately elevated [3].

There are several different methods of assessing arterial stiffness (AS), some of which are widely applicable in the clinical setting: (1) pulse pressure (the difference between systolic and diastolic pressures), which is a valuable surrogate marker for AS; (2) pulse wave velocity (the speed at which the forward pressure is transmitted from the aorta through the vascular tree); and (3) pulse wave analysis (PWA) and augmentation index (AIx) (Fig. 2) [3].

The arterial pressure waveform is a composite of the forward pressure wave created by ventricular contraction and the reflected wave. Waves are reflected from the periphery mainly at branch points or sites of impedance mismatch. Therefore, the arterial waveform varies throughout the arterial tree [3]. The velocity at which the pressure wave travels through the vasculature is influenced by the stiffness of the vessel walls: the stiffer the walls, the higher the velocity. In elastic vessels, the reflected wave tends to arrive back at the aortic root during diastole, serving to augment diastolic pressure and hence improve coronary artery perfusion. In the case of stiff arteries, the reflected wave arrives back at the central arteries earlier, causing augmentation of the systolic pressure (generating ventricular hypertrophy) and a consequent decrease in diastolic pressure (reducing coronary artery perfusion). From the applanation tonometry (also called O'Rourke PW system), the aug-

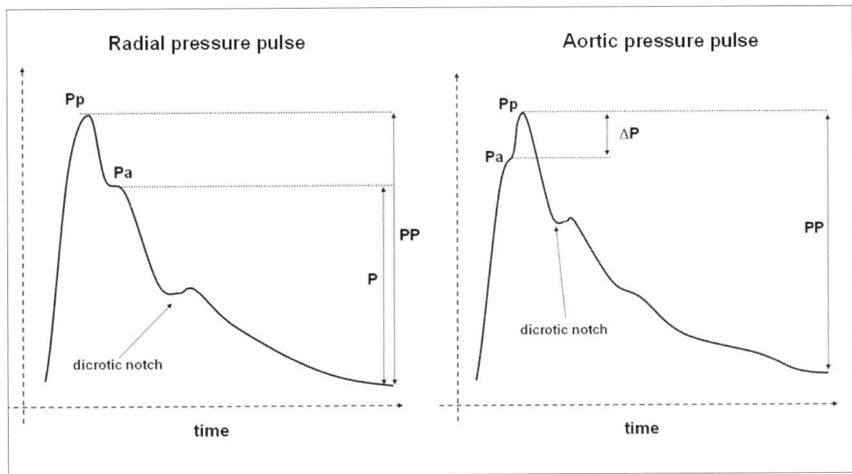

Fig. 2. Radial and ascending aorta pressure-time curves and augmentation index. The figure shows radial (left) and ascending aorta (right) pressure pulses of a same old patient. The augmentation index (AIx) is the ratio of pressure augmentation (Pa) to pulse pressure (PP). It depends on the relative amplitude and timing of the direct and reflected pressure waves that sum to produce the overall waveform. On the left, radial AIx is expressed as percentage by P/PP ratio. On the right, aortic AIx is defined as the difference between the second and first systolic peak (Pp-Pa), expresses as percentage of PP. AIx is usually negative in young healthy subjects, about zero at the age of 35, and becomes increasingly positive thereafter. The aortic pulse is synthesized from the radial pulse by using the transfer function supplied by tonometry (Millar Instruments, Houston, TX) with SphygmoCor software (PWV Medical, Sydney, Australia). (Adapted from McDonald's Blood Flow in Arteries: Theoretical, Experimental and Clinical Principles. Nichols WW and O'Rourke MF, 5th edn, 2005, Hodden Arnold, London [3])

mentation index, or AIx, which is the difference between the first and second systolic peaks expressed as a percentage of the pulse pressure, and a measure of systemic stiffness, can be derived (Fig. 2) [3]. A disadvantage of using the radial site for applanation tonometry is that the pressure pulse wave is amplified in transmission from the proximal aorta, and the wave contour is altered. This potential disadvantage can be overcome by exploitation of the (relatively) constant arterial properties in the upper limbs. These are little affected by aging, hypertension, drugs, and disease in adults. To obviate the need for central catheterization when measuring this central pulse contour, O'Rourke and associates developed a generalized mathematical transfer function that reconstructs central (aortic) waveforms from their corresponding peripheral (radial) waveforms [5]. With increased AS and wave reflections, more aggressive diagnostic as well as therapeutic strategies might be appropriate, particularly in younger patients with prematurely stiffened arteries, to prevent cardiovascular disease.

Pulse Contour Methods

Continuous measurement of arterial blood pressure is an unquestioned part of the hemodynamic monitoring of critically ill patients in the intensive care unit (ICU). However, not only blood pressure but, more importantly, blood flow, i.e., cardiac output, determines organ perfusion. This is the rationale for implementing techniques that allow measurement of cardiac output in the ICU setting. According to the hypothesis that continuous monitoring of cardiac output and other cardiovascular parameters could allow the detection of sudden hemodynamic changes which may influence patient management and outcome, different pulse contour methods (PCMs) have been utilized [6]. PCMs, unlike bolus thermodilution, which measures cardiac output over a limited time span, operate on a beat-to-beat basis, and for this reason could be suitable for the continuous monitoring of cardiac output and other cardiovascular parameters [7].

In the perioperative period, knowledge of the patient's antihypertensive treatment is important in assessing the stress-related cardiocirculatory modifications. Moreover, blood volume variations, the inflammatory response to surgery, and various compensatory mechanisms of the cardiovascular system necessitate careful control of oxygen delivery (DO_2) with respect to oxygen consumption (VO_2). Pulse pressure analysis systems allow beat-to-beat monitoring of blood flow, pressure wave changes, and vascular impedance and resistance variations. Thus, PCMs should be considered the hemodynamic monitoring techniques of choice for hypertensive patients in the perioperative period [8].

Therapeutic Strategies

There is no consensus on the ideal therapy for hypertension, but two general attitudes are presented: one based on the results of clinical trials, the other on the pathophysiologic mechanism. Diuretics and β-blocking agents have been shown to be effective in large-scale clinical trials. Their main primary action is through reduction in blood volume, venous return, and cardiac output and hence in blood pressure, even though none of these has any definite specific effect on increased peripheral resistance or on abnormal arterial distensibility as the major important secondary effects of elevated pressure. Many other drugs are employed for their ability to act on the pathophysiologic mechanisms. Prazosin, terazosin, and hydralazine are effective antihypertensive agents, but they have not been employed in studies that have shown mortality reduction. Angiotensin-converting enzyme (ACE) inhibitors, angiotensin receptor blockers, and calcium channel antagonist compounds dilate muscular conduit arteries as well arterioles, and have been shown to reduce the compliance of these arteries by a direct effect on smooth muscle. These drugs, together with nitrates, have however little or no effect on the large, predominantly central elastic arteries which are primarily concerned with cushioning pressure pulsations generated by intermittent ventricular contraction. The beneficial effects are indirect and are manifest through a reduction in wave reflection returning from peripheral reflecting sites [1, 3]. Losartan has shown a modest reduction in the primary composite endpoint (death, myocardial infarction, stroke) versus atenolol [9].

Hypertensive Crisis and Urgency

Hypertensive crisis is defined as elevated blood pressure (diastolic pressure greater than 130 mmHg) associated with evidence of acute end-organ damage. With acute damage to vital organs, such as the kidney, heart, and brain, there is a significant risk of morbidity within hours without therapeutic intervention. The absolute level of blood pressure and the rate of blood pressure elevation determine the development of hypertensive crisis. It is important to identify this syndrome early to prevent end-organ damage and to institute appropriate therapy as soon as the diagnosis is made.

The initial abrupt in blood pressure in patients with simple hypertension or normotension is probably secondary to an increase in vascular resistance. Considerable evidence suggests that mechanical stress in the arterial wall leads to disruption of endothelial integrity and diffuse microvascular lesions with fibrinoid necrosis of the arterioles [10]. Angiotensin II may injure the vascular wall directly by activation of genes for proinflammatory cytokine (IL-6) and proinflammatory mediators regulated by nuclear factor-κB (NF-κB [11, 12]. Hyperviscosity, immunologic factors, and other hormones (e.g., catecholamines, vasopressin, and endothelin) can contribute to causing an increase in peripheral vascular resistance with ischemia of heart, brain, and kidneys [13]. Patients with hypertensive crisis present with a variety of symptoms: headache (occipital or anterior), scotoma, diplopia, hemianopsia, blindness, focal deficit, stroke, transient ischemic attack, confusion, somnolence, ischemic chest pain, renal symptoms (nocturia, polyuria, hematuria), back pain (aortic aneurysm), nausea, vomiting, and intravascular volume depletion due to high levels of circulating renin and angiotensin.

During hypertensive crisis, when the blood pressure rapidly rises and central perfusion pressure exceeds the ability of the central nervous system to autoregulate, a distinct clinical syndrome appears: hypertensive encephalopathy. Autoregulation is the ability of the brain to maintain a constant cerebral flow as the cerebral perfusion pressure varies from 60 to 150 mmHg, or from 80 to 160 mmHg in chronic hypertension. If hypertensive encephalopathy is suspected, magnetic resonance imaging should be performed to seek edema in posterior regions of the cerebral hemispheres, particularly in the parieto-occipital regions [14]. Symptoms of generalized brain dysfunction tend to develop over time (12–24 h), as with an acute central nervous system bleed. Associated mental status changes improve within 24-48 hrs of antihypertensive drug treatment for antihypertensive encephalopathy.

Hypertensive urgency is defined as elevated pressure (diastolic pressure often > 115 mmHg) without evidence of acute end-organ damage and may be associated with chronic stable complications, such as stable angina, previous myocardial infarction, chronic congestive heart failure, previous transient ischemic attacks, or previous cerebrovascular accident. Complications from hypertensive urgency are not immediate, and a more gradual blood pressure reduction over hours is recommended in comparison to hypertensive emergency secondary to hypertensive encephalopathy [15, 16].

Treatment of Hypertensive Emergencies

Patients with hypertensive emergencies are best treated in intensive care with monitoring by arterial cannulation or automated blood pressure cuff measurement. The arterial pressure can have reduced by 25% within minutes to hours and normalized in 24–48 h without causing ischemia of a vital organ. In ischemic stroke there are no large clinical trials to support rapid reduction of blood pressure; in acute aortic dissection or in active unstable angina or congestive failure with pulmonary edema, a rapid reduction (15–30 min) is preferable.

The treatment of hypertensive emergency is generally associated by complex and binding pathologic conditions: ischemic cerebral infarction, subarachnoid hemorrhage, intracerebral hemorrhage, head trauma, aortic dissection, pulmonary edema, catecholamine-associated hypertension, gestational hypertension, preeclampsia, and eclampsia. Under these conditions it is necessary to appraise carefully the perfusion of the whole organism and the different regions. A hemodynamic monitoring system that is continuous, easy to use, minimally invasive, and able to appraise real-time afterload, preload, and oxygen delivery is essential. Analysis of the radial artery introduces many advantages and can also provide indications as to the action of the drugs employed (Fig. 3).

Sodium Nitroprusside

This nitric oxide donor, a vasodilator of arteriolar and venous smooth muscle, increases cardiac output by decreasing afterload. It is useful in most hypertensive emergencies. Onset of action is immediate, duration of action 1–2 min. Dosage: initial dose 0.25 $\mu g\ kg^{-1}\ min^{-1}$, maximum dose 8–10 $\mu g\ kg^{-1}\ min^{-1}$. Beware with a cumulative dose of 500 $\mu g\ kg^{-1}$, over a prolonged time. At continued infusion rates of $\geq 2\ \mu g\ kg^{-1}\ min^{-1}$ cyanide is generated more rapidly than can be taken care of. Sodium nitroprusside is con-

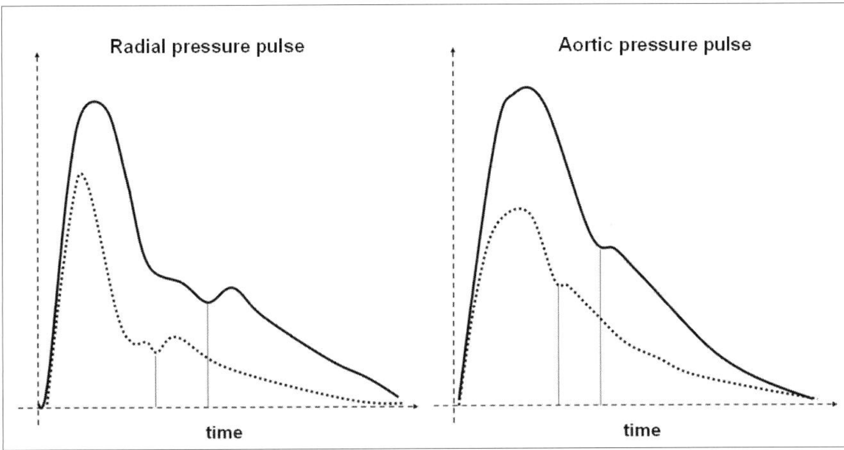

Fig. 3. *Radial and ascending aorta pressure curves.* The figure shows radial (left) and ascending aorta (right) pressure pulses measured in a same patient. The solid waves represent normal blood pressure waveforms. Dotted curves represent blood pressure waves during i.v. nitroglycerin infusion. Note the disappearance of the late systolic shoulder and the minor decrease in systolic pressure in the radial artery during vasodilator administration. During nitroglycerin infusion, both the radial and aortic dicrotic notches (vertical lines that identify the aortic valve closure) appear early on the pressure curve. The aortic pulse is synthesized from the radial pulse by using the transfer function supplied by tonometry (Millar Instruments, Houston, TX) with SphygmoCor software (PWV Medical, Sydney, Australia). (Adapted from McDonald's Blood Flow in Arteries: Theoretical, Experimental and Clinical Principles. Nichols WW and O'Rourke MF, 5th edn, 2005, Hodden Arnold, London [3])

traindicated in high-output cardiac failure and congenital optic atrophy. Anemia and liver disease are risk factors for cyanide toxicity, symptoms of which are: acidosis, tachycardia, change in mental status, almond smell on breath. Renal disease is a risk factor for thiocyanate toxicity, symptoms of which are: psychosis, hyperreflexia, seizure, tinnitus. Use with caution in patients with increased intracranial pressure. Do not use maximum dose for (8-10 μg kg^{-1} min^{-1}) more than 10 min [15, 16].

Nitroglycerin

Nitroclycerine (NTG) is also a nitric oxide danoe, bud differs from sodium nitroprusside in that it primarily dilates the venous capacitance bed, and only decreases systemic vascular (arterial) resistance at very high doses. It also dilates epicardial coronary arteries, which partly explains its efficacy for relief of angina pectoris. Use with: symptoms of cardiac ischemia, and possibly for perioperative hypertension in cardiac surgery or patients with known coronary artery disease having non-cardiac surgery or being treated for hypertension in an ICU setting. The initial dose is 5 μg min^{-1}, and the maximum dose is 200 μg min^{-1}. NTG is contraindicated with angle-closure glaucoma and/or increased intracranial pressure. Blood pressure is reduced primarily due to increased venous capacitance and reduced venous return, which leads to a secondary reduction in cardiac preload and output. Avoid use when cerebral or renal perfusion is compromised. Use with caution in patients with right ventricular infarction [15, 16].

Esmolol

Cardioselective β_1-adrenergic blocking agent used with aortic dissection, and during tracheal intubation and intraoperative and postoperative hypertension. Onset of action is 60 s, duration of action 10–20 min. Dose: 200–500 μg kg^{-1} over 1–4 min, then 50 μg kg^{-1} min^{-1} for 4 min and titer, then infuse 50–300 μg kg^{-1} min^{-1}. Esmolol is not dependent on renal or hepatic function for metabolism (metabolized by hydrolysis in red blood cells) [15, 16].

Fenoldopam

This postsynaptic dopamine-1 agonist decreases peripheral vascular resistance; it is ten times more potent than dopamine as a vasodilator. Its use may be advantageous in kidney disease; it increases renal blood flow, increases sodium excretion, and has no toxic metabolites. Initial dose: 0.1 μg kg^{-1} min^{-1} with titration every 15min, no bolus. Contraindicated in patients with glaucoma (may increase intraocular pressure) or allergy to sulfites, hypotension, especially with concurrent β-blocker. Check serum potassium every 6ase blood levels. There is a risk of dose-related tachycardia [15, 16].

Hydralazine

Primarily dilates arteriolar vasculature. Primarily used in pregnancy/eclampsia. Decrease blood pressure in 10–20 min, duration of action 2–4 h. Dose: 10 mg every 20–130 min, maximum dose 20 mg. Reflex tachycardia, give beta blocker concurrently, may exacerbate angina. Half-life 3 h, may affect blood pressure for 100 h. Depends on hepatic acetylation for inactivation [15, 16].

Phentolamine

An β-adrenergic blocker, used primarily to treat hypertension from catecholamine excess (e.g., pheochromocytoma). Onset of action 1–2 min, duration 3–10 min; dose 5–15 mg. β-blockade is generally added to control reflex tachycardia and/or arrhythmias. As in all catecholamine excess states, α_1-blockers should never be given first because the loss of α_1-adrenergically mediated vasodilation leaves α_2-adrenergically mediated vasoconstriction unopposed and results in increased pressure [15, 16].

Nicardipine

This dihydropyridine calcium channel blocker inhibits transmembrane influx of calcium ions into cardiac and smooth muscle. Onset of action 10–20 min, duration 1–4 h; initial dose 5 mg h^{-1} to maximum of 15 mg h^{-1}. Avoid with congestive heart failure or cardiac ischemia. Adverse effects include tachycardia, flushing, and headache [15, 16].

Trimethaphan

A nondepolarizing ganglionic blocking agent which competes with acetylcholine for postsynaptic receptors. It is used in aortic dissection. Dose: 0.5–5 mg min^{-1}. It does not increase cardiac output and has no inotropic cardiac effect. Disadvantages include parasympathetic blockade resulting in paralytic ileus and bladder atony, and development of tachyphylaxis after 24–96 h of use [15, 16].

Perioperative Hypertension

Perioperative hypertension is a major risk factor for the development of postoperative hypertension. To reduce this risk it is reasonable not to proceed to elective surgical interventions if the diastolic pressure is greater than 110 mmHg to exclude patients whit hypertension in whom further increased blood pressure would result in aggravation of end-organ damage.

During the induction of anesthesia sympathetic activity increases, blood pressure frequently increases, and an exaggerated response with uncontrolled hypertension can appear. As anesthesia continues, there is generally a decrease in blood pressure, with rapid and wide fluctuations more frequent in individuals with a history of hypertension. Prolonged intraoperative hypotension reduces blood flow to the vital organs, and may cause irreversible microvascular alterations causing organ dysfunction and failure (stroke, myocardial ischemia, acute renal failure, mesenteric ischemia), with increased postoperative morbidity and mortality.

In the perioperative period it is important to know the type of a patient's systemic hypertension, the severity of associated cardiovascular modifications, as well as the antihypertensive drugs the patient is taking. Some antihypertensive drugs administered before surgery should be continued intravenously when necessary. β-blockers and clonidine treatment should not be suspended before surgery. Furthermore, they must be restarted as soon as possible postoperatively to prevent rebound phenomena. Finally, optimization of anesthesia and pain control management will reduce the sympathetic response to surgical stimuli and will contribute to avoiding perioperative hypertension.

Pulmonary Hypertension

Introduction

Pulmonary arterial hypertension (PAH) is a disease of the small pulmonary arteries, characterized by vascular proliferation and remodeling. It results in a progressive increase in pulmonary vascular resistance and, ultimately, right heart failure. PAH is defined by a pulmonary artery mean pressure (PAP_m) greater than 25 mmHg at rest or greater than 30 mmHg with exercise, with a normal pulmonary wedge pressure (PWP) <15 mmHg (demonstrating precapillary PAH), and by a pulmonary vascular resistance greater than 3 mmHg l^{-1} min^{-1} (Wood units) [17].

PAH may be precapillary or postcapillary in etiology. Precapillary pulmonary hypertension can be idiopathic [IPAH—previously known as primary pulmonary hypertension (PPH)] or it may occur in association with a variety of underlying disease processes such as collagen vascular disease, portal hypertension, congenital systemic-to-pulmonary shunts, drug or toxin exposure, or HIV infection. Postcapillary causes include processes affecting the left side of the heart (e.g., left ventricular systolic or diastolic dysfunction, mitral stenosis or regurgitation, aortic valvular disease) or, more rarely, the pulmonary veins (pulmonary veno-occlusive disease). It is unclear whether the various types of pulmonary arterial hypertension share a common pathogenesis [18]. Three factors are thought to cause the increased pulmonary vascular resistance that characterizes this disease: vasoconstriction, remodeling of the pulmonary vessel wall, and thrombosis in situ [17]. Advances in our understanding of the molecular mechanism involved in this disease suggest that endothelial dysfunction plays a key role [19]. Finally, a genetic predisposition may underlie a substantial proportion of cases [20]. The classification of PAH is described in Table 1.

Table 1. Classification of pulmonary arterial hypertension (PAH)

Idiopathic

Familiar

Associated with:
- Collagen vascular disease
- Congenital left-to-right shunt
- Infection with immunodeficiency virus
- Drugs and toxins
- Portal hypertension Associated with venous or capillary involvement:
- Pulmonary veno-occlusive disease
- Pulmonary capillary hemangiomatosis

Persistent PAH of the newborn

Associated with left heart disease:
- Left-sided atrial or ventricular heart disease
- Left-sided valvular heart disease

Associated with lung disease or hypoxemia or both:
- Chronic obstructive pulmonary disease
- Interstitial lung disease
- Sleep-disordered breathing
- Alveolar hypoventilation disorders
- Chronic exposure to high altitude
- Developmental abnormalities

PAH due to chronic thrombotic or embolic disease or both:
- Thromboembolic obstruction of proximal pulmonary arteries
- Thromboembolic obstruction of distal pulmonary arteries
- Nonthrombotic pulmonary embolism (tumor, parasites, foreign material)

Miscellaneous
- Sarcoidosis, pulmonary Langerhans' cell histiocytosis, lymphangiomatosis, compression of pulmonary vessels (tumor, adenopathy, fibrosing mediastinitis)

From Humbert et al. [17] and Simonneau et al. [45]

Symptoms, Signs, and Clinical History

Because of the insidious onset of symptoms, PAH is often advanced at the time of diagnosis. Dyspnea on exertion is a common presenting symptom, but it is sometimes attributed to the patient's poor general condition of health or another cardiorespiratory ailment. Chest pain mimicking angina pectoris may occur. Patients with advanced disease may present with syncope or signs and symptoms of right-sided heart failure, including lower extremity edema, jugular venous distention, and ascites.

The clinical history should focus initially on the exclusion of underlying causes of pulmonary hypertension. Important clues to an underlying condition might include a previous history of a heart murmur, deep venous thrombosis or pulmonary embolism, Raynaud's phenomenon, arthritis, arthralgias, rash, heavy alcohol consumption, hepatitis, heavy snoring, daytime hypersomnolence, morning headache, and morbid obesity. A careful family history should be taken. Medication exposures, particularly to appetite suppressants and amphetamines, should be noted. Cocaine is a powerful vasoconstrictor and may contribute to the development of pulmonary hypertension. Intravenous drug abuse has been associated with the development of PAH. Signs of PAH may not become apparent until late in the disease. Findings such as an accentuated second heart sound, a systolic murmur over the left sternal border, jugular venous distention, peripheral edema, and/or ascites might suggest the presence of pulmonary hypertension and right ventricular dysfunction. Associated systemic diseases, such as collagen vascular disease or liver disease, may also become apparent during routine examination.

Diagnostic Methods

Laboratory Evaluation

Laboratory evaluation can provide important information in detecting associated disorders and contributing factors. A collagen vascular screen is often helpful in detecting autoimmune disease. Liver function tests may be elevated in patients with right ventricular failure and passive hepatic congestion but may also be associated with underlying liver disease. Liver disease with portal hypertension has been associated with the development of pulmonary hypertension. HIV testing and hepatitis serologic studies should be considered in patients at risk. Routine laboratory studies (e.g., complete blood cell count, complete metabolic panel, prothrombin time, and partial thromboplastin time) are recommended during the initial evaluation and as indicated to monitor the patient's long-term clinical status.

ECG and Echocardiography

The ECG may provide suggestive or supportive evidence of PAH by demonstrating right ventricular hypertrophy (RVH) and strain, and right atrial dilation. RVH on ECG is present in 87% and right axis deviation in 79% of patients with PAH. However, the ECG has inadequate sensitivity (55%) and specificity (70%) to be a screening tool for detecting significant PAH [17].

Doppler echocardiography is useful in estimating the severity of pulmonary hypertension and detecting left-sided heart disease. According to data obtained in normal subjects, mild PAH can be defined as a pulmonary artery systolic pressure of approximately 36–50 mmHg. Additional echocardiographic and Doppler parameters are important for diagnosis confirmation and assessment of severity of PAH, including enlargement of the right ventricle, right ventricular ejection, flattening of the interventricular septum, and compression of the left ventricle. Bubble contrast echocardiography may detect a right-to-left shunt, but exclusion of a left-to-right intracardiac shunt may require cardiac catheterization with an oximetry series. Echocardiography may be a useful noninvasive means of long-term follow-up [21].

Chest Radiography

Chest radiography may reveal enlargement of the central pulmonary vessels and evidence of right ventricular enlargement. Evidence of parenchymal lung disease may be apparent. When parenchymal lung disease is suspected, pulmonary function testing and high-resolution computed tomography (CT) of the chest may be indicated. Ventilation/perfusion lung scanning should be performed in an attempt to exclude chronic recurrent pulmonary thromboembolic disease, which is among the most preventable and treatable causes of pulmonary hypertension. Diffuse mottled perfusion can be seen in IPAH/(idiopathic pulmonary artery hypertension)/PPH, whereas larger segmental and subsegmental mismatched defects are suggestive of chronic recurrent pulmonary thromboembolic disease. Intermediate results on ventilation/perfusion lung scanning may require pulmonary arteriography to obtain a definitive diagnosis. Although contrast medium-enhanced CT has been popularized recently for the diagnosis of acute pulmonary thromboembolic disease, there is limited experience with this technique in chronic thromboembolic disease. Accordingly, we recommend caution at present in using contrast-enhanced CT to exclude chronic recurrent thromboembolic disease.

Hemodynamics

Right-sided heart catheterization is required to confirm the diagnosis of PAH. Left-sided heart dysfunction and intracardiac shunts can be excluded, the degree of pulmonary hypertension can be accurately quantified, and the cardiac output can be measured. Pulmonary vascular resistance can then be calculated. Acute pulmonary vasoreactivity can be assessed using a short-acting agent such as prostacyclin (epoprostenol), inhaled nitric oxide [22], or intravenous adenosine [23]. The European Society of Cardiology consensus definition of a positive acute vasodilator response in an IPAH/PPH patient is a fall of PAP_m of at least 10 mmHg to less than or equal to 40 mmHg, with an increased or unchanged cardiac output. The primary objective of acute vasodilator testing in patients with IPAH/PPH is to identify patients who might be effectively treated with oral calcium channel blockers. Unstable patients or those in severe right-sided heart failure, who would not be candidates for treatment with calcium channel blockers, need not undergo vasodilator testing.

Moreover, the assessment of pulmonary wedge pressure may allow the distinction between arterial and venous pulmonary hypertension in patients with concomitant left heart disease. Right-sided heart catheterization is important also in patients with definite moderate-to-severe PAH because the hemodynamic variables have prognostic relevance. Elevated mean right atrial pressure and mean pulmonary artery pressure, and reduced cardiac output and central venous oxygen saturation identify IPAH patients with worst prognosis [21].

Treatment

General Care

During the past 20 years treatment options for patients with the disease have evolved to help prolong their survival and improve their quality of life. Initial therapy may be directed at an underlying cause or contributing factor, such as using continuous positive airway pressure (CPAP) and supplemental oxygen for PAH associated with obstructive sleep apnea. Following the identification and treatment of underlying associated disorders and contributing factors, specific therapy for PAH should be considered. Improved survival has been reported with oral anticoagulation in IPAH/PPH [24]. The target international normalized ratio (INR) in these patients is 1.5 to 2.5. Hypoxemia is a pulmonary vasoconstrictor and can contribute to the development or progression of PAH. Most authorities agree on the importance of maintaining oxygen saturations at greater than 90% at all times. Diuretics are indicated in patients with evidence of right ventricular failure and volume overload (i.e., peripheral edema and/or ascites).

Calcium Channel Blockers

Patients with IPAH/PPH who respond to vasodilators and calcium channel blockers generally have improved survival. Unfortunately, this tends to represent a relatively small proportion of patients, comprising fewer than 20% of IPAH/PPH patients and even fewer patients with PAH from other causes. Patients who may benefit from long-term therapy with calcium channel blockers can be identified by performing an acute vasodilator challenge with the use of short-acting agents, such as intravenous prostacyclin, adenosine, or inhaled nitric oxide, during right heart catheterization. Sitbon and colleagues [25] found that less than 7% of patients with PAH had a sustained benefit from therapy with a calcium channel blockers. Furthermore, during acute vasodilator challenge, most patients who had a long-term response to calcium channel blockers had a marked improvement in their pulmonary hemodynamics (i.e., the PAP_m decreased by more than 10 mmHg, to a value lower than 40 mmHg, with a normal or high cardiac output). Long-term therapy with a calcium channel blocker is not recommended when these criteria are not met [17].

Prostanoids

Prostacyclin (prostaglandin I_2), the main product of arachidonic metabolism in the vascular endothelium, induces vascular smooth muscle relaxation by stimulating cyclic adenosine monophosphate production and inhibiting smooth muscle cell growth. It is a potent systemic and pulmonary vasodilator that also has antiplatelet aggregatory effects. A relative deficiency of prostacyclin may contribute to the pathogenesis of PAH.

Intravenous Prostacyclin (Epoprostenol)

Intravenous prostacyclin was first used to treat primary PAH in the early 1980s [26]. It was apparent that the absence of an acute hemodynamic response to intravenous epoprostenol did not preclude improvement with long-term therapy. Epoprostenol therapy is complicated by the need for continuous intravenous infusion. The drug is unstable at room temperature and is generally best kept cold before and during infusion. It has a very short half-life in the bloodstream (< 6 min), is unstable at acidic pH, and cannot be taken orally. Because of the short half-life, the risk of rebound worsening with abrupt or inadvertent interruption of the infusion, and its effects on peripheral veins, it should be administered through an indwelling central venous catheter. Common side effects of epoprostenol therapy include headache, flushing, jaw pain with initial mastication, diarrhea, nausea, a blotchy erythematous rash, and musculoskeletal aches and pains (predominantly involving the legs and feet). These tend to be dose-dependent and often respond to a cautious reduction in dose. Severe side effects can occur with overdosage of the drug. Acutely, overdosage can lead to systemic hypotension. Chronic overdosage can lead to the development of a hyperdynamic state and high output cardiac failure. Abrupt or inadvertent interruption of the epoprostenol infusion should be avoided, because this may lead to a rebound worsening of pulmonary hypertension with symptomatic deterioration and even death. Other complications of chronic intravenous therapy with epoprostenol include systemic hypotension, thrombocytopenia, and ascites. The beneficial effects of epoprostenol therapy appear to be sustained for years in many patients with IPAH/PPH [27, 28].

Subcutaneous Treprostinil

Treprostinil, a prostacyclin analog with a half-life of 3 h, is stable at room temperature. An international, placebo-controlled, randomized trial demonstrated that treprostinil improved exercise tolerance, although the 16-m median difference in 6-min walk distance between treatment groups was relatively modest [29]. Treprostinil also improved hemodynamic parameters. Common side effects include headache, diarrhea, nausea, rash, and jaw pain. Side effects related to the infusion site were common (85% of patients complained of infusion site pain and 83% had erythema or induration at the infusion site).

Oral Beraprost

Beraprost sodium is an orally active prostacyclin analog [30] that is absorbed rapidly in fasting conditions. Although several small open-label, uncontrolled studies reported beneficial hemodynamic effects with beraprost in patients with IPAH/PPH, two randomized, double-blind, placebo-controlled trials have shown only modest improvement and suggest that beneficial effects of beraprost may diminish with time [31, 32].

Inhaled Iloprost

Iloprost is a chemically stable prostacyclin analog, with a serum half-life of 20–25 min. In IPAH/PPH, acute inhalation of iloprost resulted in a more potent pulmonary vasodilator effect than acute nitric oxide inhalation. The most important drawback of inhaled iloprost is the relatively short duration of action, requiring the use of from six to nine inhalations a day.

Endothelin-Receptor Antagonists

Endothelin-1 is a vasoconstrictor and a smooth muscle mitogen that may contribute to the pathogenesis of PAH. Endothelin-1 expression, production, and concentration in plasma and lung tissue are elevated in patients with PAH, and these levels are correlated with disease severity.

Bosentan

Bosentan is a dual endothelin receptor blocker that has been shown to improve pulmonary hemodynamics and exercise tolerance and delay the time to clinical worsening in patients with PAH falling into NYHA classes III and IV [33, 34]. The most frequent and potentially serious side effect with bosentan is dose-dependent abnormal hepatic function (as indicated by elevated levels of alanine aminotransferase and/or aspartate aminotransferase). Because of the risk of hepatotoxicity, the US Food and Drug Administration (FDA) requires that liver function tests be performed at least monthly in patients receiving this drug. Bosentan may also be associated with the development of anemia, which is typically mild; hemoglobin/hematocrit should be checked regularly.

Sitaxsentan and Ambrisentan

Selective blockers of the endothelium receptor ET_A, such as sitaxsentan and ambrisentan, are being investigated for the treatment of PAH [17]. In theory, such drugs could block the vasoconstrictor effects of ET_A receptors while maintaining the vasodilator and clearance effects of ET_B receptors. Cases of acute hepatitis have been described in patients taking selective ET_A blockers, a finding that emphasizes the importance of continuous monitoring of liver function [17].

Phosphodiesterase Inhibitors

Phosphodiesterases (PDEs) are enzymes that hydrolyze the cyclic nucleotides cyclic adenosine monophosphate (cAMP) and cyclic guanosine monophosphate (cGMP) and limit their intracellular signaling. Drugs that selectively inhibit cGMP-specific PDEs (or type 5, PDE5 inhibitors) augment the pulmonary vascular response to endogenous or inhaled nitric oxide in models of pulmonary hypertension. PDE5 is strongly expressed in the lung, and PDE5 gene expression and activity are increased in chronic pulmonary hypertension.

Dipyridamole

Early studies demonstrated that dipyridamole can lower pulmonary vascular resistance (PVR), attenuate hypoxic pulmonary vasoconstriction, decrease pulmonary hypertension, and, at least in some cases, augment or prolong the effects of inhaled nitric oxide in children with pulmonary hypertension [35]. Some patients who failed to respond to inhaled nitric oxide responded to the combination of inhaled nitric oxide plus dipyridamole [35].

Sildenafil

Sildenafil is a potent specific PDE5 inhibitor that is approved for erectile dysfunction. Recent reports have shown that sildenafil blocks acute hypoxic pulmonary vasoconstriction in healthy adult volunteers and acutely reduces PAP_m in patients with PAH [36, 37]. In comparison with inhaled nitric oxide, sildenafil produces similar reductions in PAP_m; but unlike nitric oxide, sildenafil also has apparent systemic hemodynamic effects [37]. When combined with inhaled nitric oxide, sildenafil appears to augment and prolong the effects of inhaled nitric oxide [37]. As observed with dipyridamole, sildenafil appears to prevent rebound pulmonary vasoconstriction after acute withdrawal of inhaled nitric oxide [38]. Appropriately designed randomized clinical trials are needed and are in progress. Sildenafil treatment in animal models with experimental lung injury reduced PAP, but gas exchange worsened owing to impaired ventilation–perfusion mismatch [39]. Accordingly, caution is advised when using sildenafil to treat pulmonary hypertension in patients with severe lung disease.

Nitric Oxide

Nitric oxide contributes to maintenance of normal vascular function and structure. It is particularly important in normal adaptation of the lung circulation at birth, and impaired nitric oxide production may contribute to the development of neonatal pulmonary hypertension. L-Arginine is the sole substrate for nitric oxide synthase and thus is essential for nitric oxide production.

Inhaled Nitric Oxide

Inhaled nitric oxide has been shown to have potent and selective pulmonary vasodilator effects during brief treatment of adults with IPAH/PPH [22]. It is a potent pulmonary vasodilator in newborns with pulmonary hypertension (PPHN), children with congenital heart disease, and patients with postoperative pulmonary hypertension, acute respiratory distress syndrome, or undergoing lung transplantation [40]. It is of substantial benefit in PPHN, decreasing the need for support with extracorporeal membrane oxygenation (ECMO) [41]. Inhaled nitric oxide has been used in diverse clinical settings, especially in intensive care medicine and during heart or lung transplantation. In chronic PAH, the use of inhaled nitric oxide has been primarily for acute testing of pulmonary vasoreactivity during cardiac catheterization (see earlier) or for acute stabilization of patients during deterioration.

Lung Transplantation

Lung transplantation for PAH is generally reserved for patients whose condition is failing despite the best available medical therapy. While lung transplantation is challenging in general, it is even more so in the group of patients with PAH [42]. Many patients with PAH have had a single lung transplant with good long-term results. However, nearly all transplant centers currently prefer to transplant both lungs (double lung transplant), in part because there are generally fewer postoperative complications [17]. Worldwide, overall survival is approximately 77% at 1 year and 44% at 5 years [43]. Survival in PAH patients undergoing lung transplantation is 66–75% at 1 year. The higher early mortality in PAH patients may be related to higher anesthetic and operative risks, the need for cardiopulmonary bypass, and the increased occurrence of postoperative reperfusion pulmonary edema in patients with PAH undergoing single lung transplantation. In this situation, reperfusion pulmonary edema may be aggravated by the increased blood flow to the newly engrafted lung. In addition, ventilation–perfusion mismatching can be particularly severe. This is why most centers seem to prefer bilateral lung transplantation for patients with PAH [44]. The timing of transplantation in PAH is challenging. It is probably most useful in patients showing clear evidence of deterioration, such as decline in functional capacity and the development of right-sided heart failure, despite maximal medical therapy.

Treatment Algorithms

Several treatments for PAH are now approved in North America (epoprostenol, treprostinil, and bosentan) and in Europe (epoprostenol, iloprost, and bosentan). The long-term effects of new treatments are still unknown [17], and there is a need for long-term observational studies evaluating the various treatments in terms of survival, side effects, quality of life, and costs. Since no data are available from head-to-head comparisons of approved therapies, the choice of treatment will be dictated by clinical experience and the availability of drugs. A feasible and reliable algorithm for the treatment of PAH has been proposed by Humbert et al. (Fig. 4) [17].

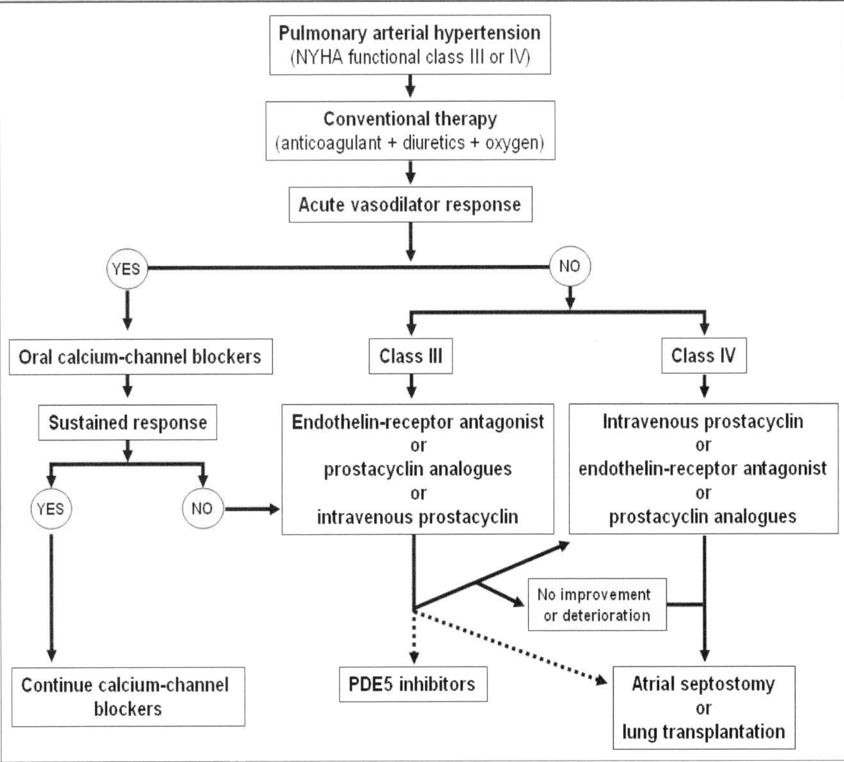

Fig. 4. Algorithm for treatment of pulmonary arterial hypertension. The figure shows the algorithm proposed by Humbert and colleagues [17]. It applies only to patients in NYHA functional class III or IV because very few data are available for patients in NYHA functional class I or II. The drugs of choice for testing of acute vasoreactivity are short-acting agents (e.g., intravenous prostacyclin, intravenous adenosine, or inhaled nitric oxide). Controlled studies are ongoing to determine the efficacy and safety of phosphodiesterase type 5 (PDE5) inhibitors, including sildenafil. Atrial septostomy is proposed for selected patients with severe disease. Lung transplantation is considered an option for all elegible patients who remain in NYHA functional class IV after three months of receiving epoprostenol. Reproduced from [17]

References

1. Hajjar I, Kotchen TA (2003) Trends in prevalence, awareness, treatment and control of hypertension in the United States 1999–2000. JAMA 290:199–206
2. Chobanian AV, Bakris GL, Black HR et al (2003) The Seventh Report of the Joint National Committee on Prevention, Detection, Evaluation and Treatment of High Blood Pressure. Latest guidelines for hypertension prevention and management. JAMA 289:2560–2572
3. Nichols WW, O'Rourke MF (2005) McDonald's blood flow in arteries: theoretical, experimental and clinical principles. Hodder Arnold, London

4. Wilkinson IB, Franklin SS, Hall IR et al (2001) Pressure amplification explains why pulse pressure is unrelated to risk in young subjects. Hypertension 38:1461–1466
5. Karamanoglu M, O'Rourke MF, Avolio AP et al (1993) An analysis of the relationship between central aortic and peripheral upper limb pressure wave in man. Eur Heart J 14:160–167
6. Cecconi M, Wilson J, Rhodes A (2006) Pulse pressure analysis. In: Vincent JL (ed) Yearbook of intensive care and emergency medicine. Springer, Berlin Heidelberg New York, pp 176–184
7. Giomarelli P, Biagioli B, Scolletta S (2004) Cardiac output monitoring by pressure recording analytical method in cardiac surgery. Eur J Cardiothorac Surg 26:515–520
8. Reuter DA, Goetz AE (2005) Arterial pulse contour analysis: applicability to clinical routine. In: Pinsky MR, Payen D (eds) Functional Hemodynamic Monitoring. Springer, Berlin Heidelberg New York, pp 175–182
9. Devereaux PJ, Leslie K (2004) Best evidence in anesthetic practice. Prevention: alpha2- and beta-adrenergic antagonists reduce perioperative cardiac events. Can J Anaesth 51:290–292
10. Beilin LJ, Goldby FS, Mohring J (1977) High arterial pressure versus humoral factors in the pathogenesis of the vascular lesions of malignant hypertension. Clin Sci Mol Med 52:111
11. Funakoshi Y, Ichiki T, Ito K et al (1999) Induction of interleukin-6 expression by angiotensin II in rat vascular smooth muscle cells. Hypertension 34:118–125
12. Muller DN, Dechend R, Mervaala EM et al (2000) NF-?B inhibition ameliorates angiotensin II-induced inflammatory damage in rats. Hypertension 35:193–201
13. Gudbrandsson T, Hansson L, Herlitz H et al (1977) Immunological changes in patients with previous malignant essential hypertension. Am J Physiol 232:F26
14. Woods JW, Blythe WB, Huffines WD (1974) Management of malignant hypertension. N Engl J Med 291:10
15. Varon J, Marik PE (2000) The diagnosis and management of hypertensive crisis. Chest 118:214–227
16. Abdelwahab W, Frishman W, Landau A (1995) Management of hypertensive urgencies and emergencies. J Clin Pharm 35:747–762
17. Humbert M, Sitbon O, Simonneau G (2004) Treatment of pulmonary artery hypertension. N Engl J Med 351:1425–1436
18. Humbert M, Morrel NW, Archer SL et al (2004) Cellular and molecular pathobiology of pulmonary arterial hypertension. J Am Coll Cardiol 43(suppl S):13S-24S
19. Runo JR, Loyd JE (2003) Primary pulmonary hypertension. Lancet 361:1533–1544
20. Deng Z, Morse JH, Slager SL et al (2000) Familial primary pulmonary hypertension (gene PPH1) is caused by mutations in the bone morphogenetic protein receptor-II gene. Am J Hum Genet 67:737–744
21. Hinderliter AL, Willis PW 4th, Barst RJ et al (1997) Effects of long-term infusion of prostacyclin (epoprostenol) on echocardiographic measures of right ventricular structure and function in primary pulmonary hypertension. Primary Pulmonary Hypertension Study Group. Circulation 95:1479–1486
22. Pepke-Zaba J, Higenbottam TW, Dinh-Xuan AT et al (1991) Inhaled nitric oxide as a cause of selective pulmonary vasodilatation in pulmonary hypertension. Lancet 338:1173–1174.
23. Schrader BJ, Inbar S, Kaufmann L et al (1992) Comparison of the effects of adenosine and nifedipine in pulmonary hypertension. J Am Coll Cardiol 19:1060–1064
24. Fuster V, Steele PM, Edwards WD et al (1984) Primary pulmonary hypertension:

natural history and the importance of thrombosis. Circulation 70:580–587

25. Sitbon O, Humber M, Ioos V et al (2003) Who benefits from long-term calcium-channel blocker therapy in primary pulmonary hypertension? Am J Resp Crit Care Med 167:440
26. Higenbottam T, Wheeldon D, Wells F et al (1984) Long-term treatment of primary pulmonary hypertension with continuous intravenous epoprostenol (prostacyclin). Lancet 1:1046–1047
27. Shapiro SM, Oudiz RJ, Cao T et al (1997) Primary pulmonary hypertension: improved long-term effects and survival with continuous intravenous epoprostenol infusion. J Am Coll Cardiol 30:343–349
28. McLaughlin VV, Shillington A, Rich S (2002) Survival in primary pulmonary hypertension: the impact of epoprostenol therapy. Circulation 106:1477–1482
29. Simonneau G, Barst RJ, Galie N et al (2002) Continuous subcutaneous infusion of treprostinil, a prostacyclin analogue, in patients with pulmonary arterial hypertension: a double-blind, randomized, placebo-controlled trial. Am J Respir Crit Care Med 165:800–804
30. Okano Y, Yoshioka T, Shimouki A et al (1997) Orally active prostacyclin analogue in primary pulmonary hypertension. Lancet 349:1365
31. Galie N, Humbert M, Vachiery JL et al (2002) Effects of beraprost sodium, an oral prostacyclin analogue, in patients with pulmonary arterial hypertension: a randomized, double-blind, placebo-controlled trial. J Am Coll Cardiol 39:1496–1502
32. Barst RJ, McGoon M, McLaughlin V et al (2003) Beraprost therapy for pulmonary arterial hypertension. J Am Coll Cardiol 41:2119–2125
33. Rubin LJ, Badesch DB, Barst RJ et al (2002) Bosentan therapy for pulmonary arterial hypertension. N Engl J Med 346:896–903
34. Channick RN, Simonneau G, Sitbon O et al (2001) Effects of the dual endothelin-receptor antagonist bosentan in patients with pulmonary hypertension: a randomised placebo-controlled study. Lancet 358:1119–1123
35. Ziegler JW, Ivy DD, Wiggins JW et al (1998) Effects of dipyridamole and inhaled nitric oxide in pediatric patients with pulmonary hypertension. Am J Respir Crit Care Med 158:1388–1395
36. Zhao L, Mason NA, Morrel NW et al (2001) Sildenafil inhibits hypoxia-induced pulmonary hypertension. Circulation 104:424–428
37. Michelakis E, Tymchak W, Lien D et al (2002) Oral sildenafil is an effective and specific pulmonary vasodilator in patients with pulmonary arterial hypertension: comparison with inhaled nitric oxide. Circulation 105:2398–2403
38. Atz AM, Wessel DL (1999) Sildenafil ameliorates effects of inhaled nitric oxide withdrawal. Anesthesiology 91:307–310
39. Kleinsasser A, Loekinger A, Hoermann C et al (2001) Sildenafil modulates hemodynamics and pulmonary gas exchange. Am J Respir Crit Care Med 163:339–343
40. Zapol WM, Falke KJ, Hurford WE et al (1994) Inhaling nitric oxide: a selective pulmonary vasodilator and bronchodilator. Chest 105:87S-91S
41. Kinsella JP, Neish SR, Shaffer E et al (1992) Low-dose inhalation nitric oxide in persistent pulmonary hypertension of the newborn. Lancet 340:819–820
42. Christie JD, Kotloff RM, Pochettino A et al (2003) Clinical risk factors for primary graft failure following lung transplantation. Chest 124:1232–1241
43. Bennett LE, Keck BM, Hertz MI et al (2001) Worldwide thoracic organ transplantation: a report from the UNOS/ISHLT international registry for thoracic organ transplantation. Clin Transpl 25–40

44. Pielsticker EJ, Martinez FJ, Rubenfire M (2001) Lung and heart-lung transplant practice patterns in pulmonary hypertension centers. J Heart Lung Transplant 20:1297–1304
45. Simonneau G, Galie N, Rubin LJ et al (2004) Clinical classification of pulmonary hypertension. J Am Coll Cardiol 43:5S-12S

16 Recent Advances in the Natural History of Dilated Cardiomyopathy: A Review of the Heart Muscle Disease Registry of Trieste

M. Moretti, A. Di Lenarda and G. Sinagra

Introduction

Dilated cardiomyopathy (DCM) is heart muscle disease characterized by left ventricular or biventricular dilatation and impaired myocardial contractility [1]. It is an important cause of morbidity and mortality, and is one of the two most frequent indications for cardiac transplantation. The prevalence of DCM in the United States has been estimated at around 0.04% [2], with an annual incidence of 0.005–0.006% [2, 3].

DCM may be idiopathic, familial/genetic, viral and/or autoimmune, alcoholic/toxic, or associated with recognized cardiovascular disease in which the degree of myocardial dysfunction is not explained by an overload condition or by extension of ischemic damage [1]. The prognosis was considered very bad in the past. Many authors have tried to identify the predictors of outcome of patients with DCM. The prevalent opinion today is that only complete evaluation of patients, using the anamnestic data and that from clinical and instrumental examinations, is useful for prognostic stratification of patients with DCM.

Patients and Methods

In collaboration with the University of Colorado, the Department of Cardiology at Trieste developed a Registry of diseases of the myocardium. The objective was to archive and analyze the data from clinical and instru-

Cardiovascular Department, "Ospedali Riuniti" and University of Trieste, Trieste, Italy

mental examinations of patients selected according to rigorous criteria and enrolled in the Registry. From 1 January 1978 to 31 December 2002 1208 patients were enrolled: 581 with DCM, 70 with myocarditis, 232 with hypertensive and ischemic cardiopathy, 95 with hypertrophic cardiomyopathy, 85 with arrhythmogenic right ventricle dysplasia, and 145 patients who could not be classified in the initial phase. At enrolment all patients underwent complete evaluation, noninvasive and invasive, including coronarography and endomyocardial biopsy. Patients underwent serial follow-ups at 6, 12, and 24 months, and subsequently every 2 years or more frequently on the basis of specific clinical necessity.

Results

The present study analyzed only the data from patients with DCM ($n = 581$) enrolled in the Registry from 1978 to 2002. The characteristics of the population are illustrated in Table 1. Mean age was 44.8 ± 15.3 years, 79% of patients were male, mean NYHA class was 2 ± 0.9, mean left ventricle ejection fraction (LVEF) was 0.31±0.108, and mean left ventricle end-diastolic diameter (LVEDD) was 67 ± 10 mm.

Table 1. Baseline characteristics of patients with DCM enrolled in the Heart Muscle Disease Registry of Trieste (1978–2002)

Age (years)	44.8 ± 15.3
Male (%)	79
HF (%)	80.9
HF duration (months)	16.8 ± 27.5
Systolic blood pressure (mmHg)	124.7 ± 16.3
Diastolic blood pressure (mmHg)	79.4 ± 10.8
Heart rate	79.0 ± 15.7
Cardiac index (ml/min per m^2)	3664.4 ± 1138.3
PCWP (mmHg)	12.0 ± 7.8
Mean PAP (mmHg)	19.4 ± 9.7
LVEDD (mm)	67 ± 10
LVEF (%)	0.31 ± 0.108
E deceleration time (ms)	164.2 ± 69.3
Mitral insufficiency (0-4)	1.1 ± 1.0
Ventricular tachycardia (episodes/h)	0.1 ± 1.0
Bycicle exercise time (s)	613.6 ± 240.4

continue →

Table 1. *continue*

β-blockers (% of patients)	54.8
Metoprolol equivalent (mg)	97.0 ± 52.8
ACE inhibitors (% of patients)	72.4
Enalapril equivalent dose (mg)	21.1 ± 12.3
Digitalis (% of patients)	69.0
Anticoagulants (% of patients)	17.8
Amiodarone (% of patients)	20.2
Diuretics (% of patients)	55.9

HF, heart failure; PCWP, pulmonary capillary wedge pressure; PAP, pulmonary artery pressure; LVEDD, left ventricular end-diastolic diameter; LVEF, left ventricular ejection fraction

Change in the Natural History of DCM in the Last 25 Years

In the past, DCM was regarded as having a very bad prognosis, with mortality rates around 50% in the first 2 years after diagnosis [4, 5]. Population studies performed in the last 50 years, such as the Framingham study, demonstrated a tendency to the reduction of mortality in patients with DCM.

In the period from 1978 to 1992 we performed a study enrolling 235 patients with DCM [6]. A continuous improvement of the survival rate was observed. At 2 years we observed 74% survival of patients enrolled in the period 1978–1982, 88% among patients enrolled from 1983 to 1987, and 90% among those enrolled in the last 4 years, 1988–1992. Survival at 4 years was 54%, 72%, and 83%, respectively, for the same groups of patients. The survival was different in the three groups, even after stratification for the clinical severity of the disease. The patients enrolled in the last years were younger, with a lower functional class, and were more frequently treated with angiotensin-converting enzyme inhibitors (ACE-I) and β-blockers.

In one more recent study we analyzed the survival of patients with DCM (n = 432) enrolled from 1978 to 1997 [7]. Patients were divided into two groups, one with 95 patients enrolled from 1978 to 1987, and the second with 337 patients enrolled in the period 1987–1997. Patients in the second group were more frequently treated with ACEI, β-blockers, digitalis, and oral anticoagulants, and less with amiodarone compared to patients in the first group. No differences in clinical characteristics existed between the patients in the two groups. Transplant-free survival at 2, 5, and 10 years was respectively 82%, 60%, and 44% in the first group and 91%, 80%, and 63% in the second ($P = 0.0001$) (Fig. 1). The improvement of the outcome in the second group was due mainly to reduction of the incidence of death due to pump failure or the necessity for heart transplantation; a reduction of the incidence of sudden death (SD) was not observed.

Comparing patients with DCM ($n = 184$) with those with ischemic cardiomyopathy (ICM) ($n = 92$), matched for age and gender, it was observed that patients with coronary artery disease (CAD) had more severe symptoms and less dilated left ventricles, although no difference existed in left ventricular (LV) function. At enrolment, patients with CAD were less frequently treated with ACE I and β-blockers, more frequently with vasodilators (particularly nitrates). The effect of the therapy on symptoms and on LV function was less evident in patients with ICM, probably due to lower reversibility of the infaction LV dysfunction (57% of cases). In addition, at 5 years, the transplant-free survival (67% vs. 79%, $P = 0.001$) was worse in patients with ICM (25% vs. 51%, $P = 0.007$) [8]. Comparing patients with hypertensive cardiomyopathy (HCM) in the absence of significant coronary disease with those with CAD and ischemic dilatative, hypokinetic cardiomyopathy (i.e., ICM as defined above), greater reversibility of LV dysfunction was observed in patients with HCM, especially if HCM was diagnosed early; namely, before the appearance of heart failure (HF). Even so, significant differences in outcomes between the two groups (those with HCM or ICM) were not observed.

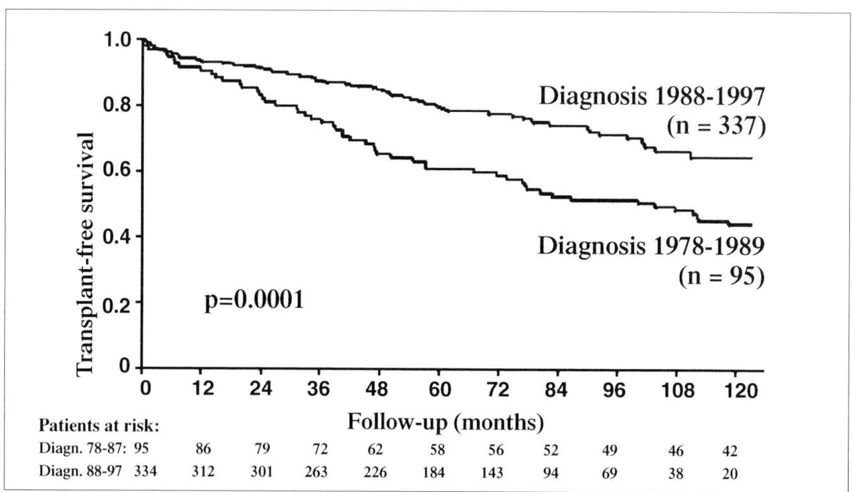

Fig. 1. Event-free survival curves for the end point heart transplantation, comparing patients enrolled 1978–1987 ($n = 95$) and 1988–1997 ($n = 337$) in the Heart Muscle Disease Registry of Trieste

Role of Early Treatment

More recently we analyzed the response to the optimized therapy and the long-term outcome of patients with asymptomatic DCM at enrolment in the Registry [9]. Of the 447 patients enrolled between 1986 and 2000, 307 (69%) were in NYHA classes II–IV, while 140 (31%) were asymptomatic and in NYHA class I (among them 71 patients, or 51%, with a previous history of HF stabilized in therapy). The asymptomatic patients were younger, with better tolerance of effort, with less dilated left ventricles, and were less frequently being treated with ACE-I and β-blockers. The transplant-free survival rates of patients in NYHA classes II–IV at 5 and 10 years were 73% and 57%, respectively; those in the NYHA class I group with a history of HF were 94% and 84% respectively; and those in asymptomatic patients without a previous history of HF were 92% and 89% ($P < 0.0001$ between NYHA classes II–IV and NYHA class I; P = NS between groups in NYHA class I with vs. without a previous history of HF). After 24 months of optimized therapy the LVEF improved in all patients, asymptomatic and symptomatic. However, after 6–8 years a greater tendency to worsening systolic function of the left ventricle was observed in asymptomatic patients [worsening by 10% of LVEF in NYHA class I (40%) vs. NYHA classes II–IV (12%), $P = 0.003$].

During long-term follow-up at least half of the patients diagnosed in an asymptomatic phase manifested progression of the disease in terms of appearance of symptoms (35%), progression of LV dysfunction (40%), hospitalizations (43%), or heart transplantation or death (13%). Within the limits of the retrospective analysis, treatment with β-blockers demonstrated effectiveness in improving transplant-free survival also in the asymptomatic patients (unpublished data).

Natural History of Familial DCM

DCM appears to be familial in 20–50% of patients [10–12]. The familial form is genetically and phenotypically heterogeneous [3]. There are 20 known mutations of genes that codify for cytoskeletal proteins in patients with DCM [13]. Recently, mutations of the sarcomere and inner nuclear membrane were identified. This discovery was the basis of the theory that alterations of power generation could also be responsible for DCM. Different mutations in genes codifying for contractile proteins could generate different intracellular transmission signals, with a consequent DCM or hypertrophic cardiomyopathy phenotype [14].

To date no clinical and morphological parameters exist that are useful to distinguish between the familial and the sporadic form of DCM. Previous data suggest that they are two different stages of a single disease rather than two different diseases [3].

In our population of patients with DCM (n = 560) enrolled in the Registry for DCM from January 1978 to June 2002, about 80% had sporadic DCM, while 20% had the familial form. At enrolment, the patients with familial DCM were younger than those with sporadic DCM and with a shorter duration of HF, lower functional class, and better stress tolerance. At echocardiography no significant differences in LV dilatation and dysfunction were found. Rate of hyperkinetic and hypokinetic arrhythmias did not differ between the groups with the familial and the sporadic form. Transplant-free and hospitalization-free survival were also similar between the two groups.

Some autosomal dominant forms of DCM are characterized by a variable musculoskeletal involvement and/or defects of the conduction system (5%). Mutations of the lamin A/C gene are responsible for this form [15]. Different mutations in this gene produce different phenotypes [16, 17]. The prognosis of this form is severe; around one-third of patients undergoes cardiac transplantation.

In our population [18] 12 patients were heterozygous carriers of mutations of the lamin A/C gene, three with an autosomal dominant form and one with the sporadic form of DCM. Manifestations of the presence of this mutation were supraventricular arrhythmias, atrioventricular block and/or necessity of pacemaker implantation, signs of muscular dystrophy, and increased levels of creatine kinase. Carriers of the lamin gene mutation had the worse outcome: 8 of 12 died, underwent cardiac transplantation, or had marked worsening of the pump function between the third and fifth decades of life. In relation to noncarriers of the mutation, carriers had a relative risk of 2.6 for cardiovascular death of (P = 0.05), 3.48 for cardiovascular death/heart transplantation (P = 0.001), and 2.2 for major events, cardiovascular death, or heart transplantation (P = 0.01).

Prognostic Significance of Left Ventricular Filling

The study of LV filling with transmitral flow Doppler analysis was one of the first clinical applications of Doppler echocardiography. The pathological features vary from an "abnormal relaxation" pattern (with the characteristic E wave velocity reduction and the prevalence of A wave) to a pattern called "restrictive", with E wave prevalence and rapid deceleration, typical of ventricular compliance reduction [19].

Many studies have demonstrated that in patients with ventricular systolic dysfunction the restrictive pattern correlates with high pulmonary capillary wedge pressure [20, 21], advanced functional class, and lower myocardial oxygen consumption on the exercise test [22, 23]. We demonstrated that the restrictive pattern has a prognostic role for the outcome of patients with

DCM [24]. Patients with the restrictive pattern (46%) had clinical and instrumental signs that suggested more advanced disease. The most interesting data of this study resulted from analysis of transplant-free survival. During a follow-up of 24 ± 12 months, all the patients who had died or received a transplant had presented the restrictive pattern at enrolment, which proved to be the most powerful independent variable.

One later study [25] analyzed the short-term evolution of left ventricular filling in patients with DCM (n = 110). After 3 months of treatment with ACE-I and β-blockers, regression of the restrictive pattern was observed. This was associated with continuous improvement of clinical findings and with excellent transplant-free survival (100% in the first 2 years, 97% at 4 years). On the contrary, patients with persistent restrictive pattern had symptomatic left ventricular dysfunction and shorter survival (65% in the first year, 46% in the second, 13% at 4 years). Persistence of the restrictive pattern during an optimized therapy was a more specific and accurate predictor than a restrictive pattern present only at the moment of diagnosis. Thus, early echocardiographic reevaluation in patients with a restrictive pattern appears very informative for the prediction of outcome. In agreement with data from other authors [26, 27], late reappearance of the restrictive filling pattern in patients from our Registry according with data from other authors [26,27] also identified a subgroup of patients at high risk of cardiovascular events.

Ventricular Arrhythmias and SD

Whether the presence of ventricular arrhythmias correlates with increased risk of SD is still debated. Although some authors have reported a significant correlation between the frequency and complexity of ventricular arrhythmias and the incidence of SD [28, 29], others have not confirmed this correlation [30, 31]. Hofmann et al. [28] and Meinertz et al. [29] demonstrated that complex ventricular arrhythmias in the presence of a left ventricular ejection fraction below 0.40 are associated with an increased risk of SD. In a previous study we sought to determine the prognostic role for SD of electrocardiographic data of 78 patients with DCM without a previous history of symptomatic ventricular arrhythmias [32]. We found that only left bundle branch block (LBBB) (61% with LBBB vs. 95% without LBBB; $P < 0.05$) and HV interval (74% HV > 55 ms vs. 98% HV ≤ 55 ms; $P = 0.01$) were predictive, while nonsustained ventricular tachycardia, inducible ventricular tachycardia at electrophysiological study, and late potentials had no impact on SD-free survival.

The severity of LV dysfunction was pointed out as an independent prognostic factor for total mortality and also for SD [33, 34]. In the ESVEM study [33] a reduction of 5 points in LVEF correlated with a 15% increase in risk for arrhythmic events. Dilatation of the left ventricle seems to identify a subgroup of patients at increased risk of dying suddenly [35]. Grimm et al. [35] reported an elevated risk of arrhythmic events in patients with LVEDD > 70 mm and nonsustained ventricular tachycardia. We analyzed data from 343 patients enlisted in the Registry from 1978 to 1997 [36]. The cumulative risk of events (death, heart transplantation, and aborted SD) was 30% at 5 years and 54% at 10 years (6.43 events per 100 patient-years). The incidence of SD was higher in the first months and after 5 years of follow-up, SD becoming the major cause of death in patients with a follow-up longer than 5 years. The presence of LVEDD $\geq$ 38 mm/m^2 and LVEF $\leq$ 30% at last follow-up were independent predictors of SD ($P = 0.01$) at 1 year. Another interesting observation in this study was that the patients who died suddenly were more frequently treated with digitalis (96% vs. 69%, P This observation is in agreement with the results from the DIG study [37].

Conclusions

The availability of data of long-term follow-up of patients enlisted in the Registry has allowed us to analyze various aspects of the natural history and prognosis of patients with DCM. The prognosis of this pathology remains severe, with a probability around 40% of death or cardiac transplantation within 10 years from diagnosis. However, in the course of last the 20 years, the availability of more effective drugs for treatment of the HF, and the initiation of treatment in the early phase of the disease, have contributed to improving outcomes, particularly in reducing the events secondary to the HF. Screening programs for the familial forms have also contributed to early diagnosis of the disease in carriers of mutations for DCM, and hence, to earlier initiation of therapy.

The extensive use of ACE-I and β-blockers contributes to complete normalization in approximately of one-fourth and improvement in approximately one-half of the patients. Response to therapy is associated with better outcomes. However, improvement is often transitory, and the majority of patients with DCM demonstrate progression of the disease by 5–8 years of diagnosis despite optimal medical management.

The risk of SD rises during the years of follow-up, particularly in patients with persistent or progressive dilatation and dysfunction of the left ventricle. The higher rate of arrhythmic events over the long term in patients with DCM is an argument for considering the implantation of an automatic defibrillator in selected patients with DCM.

References

1. Report of the 1995 World Health Organization/International Society and Federation of Cardiology Task Force on the definition and classification of cardiomyopathies (1996) Circulation 93:841–2
2. Codd MB, Sugrue DD, Gersh BJ et al (1989) Epidemiology of idiopathic dilated and hypertrophic cardiomyopathy. A population-based study in Olmsted County, Minnesota, 1975–1984. Circulation 80:564–72
3. Mestroni L, Rocco C, Gregori D et al (1999) Familial dilated cardiomyopathy: evidence for genetic and phenotypic heterogeneity. Heart Muscle Disease Study Group. J Am Coll Cardiol 34:181–90
4. Gavazzi A, Lanzarini L, Cornalba C et al (1984) Dilated (congestive) cardiomyopathy. G Ital Cardiol 14:492–8
5. Franciosa JA, Wilen M, Ziesche S et al (1983) Survival in men with severe chronic left ventricular failure due to either coronary heart disease or idiopathic dilated cardiomyopathy. Am J Cardiol 51:831–6
6. Di Lenarda A, Secoli G, Perkan A et al (1994) Changing mortality in dilated cardiomyopathy. Br Heart J 72:46–51
7. Di Lenarda A, Sabbadini G, Gortan R et al (2001) Has the prognosis of idiopathic dilated cardiomyopathy improved in the community? The Heart Muscle Disease Registry of Trieste (abstract). J Am Coll Cardiol 37:169A
8. Massa L, Vitali-Serdoz L, Di Lenarda A et al (2002) Prognostic stratification and long-term follow-up of optimally treated patients with ischemic cardiomyopathy. The Trieste HF Registry (abstract). Eur J Heart Fail 1(Suppl 1):18
9. Di Lenarda A, Sinagra G, Sabbadini G et al(2001) Long-term follow-up in asymptomatic dilated cardiomyopathy treated with beta-blockers. The Heart Muscle Disease Registry of Trieste (abstract) Eur Heart J 22(Suppl): 637
10. Michels VV, Moll PP, Miller FA et al (1992) The frequency of familial dilated cardiomyopathy in a series of patients with idiopathic dilated cardiomyopathy. N Engl J Med 326:77–82
11. Grunig E, Tasman JA, Kucherer H et al (1998) Frequency and phenotypes of familial dilated cardiomyopathy. J Am Coll Cardiol 31:186–94
12. Gregori D, Rocco C, Miocic S, Mestroni L (2001) Estimating the frequency of familial dilated cardiomyopathy in the presence of misclassification errors. J Appl Stat 28:53–62
13. Sinagra G, Di Lenarda A, Brodsky GL et al for the Heart Muscle Disease Study Group (2001) New insights into the molecular basis of familial dilated cardiomyopathy. Ital Heart J 2:280–6
14. Kamisago M, Sharma SD, De Palma SR et al (2000) Mutations in sarcomere protein genes as a cause of dilated cardiomyopathy. N Engl J Med 343:1688–96
15. Brodsky GL, Muntoni F, Miocic S et al (2000) A lamin A/C gene mutation associated with dilated cardiomyopathy with variable skeletal muscle involvement. Circulation 101:473–6
16. Jacobs PM, Hanson EL, Crispell KA et al (2001) Novel lamin A/C gene mutations in two families with dilated cardiomyopathy and conduction system disease. J Card Fail 7:249–56
17. Arbustini E, Pilotto A, Repetto A et al (2002) Autosomal dominant dilated cardiomyopathy with atrioventricular block: a lamin A/C defect-related disease. J Am Coll Cardiol 39:981–90

18. Taylor MR, Fain PR, Sinagra G et al (2003) Natural history of dilated cardiomyopathy due to lamin A/C gene mutations. J Am Coll Cardiol 41:771–80
19. Appleton CP, Hatle LK, Popp RL (1988) Relation of transmitral flow velocity patterns to left ventricular diastolic function: new insights from a combined hemodynamic and Doppler echocardiographic study. J Am Coll Cardiol 12:426–40
20. Giannuzzi P, Imparato A, Temporelli PL et al (1994) Doppler-derived mitral deceleration time of early filling as a strong predictor of pulmonary capillary wedge pressure in postinfarction patients with left ventricular systolic dysfunction. J Am Coll Cardiol 23:1630–7
21. Pozzoli M, Capomolla S, Pinna G et al (1996) Doppler echocardiography reliably predicts pulmonary artery wedge pressure in patients with chronic HF with and without mitral regurgitation. J Am Coll Cardiol 27:883–93
22. Vanoverschelde JL, Raphael DA, Robert AR et al (1990) Left ventricular filling in dilated cardiomyopathy: relation to functional class and hemodynamics. J Am Coll Cardiol 15:1288–95
23. Tabet JY, Logeart D, Geyer C et al(2000) Comparison of the prognostic value of left ventricular filling and peak oxygen uptake in patients with systolic HF. Eur Heart J 21:1864–71
24. Pinamonti B, Di Lenarda A, Sinagra G et al (1993) Restrictive left ventricular filling pattern in dilated cardiomyopathy assessed by Doppler echocardiography: clinical, echocardiographic and hemodynamic correlations and prognostic implications. J Am Coll Cardiol 22:808–15
25. Pinamonti B, Zecchin M, Di Lenarda A et al (1997) Persistence of restrictive left ventricular filling pattern in dilated cardiomyopathy: an ominous prognostic sign. J Am Coll Cardiol 29:604–12
26. Traversi E, Pozzoli M, Cioffi G et al (1996) Mitral flow velocity changes after 6 months of optimized therapy provide important hemodynamic and prognostic information in patients with chronic HF. Am Heart J 132:809–19
27. Temporelli PL, Corrà U, Imparato A et al (1998) Reversible restrictive left ventricular diastolic filling with optimized oral therapy predicts a more favorable prognosis in patients with chronic HF. J Am Coll Cardiol 31:1591–7
28. Hofmann T, Meinertz T, Kasper W et al (1988) Mode of death in idiopathic dilated cardiomyopathy: multivariate analysis of prognostic determinants. Am Heart J 116:1455–63
29. Meinertz T, Hofmann T, Kasper W et al (1984) Significance of ventricular arrhythmias in idiopathic dilated cardiomyopathy. Am J Cardiol 53:902–7
30. Diaz RA, Obasohan A, Oakley CM (1987) Prediction of outcome in dilated cardiomyopathy. Br Heart J 58:393–9
31. Keogh AM, Baron DW, Hickie JB. (1990) Prognostic guides in patients with idiopathic or ischemic dilated cardiomyopathy assessed for cardiac transplantation. Am J Cardiol 65:903–8
32. Morgera T, Di Lenarda A, Rakar S et al (2002) Substrate and prognostic impact of ventricular tachycardia in dilated cardiomyopathy (abstract). Eur J Heart Fail 1(Suppl 1):63
33. Caruso AC, Marcus FI, Hahn EA et al (1997) Predictors of arrhythmic death and cardiac arrest in the ESVEM trial. Circulation 96:1888–92
34. Cohn JN, Johnson G, Ziesche S et al (1991) A comparison of enalapril with hydralazine-isosorbide dinitrate in the treatment of chronic congestive HF. N Engl J Med 325:303–10

35. Grimm W, Hoffmann JJ, Muller HH et al (2002) Implantable defibrillator event rates in patients with idiopathic dilated cardiomyopathy, nonsustained ventricular tachycardia on Holter and a left ventricular ejection fraction below 30%. J Am Coll Cardiol 39:780–7
36. Zecchin M, Di Lenarda A, Bonin M et al (2001) Incidence and predictors of sudden cardiac death during long term follow-up in patients with dilated cardiomyopathy on optimal medical therapy. Ital Heart J 2:213–21
37. The Digitalis Investigation Group (1997) The effect of digoxin on mortality and morbidity in patients with HF. N Engl J Med 336:525–33

Subject Index